FAITH AND MENTAL HEALTH

FAITH AND MENTAL HEALTH

RELIGIOUS RESOURCES FOR HEALING

HAROLD G. KOENIG, M.D.

TEMPLETON FOUNDATION PRESS

PHILADELPHIA AND LONDON

Templeton Foundation Press
300 Conshohocken State Road, Suite 670
West Conshohocken, PA 19428
www.templetonpress.org

Designed and typeset by Kachergis Book Design

*Templeton Foundation Press helps intellectual leaders and others
learn about science research on aspects of realities, invisible and
intangible. Spiritual realities include unlimited love, accelerating
creativity, worship, and the benefits of purpose in persons and
in the cosmos.*

LIBRARY OF CONGRESS CATALOGING-IN-PUBLICATION DATA

Koenig, Harold George.
  Faith and mental health : religious resources for healing /
  Harold G. Koenig.
    p. cm.
  Includes bibliographical references and index.
  ISBN 1-932031-91-X (pbk. : alk. paper)
    1. Mental health—Religious aspects. 2. Mental illness—
Religious aspects. 3. Mentally ill—Care—Religious aspects.
4. Community mental health services--United States. 5. Church
work with the mentally ill—United States. 6. Psychiatry and
religion. 7. Pastoral counseling. 8. Spiritual healing. I. Title.
    [DNLM: 1. Community Mental Health Services—organiza-
tion & administration—United States. 2. Mental Disorders—
psychology—United States. 3. Religion—United States.
4. Religion and Psychology—United States. WM 30 K78f 2005]
  RC489.S676K64 2005
  201'.7622—dc22
                            2005006583

Printed in the United States of America

06 07 08 09 10   10 9 8 7 6 5 4 3 2

CONTENTS

Contents

13. Barriers to Research and Implementation   243

14. Identifying Possible Solutions   255

    Glossary   277
    Additional Resources   289
    References   299
    Index   333

ACKNOWLEDGMENTS

I am deeply indebted to a number of people for their help. These include Dr. Garry Crites (a theologian and Middle Ages historian at Duke University), Dr. Keith G. Meador (a psychiatrist and professor at Duke Divinity School), and Dr. Daniel E. Hall (a theologian and graduate of Yale Divinity School), who provided their expertise to help shape the theological content of this book. Support was provided by the Substance Abuse and Mental Health Services Administration, U.S. Department of Health and Human Services.

INTRODUCTION

This book is not a profound theological treatise on mental illness. I am not an expert in any world religion and therefore cannot speak with authority on Islam, Judaism, Hinduism, or Buddhism, or even on my own Christian tradition. You will not find here a book that brings out the nuances of different ideological views within particular religious traditions and explores their impact on mental health. You will, however, discover an unprecedented source of practical information about the religion-mental health relationship and a detailed examination of how Christianity and other world religions deliver mental health services every day.

My credentials are as a psychiatrist who has spent years in the trenches with those who struggle with emotional problems or severe mental illness, people whom I have come to love and deeply appreciate. For the past twenty years I have also been involved in conducting research on how religion affects mental health and well-being. As a result of this work, the Substance Abuse and Mental Health Services Administration of the U.S. Department of Health and Human Services asked me to investigate the role that faith-based organizations play in delivering mental health and substances abuse services to those in need. It is through such experiences, then, that I come to write this book.

Although not a theologian, I recognize and respect the role that theology plays. Theology ("the study of God and the relations between God and the universe"[1]) has influenced almost every social and political movement in the United States since early colonial days. The influence of Christianity, particularly Protestant Christianity, on our government, political parties, social values, medical care system, and even scientific establishment is enormous, whether recognized or not. Understanding the different theological streams is essential, then, to appreciate the role that religious organizations have played and continue to play in providing for the poor, the sick, and those with severe and persistent mental illness. Patterns of mental health care delivery by different religious groups can be directly traced to differences in theological emphasis (see chapter 7). For that reason, and because of my theological naïveté, I have consulted with experts in this area. In the end, though, what you read here will be relatively light on theology.

Who then might be interested in reading this book? A brief description of the two primary audiences will help the reader decide.

The Health Care Community

This book is for mental health providers, public health service planners, researchers, university or medical school faculty involved in the training of mental health practitioners, and other health professionals who desire to understand better the role of religion as a resource (or liability) for those with emotional or mental problems. Especially useful to these readers will be the summary of past research on the relationships between religion and positive emotions, psychiatric illness, and severe and persistent mental disorder, as well as a recent update on the latest studies carried out since the year 2000 (chapters 3, 4, and 5). A description of ways that religion can influence mental health and a discussion of religious interventions (chapter 6) will interest both clinicians and researchers. Those delivering or coordinating the delivery of mental health services will be attracted by the comprehensive description and categorization of Christian and non-Christian faith-based organizations that provide mental health services (chapters 7 to 12)—this information, to my knowledge, is not yet available elsewhere. Finally, chapters on barriers and solutions to research on and implementation of faith-based services (chapters 13 and 14) will serve those planning future mental health services at a time when mental health resources for high-risk populations are rapidly dwindling, especially at the state level.

Religious Professionals

This book is also written for pastoral counselors, chaplains, seminary professors, and other religious professionals who either feel called to serve those with emotional illness or to train others to do so. Of particular interest will be chapters on persons and communities of faith (1 and 7–11); the fascinating historical connections linking mental health care and religion (2); the latest research on religion and mental health (3, 4, and 5); and a discussion of barriers that prevent faith-based organizations from delivering services (13 and 14). Toward the end of the book are additional resources for religious professionals and faith communities wanting more information on how to design programs to meet their local needs.

I use several terms here that need definition. By *emotional problems* I mean short- or long-term struggles with depression, anxiety, or other difficulties with mood or happiness. By *mental illness* I mean schizophrenia, bipolar disorder, and other long-term psychoses or severe personality disorders (more detailed definitions of other terms are found in a glossary at the end of this book). Emotional problems and mental illness trap people in prisons of fear, despair, confusion, and loneliness. Throughout history people of faith (whether faith is acknowledged or not) have sought to free these captives or at least walk alongside them on their difficult journeys. Those afflicted with these conditions did not choose them, nor did most commit such horrible crimes that they would deserve such suffering. No, more likely it is their genes, childhood experiences, or severe adult trauma that have thrust them onto these precarious, painful paths. Many see it as a cruel stroke of fate. Or is it?

What if having such a life meant something else, something not completely senseless but rather was evidence for—and I say this a bit cautiously—a type of unique "calling"? Is it possible that those with mental illness provide others with the *opportunity* to care, to love, to reach out to them, an opportunity that otherwise would not exist? What if their pain caused people of faith to sacrifice their comfort and smug way of life to reach out and minister to them? Who, then, would really be the receiver of ministry and who would be the giver? Could those struggling with mental illness serve as beacon lights illuminating the "narrow" way to real life that few ever find? Could they be pointing the way for people of faith and others to follow, so that the care, love, and service provided to the mentally ill by them would demonstrate to the world the best of what it is to be human? Would that be possible without the help of those with mental illness, without their pain? Does this mean that religious congregations need persons with mental illness in their midst in order to be fully functional caring communities? It's worth thinking about.

Might such a calling for those in mental distress require the experience of suffering and pain in order to give these "wounded healers" the insight and compassion necessary to truly help others with similar afflictions, a special kind of training that prepares them to really know, to really understand what others are going through? For those who must live day in and day out with the demon of despair, who must bear the heavy burden of mental anguish despite the best treatments that modern medicine can offer, this "calling" is indeed a tough one.

If you are interested in the plight and the potential of those who struggle with emotional problems or mental disorder, and in what religion has done and continues to do both for and against them, then you will enjoy reading this book. Please join me now in learning about caring individuals and communities of faith, in discovering the historical connections between religion and mental illness, in exploring how religion causes or cures mental distress, and in discussing what people of faith are now doing to meet the needs of the mentally ill—and what *more* they might be doing.

PART I

HISTORICAL
CONSIDERATIONS

CHAPTER I

PEOPLE AND COMMUNITIES
OF FAITH

Both individuals and entire religious communities have long been involved in caring for the emotionally or mentally ill. These efforts have often been truly heroic, although at other times they have been less than so. The following five accounts illustrate such contributions at different times and in different places.

Granada, Spain (16th Century)

The first three-quarters of John Cuidad's life were not very remarkable. Not until he was forced to confront mental pain himself was his heart transformed over the plight of those similarly affected.

John was born to devout religious parents in Monternor-o-novo, Portugal, in 1495 during the early Renaissance period.[1] At the age of nine, he left his family home and followed a Spanish priest to Oropeza, Spain, where he was placed in the care of a local shepherd. There he learned discipline, commitment to hard work, and a deep faith in God. As he grew into manhood, the shepherd encouraged him to marry his daughter, an idea that was not to John's liking. To escape this fate, he enrolled in the army of Charles V and traveled to Austria to fight the invading Turks. When he returned to his home in Portugal, he discovered that his mother had died. Greatly saddened by this news, he went into seclusion. After getting his life back together, John took a job as a shepherd in Seville and later took up a similar occupation in Gibraltar, working his way towards the

3

coast. There he planned to catch a ship to Africa to help free Christians living under Moorish domination. He eventually succeeded in getting to Africa by winning the support of a Portuguese family. However, he was soon expelled and returned to Gibraltar. There he went about as an itinerant book peddler selling religious books and pictures, often giving them away for free.

Around this time he had a vision of the infant Jesus whom he heard call him "John of God." Soon he was led back to the Spanish city of Granada, drawn by the teachings of a man called John of Avila who was preaching there. John was so inspired by this man's teachings that he gave away all of his earthly belongings and went through the streets "beating his chest and calling on God for mercy." He was diagnosed with an acute psychological breakdown and hospitalized in the psychiatric wing of Granada's Royal Hospital in 1538. He was forty-three years old at the time.

On discharge from the hospital, John was released to the streets where he remained homeless and disillusioned. One of his friends allowed him to find shelter from the bitter winter cold under the porch of his house. These experiences deeply affected John, sensitizing him to the suffering of the poor, the homeless, and those marginalized from society. Soon he began to invite the sick, the weak, and the mentally ill to share with him the small porch of his friend's house. He worked alone in his care of the sick, begging by night for necessary medical supplies from local merchants and caring for the needs of his sick guests during the daytime.

As word got out about his selfless, charitable ministry to the weak and needy, however, he began to receive help from local priests and physicians. Rumors about him spread rapidly. John developed a reputation for giving his overcoat to needy beggars on the street. Learning about these kind acts, the Bishop of Tuy had a special tunic and cloak made for him (the garb later adopted by his followers), and officially gave him the name John of God. Over the next few years, a hospital emerged out of the small house porch in Granada and was to become one of the first psychiatric facilities in that area of the world.

In 1550, after twelve years of devotion to his patients, John of God died at the age of fifty-five from an illness that—according to legend—resulted from an attempt to save a young man from drowning. Soon, a movement of compassion for the sick, poor, and mentally ill spread across Spain. During the last days of John's life, the leaders and nobility of Granada came to express their gratitude for his services to the needy of the town. After his death, John of God was buried with the pomp and ceremony reserved for princes. Pope Alexander VIII canonized him in 1690, and several centuries later, Pope Leo XIII designated him the patron saint of hospitals, psychiatric nurses, and hospital workers.

Two religious orders emerged from the group of employees, volunteers, and benefactors that helped John in his work at the Granada hospital. An order of brothers, called "The Hospitaller Order of St. John of God," formed the nucleus of a wider group of followers that today number around 35,000. The Brothers have come to staff over 250 hospitals in 48 countries around the globe, caring every day for thousands of poor, homeless, mentally ill, and emotionally distraught persons.[2]

Years later, an order of sisters of St. John of God was also started. It began in Ireland in 1871, in response to widespread hunger and famine at that time.[3] Thomas Furlong, the bishop of Ferns, helped institute this order of nursing sisters whose purpose was to meet the needs of the poor, sick, and mentally ill of the region, thus carrying on the tradition of St. John of God.

From the care and welcome that John gave the poor in the city of Granada nearly 500 years ago, some say, came the word *hospitality*. Huddling together with his cold, hungry, and sick companions during the early days of his ministry, little did he know that someday his life would inspire a movement that would reach around the world. The following prayer by John of God is often used to summarize his mission:

May Jesus Christ give me the grace to run a hospital where the abandoned poor and those who suffer mental illness may have refuge, so that I may be able to serve them as I wish.[4]

John's story is in some ways the story of every person of faith—Christian or non-Christian—who feels compassion for those who suffer with emotional problems or mental illness. Such a person is moved to do something to make a difference. Indeed, there is much that can be done by those both inside and outside of religious organizations.

Worchester, Massachusetts (20th century)

Born in 1876 in Bloomington, Indiana, Anton T. Boisen was raised in a family of teachers and ministers.[5] He began a career as a language teacher, but then later switched and completed a three-year forestry degree at Yale University. In 1905 Boisen experienced a call to the ministry and in 1908 entered Union Theological Seminary. It was there that he was influenced by the writings of William James (about religious experience and "the sick soul"). After graduation from seminary and ordination in 1911, Boisen worked several years for the Presbyterian Board of Home Missions. He then served as a rural Presbyterian pastor for five years and after that traveled overseas with the YMCA during World War I.[6]

Always a shy and introverted man, Boisen lost his father when he was only seven years old. Throughout his life he would struggle with mental problems. After a failed relationship with a young woman, Boisen developed a fear of emotional intimacy, an experience from which he would not completely recover that would soon lead to even worse problems. At the age of twenty-two, Boisen had his first psychotic break, described in his own words: "The tension reached the breaking point on Easter morning of 1898. I got up early that morning after a sleepless night and went into the garden where Mother's hyacinths and daffodils were in full bloom. It was a beautiful day, but there was no sunshine there for me, no beauty, only dark despair. I came back to my room and threw myself on my knees with an agonized cry for help. And help came!"[7] But not in the way he wanted.

Boisen managed to cope with his mental condition without treatment until the age of forty-four. In October 1920, however, he was admitted for three weeks to the Boston Psychopathic Hospital. Plagued by distressing delusions and fantastic hallucinations, he was diagnosed with "dementia praecox, catatonic type" (i.e., schizophrenia), but this diagnosis is highly questionable given his subsequent course.[8] Boisen describes his experience: ". . . feelings of world catastrophe, followed by environmental and natural resource shortages. The presence of forces of evil was made known to him. He felt terror. Time became compressed."[9]

These personal experiences motivated him to study his own mental illness, convinced that this was somehow connected to his spiritual life. Boisen believed that schizophrenia could be understood as an attempt to solve the problems of the soul, and that mental illness involved both a psychological and a spiritual crisis. He wrote that ". . . certain types of mental disorders and certain types of religious experiences are alike attempts at re-organization."[10] When such attempts at reorganization were successful, they were recognized as religious experiences and could be transforming. When unsuccessful, however, they led to insanity. Thus, Boisen argued that symptoms of mental illness had both the potential for good and for bad:

[T]o be plunged as a patient into a hospital for the insane may be a tragedy or it may be an opportunity. For me it has been an opportunity. It has introduced me to a new world of absorbing interest and profound significance; it has shown me that world throughout its entire range, from the bottommost depths of the nether regions to the heights of religious experience at its best; it has made me aware of certain relationships between two important fields of human experience, which thus far have been held strictly apart; and has given me a task in which I find the meaning and purpose of my life.[11]

In July 1924, after hospitalization for another acute psychosis at Worcester State Hospital, Boisen was hired by superintendent Dr. William A. Bryan to become that hospital's first chaplain. Boisen attended a class at Harvard taught by well-known Boston physician Richard C. Cabot, who taught that the minister and physician should work together when treating patients. For the next five years Boisen, Cabot, and Bryan developed a new form of theological education for student chaplains that would accomplish Cabot's goal. In 1930, these men organized the Council for Clinical Training of Theological Students, which was later to become the Association for Clinical Pastoral Education. Boisen became the first ordained minister in the United States to supervise theological students in a clinical setting.[12] Although chaplains had served in the military for quite some time, there had been no attempt to integrate them into the health field.[13] This was the beginning of chaplains serving in health care settings.

Life continued to be difficult for Boisen as he battled with his own chronic mental illness. In the early 1930s, after his mother died, Boisen experienced another psychotic episode, which forced him to leave Worcester. He took a position as chaplain at Elgin State Hospital in Illinois and served part time on the faculty of the Chicago Theological Seminary, where he continued to train students to minister to those with physical, mental, or emotional illness.[14] Before his death at the age of eighty-nine in 1965, Boisen would help to usher in a completely new field—pastoral counseling. Just as with St. John of God, here was a man who himself struggled with mental illness, but whose religious faith enabled him to use these experiences to make lasting contributions to the care of those with similar problems.

Gheel, Belgium (13th century)

Besides the work of individuals such as John of God and Anton Boisen, communities have likewise played a role in easing the burden of those with mental illness. Imagine an entire town where mentally ill children and adults are not only supported by the faith community, but are cared for in private homes and included in family life.[15] This is the story of Gheel, Belgium, where the people actually do this and where what we now know as foster family care had its origins.[16] The motivation of the people here was again religious, an act of Christian charity. It was thought that "if we take care of these people and treat them as family members, we will be rewarded in the hereafter."[17] For nearly eight hundred years the tradition has continued. For the past two hundred years, Gheel has served as a model for initiatives in foster family care for the mentally ill in Europe, Canada, Japan, and the United States.[18] Today, as many as two thousand patients live with families in this small town of thirty thousand located in Belgium, thirty miles southwest of Antwerp.[19]

The story of how an entire community came to care for and involve the mentally ill in their daily lives is fascinating, although probably based more on fiction than on fact. The first record of this tradition comes from 1200 CE, although some accounts date it back to the seventh century. According to local oral history, a fifteen-year-old girl named Dymphna (secretly baptized by her Christian mother) ran away from her pagan chieftain father in Northern Ireland around 650.[20] After the death of her mother, the chieftain father became grief-struck, mentally ill, and lost his reason. He decided to marry his daughter Dymphna to replace her mother. On learning of his plans she ran away from home, accompanied by an elderly priest (named Gerebran) and a court jester and his wife. Living as hermits, the four hid in Belgium near a small chapel dedicated to St. Martin of Tours (present day Gheel). Her crazed father was persistent, though, and sent spies out to search for her. After learning her whereabouts, he led his troops from Ireland to Belgium to bring her back home. When Dymphna and her friends were found, her father begged her to return with him. Based on her religious faith and dedication to Christian purity, however, she refused. Enraged at her decision, he had Dymphna, the priest, and her friends killed. During the short time between her arrival and the time of her execution, Dymphna had gained a reputation for holiness because of her care for the poor and suffering in the area.

Six hundred years later, the bones of an unknown man and woman were discovered in Gheel.[21] The name "Dymphna" was found on a brick alongside two marble coffins. This is likely the source (rather than the proof) of the story about Dymphna and the elderly priest Gerebran. Soon after this discovery, according to the legend, five mentally ill persons were wandering about the countryside and bedded down for the night at the spot where the coffins were found.[22] When they awoke the next morning, they were completely cured of their mental disorders. News quickly spread throughout the region. Soon, others with mental illness who visited or slept at the site reported similar miraculous cures.

As a result, a shrine-hospital was built over Dymphna's purported gravesite around 1215. Today the shrine houses the two coffins and the brick with her name inscribed on it.[23] After being destroyed by fire in 1489, the shrine was rebuilt in 1532 and has been maintained to this day. The veneration of Dymphna as the patroness of the mentally ill grew rapidly, and soon the bishop of Cambrai had her biography written down from the oral tradition. Not long after this, she was declared a saint.[24] Today on her feast day (May 15) hundreds of people with mental illness are brought to her shrine for healing. The most common image of St. Dymphna depicts her as a young girl, a virgin (a lily across her arm), with an Irish shamrock on the Bible she is holding. This is likely an example of a folktale adapted as the life story of a saint. Whether a folktale, legend, or truth, its impact on the local community cannot be denied.

As news got out, people with mental illness were brought from all over, even from foreign countries, for healing at St. Dymphna's shrine. The local hospital was soon overflowing with chronic sufferers who were often left there, sometimes chained to trees near the shrine. Religiously motivated local peasants began to offer lodging to the mentally ill. They were absorbed into local families and worked in the town, on farms, or in private domiciles. Thus, the mentally ill were integrated not only into families but also into the community at large.[25] In this way, Gheel became the oldest community care program on record—the forerunner of today's community mental health programs, the concept of "transitional facilities," and the symbol for family home care.[26] During the eighteenth and nineteenth centuries, Gheel was visited by leading psychiatrists from both Germany and France, who started models of family care in their own countries.

In 1850, the Belgian "general lunatic law" became effective.[27] This gave the "colony of the mad" (as Gheel became known) a special status. Patients in locked asylums were given permission to be placed in foster families there. This eventually led to a declaration of the entire province as a kind of infirmary for the mentally ill.[28] Inspections of homes where the mentally ill stayed were made by supervisors and occasionally by physicians from the local asylum. Although some sources indicate that a section of the ordinance (Article 27) prevented anyone except the harmless insane from entering into this community, other records suggest that this rule was hard to follow and sometimes those with violent tendencies ended up in foster families (often with good results).

Bear in mind that the people of Gheel were reaching out to the mentally ill at a time in history (thirteenth to eighteenth centuries) when they were almost universally neglected or treated harshly. This system of care would survive changes in government and sovereignty and even wars that devastated the area. Today, Gheel has a state mental hospital that is one of the largest and most efficient in the world.[29] It is associated with a community program where the mentally ill board in the homes of local farmers or residents and help with work and family life. In the United States, a shrine to St. Dymphna was built in 1939 in Massillon, Ohio, next to a large modern hospital. It is maintained by the Franciscan Mission Associates, who do their work in the name of St. Dymphna among the poor in Central America and elsewhere.[30]

Ramsey, Minnesota (21st century)

Although it is not likely that an entire town would devote itself to caring for those with mental illness today, religious communities might be expected to help in some way. The following story was published in the *Minneapolis-St. Paul Star Tribune*,[31] and illustrates the role that modern-day faith communities can play in helping persons with severe, persistent mental illness. Unfortunately, it also illustrates how some faith communities can neglect their wounded, and how important it is for someone in the congregation to stir up interest by serving as an advocate.

When Brian Haberle was hospitalized shortly after his schizophrenia diagnosis 20 years ago, he told his mother, Bonnie, that he'd like a visit from their parish priest. The response she got at the rectory would break her heart and seal her fate.

"His first question to us was, 'Is he violent?'" said Bonnie Haberle of Ramsey, Minnesota. Her son, in other people's eyes, had been instantly re-categorized from "kind, neat young man to someone you need to be afraid of."

About the same time, [Bonnie] Haberle's mother was diagnosed with cancer. "Her help from her faith community and friends was 180 degrees different from what we were experiencing with our son," Haberle said. "We had people coming from the church to our house for her, prayers, the whole nine yards. We received not a fraction of that for our son. Nothing.

"People seemed to be stunned. They just couldn't make any sense of it and didn't even ask how he was. . . . It was just totally, totally different."

Fear, ignorance and shame often prevent people from talking about mental illnesses, although disorders such as depression, anxiety, bipolar disorder and schizophrenia affect as many as one in four Minnesota families.

Still, the myths that mental illness is caused by bad parenting, and that people who have mental illnesses are prone to violence, prevent people from talking about it. Sometimes the prejudices are rooted in religion, such as the belief that people with mental illnesses are possessed by demons or being punished by God.

Haberle made a mission of educating congregations about mental illness and the needs of mentally ill people and their families. She is chairwoman of the Faithways program of the National Alliance for the Mentally Ill, which offers training and other resources for religious communities.

The benefits of open communication are tangible, according to Faithways director Mary Jean Babcock.

"It's the people who talk about it, who bring it out into the light of day, who make it easier for other people to go out and get help for their own situations," Babcock said. "Then other people can feel like, 'Well, I can talk about it. I can start looking at it, and I can start dealing with it.'"

Networks of advocacy groups, families and people who live with mental illnesses are working hard to educate clergy and congregations and help them see people with mental illnesses as parishioners who may need their help and deserve their compassion.

"One of the most important things to do is to educate everybody in the community," said Laurie Kramer, director of the Mental Health Education Project, a collaborative program of the Twin Cities Jewish community. "It's great to say we welcome everybody, which we do, but we have to know what the needs are and how to meet those needs so people will be truly welcomed."

Support from religious communities is vital. After the doctor's office, the church or synagogue often is the first place people go for support.

"Oftentimes people who are struggling with mental illness issues are in need of a sense of community," said Rabbi Morris Allen of Beth Jacob Congregation in Mendota Heights. "There's a need of feeling affirmed, knowing that God's affirmation of them is expressed through a community of shared faith. . . . Often these are the same people who are shunned by the community, and they feel that they are shunned by God."

The Rev. Linda Koelman, pastor at North United Methodist Church in Minneapolis, was one of several clergy who said that churches by nature must take extra steps to be inclusive.

"If we say we are a welcoming place in Christ's name, yet we shut out a large group, we are not living up to what we are called to do," she said. "What people look for is a place that will be safe and that will accept them where they are."

In providing such a haven, religious communities get back more than they give, Koelman said. "By looking at other people and the gifts that they have to bring, it helps open a church up and make it far richer in diversity and in the caring and support that a church can give."

Although leadership from the clergy is key, the change often begins within the congregation.

"What it really takes is someone who has experienced mental illness in their family to go to the pastor or rabbi, get the pastor or rabbi on board, and get a group of people together who really care about this issue," said Barbara Holmquist, director of caregivers at Mount Olivet Lutheran Church in south Minneapolis.

In the late 1970s, Mount Olivet member Joanna Kuehn was diagnosed with a schizo-affective disorder and hospitalized for two months. It was a year before she felt able to rejoin her church choir, and two years before she started feeling like herself again.

A few years later, she approached her pastor to suggest a task force on mental illness. "My pastor and my church were willing to listen to me, which validated me as a person with mental illness, and so I am so grateful," Kuehn said.

"It's been one of the most therapeutic things of my experience, to be able to share something that I never would have wished for, but when I think of all the people I've met, and the opportunity to find meaning in what I had gone through, I think, what a blessing in my life."

In 1986, Kuehn and a group of supporters founded the Task Force on Mental Illness/Brain Disorders. Over the years, their mission has grown roots into all parts of Mount Olivet's ministry. Mental-health education is part of Sunday services, and part of training for all outreach volunteers. The church sponsors a group home for people who live with severe and persistent mental illnesses. There is a psychologist and a psychiatrist on the church staff. The group sponsors interfaith training sessions.

"God calls us to stand by people with mental illness, just like he calls us to stand by people who are homeless," Holmquist said. "This is part of our Christian faith, bringing that cup of cold water to someone who is in need."[32]

Durham, North Carolina (21st century)

The fifth story comes from my own caseload.[33] One evening in the fall of 2002, I received a call from "Sally," who was a patient of mine whom I had been treating for several years. She had a diagnosis of schizo-affective disorder (schizophrenia with periods of severe depression). I really liked Sally. She was a kind and caring lady who had a terrible disease that devastated her quality of life. When Sally called that evening, she asked me if I knew anyone who might give her a little emotional support once or twice a week. She said she was going through a rough time. I knew that the medication I prescribed was not controlling her symptoms very well, and she was having lots of guilt and shame and feeling generally overwhelmed.

Sally was in her mid-fifties and had been hospitalized several times during the past four decades to treat episodes of psychosis and/or severe depression. However, when not acutely ill, she was deeply religious, regularly attended her church, and tried to become involved in the congregation's ministries. I heard from someone at her congregation that during the church services she would become totally involved, singing passionately and sometimes crying with joy or weeping with sorrow. Sally was always there at special church meetings, and often would be the first person to volunteer when help was needed (although was seldom taken up on her offers).

I asked Sally why she hadn't contacted someone in her church to meet with her and provide support. She had contacted the minister and met with him several times, but his time was always short and she needed someone to talk with and confide in as a friend. She was having difficulty finding a person to support her even though her congregation consisted of nearly one thousand members. Her church, she said, tended to focus on the youth and on evangelism, and really didn't put much emphasis on ministry to those who were older or had chronic mental problems. To their credit, they promised to enroll her in a women's mentoring program that was to start up in the spring. That, however, was still six months away, and she needed help now. So, in desperation, she decided to call me, her doctor.

I agreed to make some phone calls and see what I could do. I thought it would be a snap to locate someone to help her, someone eager to minister to this poor soul who was a committed Christian. Little did I know that it would take months and several dozen e-mails and phone calls before I could locate that someone. One person after another gave excuses why they couldn't do it and referred me to someone else. Phone calls and e-mails wouldn't be returned for weeks. I even tried to go outside the state to tap into church-related mental health networks that might know of someone locally.

Here I was, a well-known and respected psychiatrist with many, many contacts in the Christian community. If I was having this much trouble, I couldn't imagine how difficult it would be for Sally to find support on her own. I thought, "Why is this so hard? Why won't a person of faith—perhaps someone who is retired—give a few moments of their time each week to provide love to a hurting neighbor?" It just didn't make sense to me. I would have thought my phone would be ringing off the hook with offers of help. After nearly two months, I finally found an older lady from a local church who was willing to meet and talk with Sally. "Karen" was wonderful, just the kind of person that Sally needed—a friend to talk with once in awhile, who made her feel loved and cared for. But this whole experience disturbed me. Why was it so difficult to find someone in the faith community willing to support and walk alongside Sally in her struggles?

So I talked about the situation with friends, colleagues, and religious people I knew, and this is what I learned. Everyone is busy, preoccupied with their own work, ministries, families, and friends. Many don't want to get involved with someone who isn't a member of their church. Some judge the person with emotional or mental problems, blaming them for their condition. Many people are just plain scared of making contact with a person who has severe and persistent mental problems, afraid of the unpredictability of entering into such a relationship. What if the person becomes overly attached, doesn't understand limits, wants to become too involved in my life, or becomes too emotionally draining? What if the person gets violent or angry? What about my safety and the safety of my family? What if the mentally ill person gets into trouble with the police, or hurts him or herself, or hurts someone else? What if . . .

No question, the "what ifs" are a lot to overcome—even for many deeply religious people with the sincerest of intentions. This is especially true if the helper doesn't know much about the person's mental condition or about severe mental disorders in general. Lack of knowledge is a huge barrier to feeling comfortable enough to get involved.

Summary

People of faith, whether they are from Christian, Jewish, Muslim, Hindu, or Buddhist religious orientations, have a duty and responsibility to care for those who are sick, weak, poor, or in some other way troubled or in need. The founders of every great religious tradition and their sacred scriptures urge followers to care for the needy and to regularly perform acts of charity and kindness. When it comes to mental illness, however, there are many factors that prevent religious persons from reaching out as they normally would to others.

Personal experience with mental illness, either one's own or that of a loved one, can either be paralyzing or can serve as a powerful motivator to get involved. John of God was a role model of the latter. His faith and personal pain helped him to initiate an entire movement. This resulted in the creation of a religious order devoted to meeting the needs of the mentally ill and poor. The same applies to Anton Boisen, the founder of clinical pastoral education, pastoral counseling, and to some extent, hospital chaplaincy. This was also true for Joanna Kuehn, who after recovering from her bout of mental illness began a ministry in her congregation at Mount Olivet Lutheran Church that included mental-health education, training of outreach volunteers, and sponsorship of a group home. These stories illustrate what people can do even if they are struggling with mental illness. They also illustrate how the power of religious faith can fuel such actions.

Family members of persons with severe and persistent mental illness can also transform their pain into advocacy, as Bonnie Haberle did after discovering her church's lack of response to her son's needs. She now serves on a national board that focuses on providing resources to religious communities so that they can better understand and meet the needs of those with mental illness. People like Karen, who agreed to be a friend to Sally, are also critically needed—those who are willing to take a leap of faith to risk loving a needy stranger.

These cases illustrate how individual persons and communities of faith can help those with emotional and mental problems bear their burdens, which is a major focus of this book. The next chapter will give the reader a historical perspective across time that will illustrate how attitudes of faith communities and their contributions toward the care of persons with mental illness evolved through the centuries.

CHAPTER 2

HISTORY OF MENTAL
HEALTH CARE

Attitudes of faith communities toward the mentally ill today are based on a long and complex history of care, compassion, and persecution. Having examined the life of John of God, Anton Boisen, the community of Gheel, and several modern religious communities, let us now take a broader and more detailed view of the historical relationship between religion and care of the mentally ill from both Western and Eastern perspectives.

Pre-Middle Ages

From the dawn of recorded history comes information about the first medicine man—the shaman. The shaman was often distinguished by having mental illness. This allowed him to have visions and, it was thought, enabled him to communicate with the spirit world, which was believed to be the cause of all disease and physical illness.[1] Drinking alcohol or ingesting hallucinogenic herbs might further enhance these "powers." As a result, mental illness was often highly regarded and respected in primitive societies.

As civilization advanced, severe mental illness (also called "madness" or "insanity") came to be understood as resulting from a disordered physiological condition. The Greeks in the fifth century BCE argued that hallucinations, delusions, or unusual mental excitement were due to an imbalance of the four humors (yellow bile, black bile, blood, and phlegm), not the work of gods or spirits. Mental illness, along with epilepsy, was called

17

the "sacred disease" in the Hippocratic tradition: "those maddened through bile are noisy, evil-doers and restless, always doing something inopportune . . . But if terrors and fears attack, they are due to a change in the brain."[2]

Graeco-Roman law made provision for the care of the mentally ill (largely by secluding them) to keep them from harming themselves or others. Nevertheless, care for the insane was generally considered a family responsibility, since there were no asylums or places to house the mentally ill. If severely disturbed, they might be restrained at home or, failing that, allowed to wander in the streets.

From the public's perspective, the mentally ill person in Greek and Roman times was no longer seen as special and gifted (as the shaman had been in early antiquity). Instead, he or she was viewed as strange and deranged, someone to be feared. A popular belief was that evil spirits were causing the illness and might fly out and possess others around the person.[3] Consequently, such individuals were avoided and shunned. If the mentally ill person had no family or if the family refused to provide care, a town might either assign a caretaker or have the person held in a jail or a dungeon.[4]

Christians prescribed religious treatments in the mid-fourth century CE, since at least some cases of mental illness were thought to be due to possession by demonic spirits. According to Ronald Numbers and Darrell Amundsen,[5] prayers were included in the *Canones Ecclesiastici* and *Bishop Serapion's Prayer Book* to be used with the application of holy oil to heal those with fever, sickness, or those possessed by demons, and both sacramental healing and exorcism were mentioned in other sacred writings as early as the mid-second century. Origen (185–254 CE) was particularly influential in forming early Christian thinking about mental illness and demonology. In *De Principiis* he articulated his belief that demons could completely take over the mind, removing the power of reason and emotional control. He used the terms "possession" and "insanity" as referring to similar states, and emphasized that Jesus healed the insane by exorcism—the casting out of demonic spirits.

The establishment of large hospitals for care of the sick in the general population, according to historians Sarton, Granshaw, and Porter, was a Christian notion that developed in the fourth century.[6] Inspired by biblical teachings to clothe the poor and heal the sick, Christians extended the long-held Jewish tradition of care for the sick. By 250 CE, the Christian church in Rome had developed an outreach to the poor and ill of all faith backgrounds, including the mentally ill. When Constantine declared Christianity the official religion of the Roman Empire, this charity "found expression in bricks and mortar."[7] Between 344 and 358, the bishop of Antioch set up several hostels. In 360, the bishop of Sebasteia built a poor house. In 372, the bishop of Caesarea (in present-day Turkey) established the first great hospital, called Basileias, described as "almost a new city" for the treatment of the sick, the poor, and those with leprosy. This hospital had both nurses and medical attendants.[8] Hostels, poor houses, and these early hospitals often addressed the mental health needs of patients right alongside their physical needs.

Soon, the Christian church began building hospitals throughout Western Europe. Around 390 a facility was built in Rome to care for the sick poor. These Christians "personally tended the unhappy and impoverished victims of hunger and disease . . . washing wounds which others . . . could hardly bear to look at . . . gathered sufferers from the streets . . . carried home, on [their] own shoulders, the dirty and poor who were plagued by epilepsy! [or mental illness, which epilepsy was often confused with] . . . washed the pus from sores which others could not even behold!."[9] Comparing these activities with attitudes in the surrounding populace, historian Roy Porter remarks, "Greek and Roman paganism had acknowledged no such duties." Numbers and Amundsen also note, "In general there was no religious or ethical motivation for charity in the pagan classical world. Among the Greeks and Romans, benevolence manifested itself in civic philanthropy on behalf of the entire community rather than in private charity undertaken for individuals in need, such as the sick, widows, or orphans."[10]

Middle Ages

The Middle Ages covers the period between around 500 and 1500 CE. By the fifth century, there were clear records of the Christian church helping the mentally ill. One of the first hospitals devoted to treating those with mental illness was established in Jerusalem in 490.[11] In the sixth century, the mentally ill were cared for in monasteries run by the Christian church, although these tended to focus on the care of their own members.[12] Between 1225 and 1230, a Franciscan monk and professor of theology named Bartholomaeus wrote an encyclopedia that dealt with mental illness in terms of natural causes, not supernatural ones.[13]

In 1247, Europe's first psychiatric hospital, the Priory of St. Mary of Bethlehem, was established in London on the Thames River.[14] It was originally designed to house "distracted people." Three centuries later in 1547, after the land of the priory was given to the city of London, St. Mary's was torn down and replaced by Bethlehem or Bethlem Hospital.[15] The common name for the hospital was "Bedlam," which became famous for its inhumane treatment. Patients were often chained to walls[16] and dunked in water or beaten if they misbehaved. The hospital housed about sixty patients at a time. In 1676 a new hospital was built on the original site. Larger and more modern, it held about 150 patients. Bedlam soon became a popular tourist attraction, since people from London often came to observe and be entertained by the patients. The admission in 1753 was two pence. This was such a lucrative venture for the hospital that they continued to "show" patients until the end of the eighteenth century.[17]

In 1409, another religious-sponsored hospital in Europe was built specifically to care for persons with mental illness. It was established in Valencia, Spain, directed by a priest, and both supported and operated by a religious order of brothers.[18] Mentally ill persons were also admitted to the Hotel-Dieu (Hospital of God) in Paris, the largest hospital in Europe and the center of medical training throughout the Middle Ages. A common treatment at the Hotel-Dieu was to arrange for the insane to be taken to various healing shrines in the area (including the Dymphna shrine at Gheel), since there were no other treatments.[19] The care provided in religious-sponsored hospitals like these, administered under the direction of priests and sisters, was reported to be much better than that provided by state-supported mental asylums centuries later.[20]

The Christian church, however, did not always behave compassionately toward the mentally ill. A common explanation in the general population was that mental illness was due to demonic possession, which led to persecution of the insane (whose numbers in Europe increased dramatically after 1300). However, historical evidence suggests that the role of the church in persecuting the so called demon-possessed has been widely exaggerated.[21] The Inquisition, established in 1233, was an institution in the

Christian church whose purpose was to eradicate heresies, not combat witchcraft or demon-possession, which was of secondary interest only. Not until 1487, with the publication of *Malleus Maleficarum* that describes the diagnosis and treatment of those thought to be demon-possessed, did the Christian church's persecution of sorcerers and witches (and sometimes the mentally ill) become widespread. Prior to that time, natural and folk remedies were used extensively for the treatment of mental and what were considered "spiritual" illnesses. After that, torturing and burning "the possessed" became a more regular occurrence.[22] This continued for nearly two hundred years with thousands of persons being burned at the stake or decapitated.[23] The last witch-hunts in the United States occurred in Salem, Massachusetts, in 1692, with nearly one hundred persons accused and nineteen executed.[24]

As psychiatrist and historian Jerome Kroll points out, however, "mental and spiritual illnesses were attributed as much to overwork, overeating, and overindulgence in sexual activity as to climatic conditions, magic spells and demon possession."[25] Over time, sin became viewed less and less as the cause of mental illness. A systematic review of persons diagnosed with mental illness reported during the Middle Ages indicates that writers of the day attributed sin as the cause for only 16% of cases.[26]

Suzanne Phillips from the department of psychology at Gordon College (Wenham, MA) also notes that, "Present-day psychology reports an inaccurate history of the European witch-hunts as a history of cruelty toward people with mental disorders at the hands of the church. In actuality, people with mental illness were not believed to be witches, nor were they executed. Throughout the medieval period, people with mental illness were cared for by the church and by society more generally; this care was rooted in a richly integrated understanding of mental disorder as simultaneously biological, psychological, and spiritual in nature."[27] Thus, historians disagree on the extent to which mentally ill persons were persecuted during this time. No doubt, such persecutions did occur to some extent and resulted in many deaths, but exactly how many and over what period of time remains controversial.

Renaissance and Reformation

The Renaissance was the period in Europe beginning in the mid-1300s following the Black Death (which killed one-third of the population) and ended in 1517 with the Protestant Reformation, when Luther nailed his ninety-five theses on the church door at Wittenburg. The Reformation era lasted until the close of the eighteenth century.

I draw heavily here on the work of psychiatrist and historian Samuel Thielman, who has summarized the events that occurred during these periods.[28] Between the mid-fourteenth century and the end of the eighteenth century, ideas about mental illness in both the medical profession and the Christian church did not change much. These views oscillated back and forth between biological and spiritual causes. Both Catholics and Protestants believed that some mentally ill people were possessed by demons, even though others might simply have diseases of the brain. St. John of the Cross (1542–1591) described two types of depression in his book *Ascent of Mount Carmel*. One type he thought was spiritual and described as the "dark night of the soul" that led to spiritual growth and deeper understanding. A second type, which he characterized as melancholy, led to further despair and loss of hope. He instructed priests who took confessions to try to distinguish between these two conditions.[29]

On the one hand, even well-known mental health professionals of the day attributed some kinds of depression to religious forces. In his famous *The Anatomy of Melancholy* (1621), Robert Burton described religious melancholy as being due to both natural and supernatural causes. On the other hand, religious professionals such as St. John of the Cross, who themselves had experienced depression, refuted arguments that demons caused depression, maintaining that those with melancholy should receive compassionate care and see doctors who might help ease their burdens. Protestant minister Timothy Rogers emphasized in 1691 the need to address the melancholic's spiritual, medical, and psychological concerns in a balanced fashion: ". . . it is a very overwhelming thing to attribute every action almost of a Melancholy man to the Devil, when there are some unavoidable Expressions of sorrow which are purely natural, and which he cannot help."[30]

During the late seventeenth and eighteenth centuries, as the scientific revolution gained momentum, references in the medical literature to demons as a cause for mental illness became less and less common. Physician George Cheyne argued forcefully in his 1733 publication, *The English Malady*, against the notion that mental disorders were caused by witchcraft or possession, using his own case of mental illness to illustrate his points.[31] As a religious person, he described both the comforts of religious faith and the religious preoccupations that created turmoil and anxiety. The fact that many well-known religious men throughout the Renaissance and Reformation periods experienced severe bouts of depression, including Martin Luther himself,[32] helped to discredit the notion that demonic possession or a weak religious faith was at the root of melancholic or neurotic disorders.

The Age of Reason and Enlightenment

The Age of Reason followed soon after the Reformation era and was characterized by a decline in tolerance for religious beliefs. This period culminated with the arrival of the Enlightenment in 1800, as the French Revolution came to a close. The appearance of nonreligious explanations for mental disorders increased rapidly, as scientific explanations were sought for these conditions and all other illnesses. Since there were still no proven treatments for mental disorder, attention turned to asylum reform. Indeed, there was much to reform.

London's Bethlem Hospital (Bedlam) is a case in point. To this day, books and horror movies display the cruelty and neglect, the whips and chains used to control and dehumanize the mentally ill. Consider the description below:

A stout iron ring was riveted around his neck, from which a short chain passed through a ring made to slide upwards and downwards on an upright massive iron bar, more than six feet high, inserted into the wall. Round his body a strong iron bar about two inches wide was riveted; on each side of the bar was a circular projection; which being fastened to and enclosing each of his arms, pinioned them close to his sides.[33]

The new asylums of the nineteenth century tried to eliminate such abuses. The French physician Philippe Pinel, a religious man who had at one point planned to become a priest, was made head of an asylum in

France in 1793. Upset by the way that patients were being cared for there, he tried releasing them from their restraints and treating them with compassion. To everyone's amazement, this action met with great success, especially for those suffering from melancholia (depression) or mania. Pinel emphasized that mental illnesses were influenced by psychological and social factors as well as by physical causes, and therefore needed psychological treatments. He called his new method *traitement moral* or "moral treatment," which emphasized kindness and "ways of gentleness."[34] The idea that mental illness might be curable using this new form of treatment spread quickly across Europe. This led to the reformation of asylums and the development of more humane methods of managing mental patients. Restraining with chains and beatings were soon done away with.

At almost the same time, another form of moral treatment was being developed in England independent of what was happening in France. An English merchant and devout Quaker named William Tuke established the York Retreat in 1796.[35] He was motivated by the death of a Quaker patient in a New York asylum due to abuses that were still common there. As a result, Tuke and the Quaker community decided to set up their own asylum. Rather than restraining and isolating patients, treatment involved intelligent and humane care. At the York Retreat they instituted a regimen of exercise, work, and recreation, treating the insane with compassion. Tuke saw the mentally ill as brothers capable of living a moral, ordered existence if treated with kindness, dignity, and respect in a comfortable setting. As a result, patients lived, worked, and had their meals together in a family-like atmosphere. The goal was restoration of self-control. The Quakers argued, as Pinel had in France, that insanity was a disruption of the mind and spirit, not just the body. Tuke testified before English Parliament in 1815, contrasting the "hell"-like atmosphere of Bedlam with the "heaven"-like setting at the York Retreat. Soon moral treatment was adopted throughout England.

Origins of American Psychiatry

Early American psychiatry was heavily influenced by developments in England at the time. The Quakers brought moral treatment to America in the early 1800s and this soon became the dominant form of psychiatric care in the United States.[36] Friends Hospital (or Friends Asylum), established in Philadelphia in 1813, became the nation's first private institution dedicated solely to the care of those with mental illness.[37] In 1818, the McClean Hospital was established in Boston; in 1821, the Bloomingdale Asylum in New York; and in 1824, the Hartford Retreat in Connecticut—all modeled after the York Retreat in England and implementing moral treatment as the dominant therapy.

Insane asylums in early and mid-nineteenth-century America, then, involved a mixture of science and religion.[38] Patients in some institutions were rewarded for self-control and good behavior by allowing them to attend religious services.[39] According to Amariah Brigham, the superintendent at the Hartford Retreat and founding editor of the *American Journal of Insanity* (later to become the *American Journal of Psychiatry*), "No doubt that these services are beneficial to our patients. Permission to attend them is solicited by nearly all and many are induced to exercise their self-control in order to enjoy this privilege."[40] Even Samuel Woodward, superintendent of the Worcester State Hospital in Massachusetts and founder of the Association of Medical Superintendents of American Institutions for the Insane (later to become the American Psychiatric Association), observed, "By our whole moral treatment, as well as by our religious services, we try to inculcate all of that which is rational."[41] Clergy were routinely hired to live on the grounds of these early psychiatric hospitals, both holding religious services and providing spiritual counsel.[42]

In the mid-1800s, Dorothea Dix championed the cause for humane care of the mentally ill in America and Europe.[43] Raised in a religious family that instilled strong moral values, Dix was outraged at finding mentally ill prisoners locked away in unheated jail cells in Cambridge, Massachusetts. She spent several years investigating the conditions of the mentally ill in jails and almshouses, and then spoke out for the building of asylums where proper treatment could be delivered. Within a decade, seventeen states had built or enlarged hospitals for the mentally ill. Traveling to Europe, Dix influenced the care of the mentally ill in England and Scotland during that period also.

Thus, those who crusaded for better treatment of the mentally ill and asylum reform were often people of faith: Philippe Pinel, William Tuke, and Dorothea Dix. The close relationship between religion and psychiatry, however, was to change dramatically over a period of little more than fifty years. Sigmund Freud would have an enormous influence on psychiatry's attitude toward religion and lead to a near complete separation of the two within a few decades.

Modern Times

Freud described religion as an "obsessional neurosis" based on illusion and projection. In his first paper on the topic in 1907, *Obsessive Acts and Religious Practices*, Freud compared the act of prayer to the obsessive-compulsive actions of the neurotic.[44] Over the next thirty years, he would write five more treatises underscoring the destabilizing effects of religion on the psyche.[45] In *Future of an Illusion*, Freud wrote:

Religion would thus be the universal obsessional neurosis of humanity. . . . If this view is right, it is to be supposed that a turning-away from religion is bound to occur with the fatal inevitability of a process of growth. . . . If, on the one hand, religion brings with it obsessional restrictions, exactly as an individual obsessional neurosis does, on the other hand it comprises a system of wishful illusions together with a disavowal of reality, such as we find in an isolated form nowhere else but amentia, in a state of blissful hallucinatory confusion. . . .[46]

By 1980, psychiatric wards at a number of prominent academic teaching hospitals in the United States had completely removed any religious influences from the treatment of psychiatric patients. Even at Methodist-affiliated institutions such Duke University and its adjoining hospital, the attending physician on the psychiatry ward had to explicitly authorize a visit by a clergyperson or even by a hospital chaplain. Psychiatrists and psychologists often interpreted religious beliefs as emotionally disturbing and harmful for patients.[47] Professor of psychiatry Wendell Waters at McMaster's University said it this way:

Evidence that religion is not only irrelevant but actually harmful to human beings should be of interest, not only to other behavioral scientists, but to anyone who finds it difficult to live an unexamined life. Finally, the argument advanced in this volume should stir the political decision makers who complain about the high cost of health care even while continuing to subsidize that very institution that may be actually making the public sick.[48]

Psychologist Albert Ellis, the founder of rational emotive therapy (a forerunner of cognitive-behavioral therapy), also emphasized that:

Devout, orthodox, or dogmatic religion (or what might be called religiosity) is significantly correlated with emotional disturbance. . . . The emotionally healthy individual is flexible, open, tolerant, and changing, and the devoutly religious person tends to be inflexible, closed, intolerant, and unchanging. Religiosity, therefore, is in many respects equivalent to irrational thinking and emotional disturbance. . . .[49]

By the close of the twentieth century, the negative attitude toward religion expressed by Freud and more contemporary mental health professionals such as Watters and Ellis had impacted the personal views of many practicing psychologists and psychiatrists. Surveys in the 1980s and 1990s found that 57% to 74% of psychologists[50] and 24% to 75% of psychiatrists[51] did not believe in God, compared to only 4% of nonbelievers in the general U.S. population.[52] Psychiatrists in England were even less likely than those in the United States to have religious beliefs. Neeleman and King studied 231 psychiatrists at general and psychiatric hospitals in London. Investigators found that 73% of psychiatrists reported no religious affiliation and 78% attended religious services less than once a month. Among female psychiatrists, 39% believed in God, whereas only 19% of male psychiatrists did so. Although over 90% believed that religion and mental illness were connected and that religious issues should be addressed in treatment, 58% of psychiatrists in that survey *never* made referrals to clergy.

The gap between mental health professionals' personal religious beliefs and the beliefs of their patients no doubt affected the kinds of treatments prescribed. In fact, until 1994 the *Diagnostic and Statistical Manual of Mental Disorders* (DSM) commonly used religious examples to illustrate serious cases of mental illness that included illogical thinking, incoherence, poverty of content and speech, poverty of affect, catatonic posturing, delusions of being controlled, hallucinations, magical thinking, and psychotic delusions. A systematic review of the religious content of DSM-III-R found that over 22% of all cases of mental illness included religious descriptions.[53]

Trainees graduating today from psychiatry residency programs, however, may be more informed about both the positive and the negative effects that patients' religious beliefs and practices may have on mental health. The American College of Graduate Medical Education now includes in its *Special Requirements for Residency Training for Psychiatry* that all programs provide training on religious or spiritual factors that influence psychological development.[54] At least the official word, then, is that psychiatrists should be aware of these issues. Research suggests that recent graduates may be more open to discussing the religious or spiritual beliefs of patients. In a study of 96 psychiatric residents, 40% reported a substantial degree of religiosity [high belief (74%), high practice (50%), high priority (71%)], and indicated that it was particularly important to know about the religious beliefs of psychotherapy patients.[55]

At least sixteen psychiatric residency programs in the United States now offer formal training in religious and spiritual issues,[56] and there is evidence that similar training is occurring in some Canadian residency programs as well. Grabovac and Ganesan surveyed fourteen of the sixteen psychiatry residency programs in Canada to determine the extent of training they provided in religion and spirituality.[57] Investigators discovered that four of the fourteen programs had no training whatsoever on the topic. Four others had mandatory lectures and nine offered at least some degree of elective or case-based supervision on the interface between religion, spirituality, and psychiatry.

More recent studies of practicing psychologists also suggest changing attitudes toward religion. Bilgrave and colleagues examined religious beliefs and psychotherapeutic orientations of a national sample of 237 clinical and counseling psychologists.[58] Two-thirds (66%) believed in the transcendent, 72% indicated that their religious beliefs influenced their practice of psychotherapy, and 66% claimed that their practice of therapy influenced their religious beliefs. Psychology training programs are now required to "include exposure to theoretical and empirical knowledge bases relevant to the role of cultural and individual diversity," which includes religion.[59] Nevertheless, it is still true that many psychologists and psychiatrists in the United States still do not inquire about the religious or spiritual beliefs of patients, and it is even less common for them to address spiritual needs or utilize the spiritual resources of patients as part of therapy (see chapter 6).

History of Mental Health Care in Non-Western Cultures

In many if not most non-Western cultures, mental health care developed within a religious framework. This is especially true for areas of the world where Islam, Judaism, and the great Eastern religions of Buddhism and Hinduism predominate. Historical information, however, is more difficult to obtain on these developments.

ISLAM

Islam has a long tradition of compassion for those with mental illness.[60] Muslims played a key role in setting up some of the first hospitals built for the care of persons with severe mental illness, since the Qur'an emphasizes the need to provide humane care for those with mental problems. The first major Islamic medical hospital was built in Baghdad in 805. During the Middle Ages, the Islamic hospital served several purposes beyond that of providing medical care alone. It also served as a convalescent home for those recovering from illness or accidents, a retirement home that met the basic maintenance needs for the aged and infirm, and, in some cases, an insane asylum.[61]

According to historical record, the earliest hospital providing care to the insane was in Cairo, built in 872 by Ahmad ibn Tulun, the governor of Egypt. These hospitals, called *maristans*, developed a worldwide reputation for their humane care of those with mental illness.[62] The most famous of the Middle Ages Islamic hospitals was also located in Cairo. Built in 1283, it was dedicated to the rich, the poor, and people of all faiths. This hospital had special wards for persons with mental diseases (and remarkably, it had a chapel for Christians as well as a mosque).[63] Muslims also established one of the first hospitals in Europe that was designed specifically for treatment of the mentally ill. This was built in 1365 and located in Granada, Spain.[64] (Muslims ruled Spain from 711 until 1492, when it was reconquered by Christians.[65])

Persons with mental illness were hospitalized because influential Muslim physicians of the period considered it a medical condition (in contrast to the more widespread popular Arab belief that attributed such illnesses to demons or spirits). These hospitals were supported by rulers who believed that caring for the mentally ill was one way to fulfill their religious obligation of charity to the needy,[66] based on Sura 4:5 in the Qur'an, which states, "Do not give to the incompetent [mentally ill] their property that God has assigned to you to manage; provide for them and clothe them out of it; and speak to them honorable words."

Ihsan Al-Issa describes how mental illness was treated in medieval Islamic society.[67] Islamic psychiatry dates back to the seventh century when Islamic civilization started to grow and spread across the near East and northern Africa. Islamic beliefs about mental illness were themselves affected by the ideas and folklore of countries into which Muslim influence expanded. While Muslim physicians did much to preserve Hippocratic and Galenic theories, Islamic beliefs provided alternative views from the classical Greek perspective. In the tenth century, Islamic physician Al-Razi reformulated the work of Galen and added his own ideas in the renowned encyclopedic work called *Continens* (or *Al-Hawi*). Considered the Father of Islamic Psychiatry, Al-Razi was the first Islamic physician to write about neuropsychiatric disorders and suggest treatments for them. Rather than being due to evil spirits, he claimed they were due to a nervous breakdown or other problems with the mind.

In *Continens*, Al-Razi included an entire chapter on melancholia, describing the symptoms of depression, and drugs for eliminating its root cause (thought to be black bile). He described drugs for treating insomnia and calming agitation, and wrote about a condition called lycanthropy (the delusion that one is a wolf) associated with mental confusion, social withdrawal, and reclusion. He was also the first Muslim physician to refer to the benefits of psychotherapy *(Al-Ilaj Annafsani)*, recommending that physicians provide patients with suggestions of good health and with psychological support. Al-Razi believed that changes in the mind preceded changes in the body, providing the basis for psychosomatic medicine in the tenth century.[68] Another Islamic physician, Al-Majusi, wrote in a tenth-century medical textbook called *Kitab al-Malaki* that "persuasion" together with music and potions should be used to treat the mentally ill. There is little doubt that Al-Razi, Al-Majusi, and other Muslim physicians of their day firmly believed in a medical and psychological model for treating mental illness.

During the same time and long thereafter, however, popular approaches to the treatment of mental illness thrived in the general Muslim population. Some mental conditions, in fact, were redefined as normal, precluding the need for treatment. For example, the insane might be seen as "holy fools" or "wise fools." The holy fool was someone whose love for God or adherence to religious ideals bordered on the abnormal. The wise fool had poetic or mystical gifts, but who nevertheless showed little concern for appearance and might disregard social conventions by appearing naked in public. Religious or spiritual qualities were attributed to such people who today would be considered mentally ill. Thus, Islamic society had a broad concept of mental illness and was relatively tolerant of deviant behavior.

Although the Qur'an gives little advice about medical matters, *Prophetic Medicine*, written by Ibn Qayyim Al-Jaziya in the fourteenth century, summarizes the teachings of the Prophet that relate to medical care (combining this with aspects of Arab folk medicine). Illness, including mental illness, was viewed as a trial or a blessing for believers, and those who endured these conditions to the end were thought to enter into a special place in paradise after death. The idea that original sin and the inherent sinfulness of mankind was the cause for illness did not exist in Islamic teachings, since the Qur'an states: "there is no fault in the blind, and there is no fault in the lame and there is no fault in the sick . . ." (Sura 24:61). Prayer, however, was widely recognized as a valid method for treating the sick.[69]

While exorcism is not part of Islamic teachings, evil spirits *(jinni)* are acknowledged in the Qur'an and exorcism was allowed to treat various conditions—as long as it was practiced in the name of Allah to help others. Belief in the "evil eye" was present in Islamic society and thought to be the cause of suffering in many persons with mental disorder. A person with the evil eye was believed to have the power to harm others using negative spiritual powers.[70] Ways to protect oneself from the evil eye included reciting the opening verse of the Qur'an (called the *Fatiha*) or other verses (the Throne Verse). Alternatively, one might write out these verses on paper, soak the paper in water, and drink the water. As in Christianity, visits to the tombs of Muslim saints such as Sidi 'Ali ben Hamdush or Sidi Ahmed Dghughi were a common way for the mentally ill to seek healing.[71]

Today, native healers in many Islamic countries utilize traditional healing methods based on understandings of mental illness that date back to this historical era. These include treatments for conditions such as *Wishrah*, demonic possession, the evil eye, Sihr, and Zar.[72] *Wishrah* is a condition characterized by incoherence or senseless speech. It is thought to involve a lack of healing of the skull bones, which is identified by slowly moving the fingers over the patient's scalp. *Sihr* involves the belief that witchcraft (strictly forbidden in Islam) is responsible for a problem. Marital difficulties or sexual problems are often attributed to this condition. *Zar* is a special form of demonic possession that is emphasized in a cult widespread in Saudi Arabia. Recitation of the Qur'an continues to be a key aspect of healing rituals designed to treat these maladies, along with herbs, dietary restriction, seclusion, and occasionally, electricity.

JUDAISM

In the Jewish tradition, God is seen as passionate, deeply caring about his people and their relationship with him, and at times jealous and angry. God is also viewed as good, a God who wants to be involved in human affairs. Because God is good, all of his creation was also seen as good. Out of this belief arose a strong emphasis on social services and humanitarian activities ("... thou shalt love thy neighbour as thyself: I am HaShem").[73]

A careful examination of the Jewish Bible and the Talmud (which takes the rules listed in the Torah and describes how to apply them to different circumstances in life) reveals many references to mental health and its preservation. For example, Rabbi Hunah wrote that it was common for good men to have bad dreams because dreams served as a psychological safety valve for natural human desires that were repressed by moral laws.[74] Likewise, Rabbi Asi recommended that if mentally ill patients would talk freely about their worries, then this might help them. Centuries later the Jewish psychiatrist Sigmund Freud would encourage patients to talk about their problems and help to interpret their dreams.[75] This became part of his psychoanalytic theory that would revolutionize and define the practice of modern psychiatry.

However, in early Hebraic times dating back at least to the time when Deuteronomy was written (1420–1220 BCE), mental illness was often understood as a consequence of divine retribution for sin: "HaShem will smite thee with madness, and with blindness, and with astonishment of heart."[76] For example, when King Saul disobeyed the prophet Samuel, he developed what sounds like a mental illness: "Now the spirit of HaShem had departed from Saul, and an evil spirit from HaShem terrified him."[77]

Similarly, "And it came to pass on the morrow, that an evil spirit from G-d came mightily upon Saul, and he raved in the midst of the house. . . ."[78] David's playing the harp was the only activity capable of soothing King Saul's disturbed emotions. That mental anguish may have contributed to Saul's suicide after an unsuccessful battle: "And the young man that told him said: 'As I happened by chance upon mount Gilboa, behold, Saul leaned upon his spear.'"[79]

Another example of mental illness as a punishment for sin involved the Babylonian king Nebuchadnezzar, who became psychotic after refusing to acknowledge and worship God: "The same hour was the thing fulfilled upon Nebuchadnezzar; and he was driven from men, and did eat grass as oxen, and his body was wet with the dew of heaven, till his hair was grown like eagles' feathers, and his nails like birds' claws."[80] It was not until he acknowledged and honored God that his sanity was restored: "'And at the end of the days I Nebuchadnezzar lifted up mine eyes unto heaven, and mine understanding returned unto me, and I blessed the Most High. . . .'"[81]

A consequence of the Jewish view in one God was that many of the magical ideas concerning mental health of the pagan cultures of the day were discarded and replaced by the belief of punishment and reward by a single God (who ultimately loved and cared about his people and punished them in order to enable them to fulfill their destiny). The Hebrews would later go beyond what many cultures of the day (particularly Western cultures) did in terms of caring for those with mental illness. These more compassionate ideas, however, were constantly in tension with the widespread belief since early Hebraic times that evil spirits were a cause of mental disturbance. Those beliefs persisted for many centuries afterward as part of folk medicine. As a result, the mentally ill were often treated as if controlled by evil spirits or demons, including the use of exorcism at times (as Christians did).[82] This reflected the writings of religious Jews who were often skeptical of secular healers, and emphasized that cures were only brought about either directly by God or by God's prophets.[83]

Despite skepticism with secular healers, notable Jewish scholars, such as Ben Sira in the second century, advised, "Honor the physician." In fact, the Talmud prohibited Jews from living in a city in which there was no physician.[84] Over time, Jews began to see mental illness less and less as a moral fault for which persons should be punished, and more as an illness that needed treatment.[85] Jewish scholar and physician Maimonides wrote in the twelfth century, "When one is overpowered by imagination, prolonged meditation and avoidance of social contact, which he never exhibited before, or when one avoids pleasant experiences which were in him before, the physician should do nothing before he improves the soul by removing the extreme emotions."[86] Maimonides believed that mental health was as important as physical health, earning him distinction as the father of psychosomatic medicine.[87] He emphasized the prevention of illness of all kinds, mental or physical, since they interfered with the person's ability to serve the Lord.[88]

While the Jewish tradition in later years was not known for establishing mental hospitals, Jews generally sought to prevent and cure mental illness. Rather than isolating the mentally ill, their legal capacities were limited as much as possible to prevent them, for example, from becoming empowered as someone else's legal agent. Rather, it was the obligation of the family or community to care for those with mental problems.

Following the Enlightenment period in Europe, which helped to decrease discrimination against Jewish professionals, Jews began entering medical schools. After another one hundred years, they comprised a high percentage of medical professionals in the West, and were often at the forefront of their fields. Sigmund Freud was among them. Freud received his M.D. in 1881 from the University of Vienna, specializing in clinical neurology. Heavily influenced by Josef Breuer and Jean Charcot, Freud wrote prolifically on the origins of hysteria and other neuroses. Freud believed that neuroses developed from diverse mental energies that were in conflict with one another (especially sexual and aggressive instincts vs. moral instincts). The notion of competing mental energies led to his elaboration of constructs such as the id, the ego, and the superego. These ideas became the basis for his theory on how to treat neurosis (psychoanalytic theory), and eventually broadened to explain the psychic origins of art, religion, and even human society. Freud and his closest Jewish colleagues, including Sandor Ferenczi, Karl Abraham, and Otto Rank, were to become the leading thinkers in European and American psychiatry for three-quarters of a century, and their influence remains widespread today in the field of mental health.

After the turn of the twentieth century, medicine, and the mental health professions in particular, soon became a favored occupation for many American Jews. In 1969, a survey of 1,371 psychiatrists, 1,465 clinical psychologists, and 1,154 psychiatric social workers in the United States revealed that 34% were Jewish, compared to 2.5% Jews in the general population.[89] Twenty years later, a national survey of psychotherapists in the United States revealed that 12% of marriage and family therapists, 22% of clinical social workers, 14% of psychiatrists, and 24% of clinical psychologists were Jewish.[90] Jews are also more likely to value mental health care and to seek such care for psychiatric problems. Those with a Jewish affiliation make up a considerably higher proportion of psychiatric inpatients and outpatients (14.8%), compared to their representation in the general population (2.5%).[91] Jewish clients may feel easier about seeking such care in part because a significant proportion of mental health professionals come from this religious or ethnic background.

HINDUISM AND BUDDHISM

Prior to 1500 BCE, all illness (including mental illness) in India was understood in terms of evil spirits and demons. During the Vedic period between 1500 and 500 BCE, prayers and charms were used to fight off evil spirits. After that, Hindus began focusing less on gods and more on the role of humans and human deeds. The sacred text dealing with these matters and other Hindu religious beliefs is called the Upanishads.[92] The Upanishads, together with the Vedas and the *Bhagavad Gita*, are the major scriptures of Hinduism. These writings, especially the Upanishads, focus on the existence of one creator and supreme reality that is called Atman, Brahma, or Self. This Self is one and the same in everyone and in all creatures, and is the Ultimate Reality or God.[93] Hindus look upon Krishna, Rama, Buddha, and Vishnu as divine incarnations of God. "Whenever righteousness declines and the purpose of life is forgotten, I manifest myself on earth. I am born in every age to protect the good, destroy the evil and re-establish the truth" (from the *Bhagavad Gita*).[94]

Karma involves all deeds or actions of human beings, and the law of Karma says that every event is both a cause and an effect (and includes the idea that a person's present life is a moral consequence of actions in previous lives). Yoga is a method of training that enables a person to more fully connect with and manifest Brahma (God), thereby improving karma. It involves reflection, love, work, and exercises that in the West we call meditation. The caste system, to some extent a consequence of karma, is a relatively rigid social hierarchy that places individuals in different social classes, from outcasts or untouchables to those in the highest class of religious leaders. Through reincarnation, or repeated rebirths, a person can move up the caste system by doing good works and connecting more fully with Brahma in each lifetime. The goal is to ultimately achieve enlightenment, union with God, and thereby reach Nirvana.[95]

The emphasis in Indian writings has not focused as much on psychopathology, psychosis, or neurosis, as it has on consciousness, identity, and motivation. Indian medicine began in the first or second century BCE with the work of Caraka, who attributed mental illness to two major causes: either an imbalance of bodily fluids (from Greek medicine) or a consequence of human action, divine punishment, or karma. Psychological methods (to show sympathy for, or sometimes even scare a patient) were among the treatments suggested for mental illness in early India.[96] In the thirteenth century CE, Unani medicine began to take root (based upon the teachings of Hippocrates and Greek medicine). At this time Indian physicians described several types of mental disorder: *Sauda-a-Tabee* (schizophrenia), *Muree Sauda* (depression), *Ishk* (delusional disorder), *Nisyan* (organic mental disorder), *Haziyan* (paranoia), and *Malikholia-a-maraki* (delirium). Various concoctions might be prescribed to help correct the imbalance of humors thought to underlie these disorders. There was even a primitive type of psychotherapy called *Ilaj-I-Nafsani* that was used to treat the mentally ill in some areas.[97]

Describing the history of psychiatry in India, S. R. Pakar and colleagues note that hospitals for the mentally ill were first established in India during the reign of King Ashoka (circa 300 BCE).[98] A temple of Lord Venkateswara in the Chingleput District dating to this period of Indian history contains an inscription on its walls indicating that a fifteen-bed hospital and school existed at this location. The first true mental asylums in India, however, were probably not built until the fifteenth century CE (Mandu Hospital). Several centuries would pass until the first modern Indian asylums were established in Bombay, Monghyr, and Madras in the late eighteenth century. Progress, however, would be slow for the next two hundred years. Many of the mentally ill were still segregated from those in the general population by placing them in stables, barracks, or prisons.[99] In 1912, the Indian Lunacy Act resulted in the opening of many new asylums and improvement of conditions in existing ones, and in 1920, the name of these hospitals was changed from lunatic asylums to mental hospitals. In 1953 the concept of a "therapeutic community" was introduced into Indian mental hospitals, resulting in considerable improvement in conditions. Occupational therapy, recreational facilities, and outdoor games were all introduced as part of this movement. Although recent years have brought about substantial changes, the gap between the mental health needs of a population of over one billion and available mental health services remains large.[100]

Buddhism, an offshoot of Hinduism in the sixth century BCE, began with the teachings of Siddhartha Gautama, a wealthy prince living on the Indian-Nepalese border. After six years of spiritual searching between the ages of twenty-nine and thirty-five, Siddhartha experienced a "great awakening" and became Buddha. The Buddha's preaching and teaching focused on condemning the meaningless rituals and traditions he saw in Hinduism. Instead, he emphasized a belief system that minimized authority, ritual, and the supernatural, and instead focused on the Four Noble Truths about the nature of existence: (1) that suffering is what life is all about *(dukkha)*, (2) that suffering is a consequence of human desire or craving *(samudaya)*, (3) that suffering can be relieved by relinquishment of desire and by detachment to things of this world *(nirodha)*, and (4) that the end of desire or craving can be accomplished *(magga)* by following the Eightfold Path: right understanding, right thought, right speech, right action, right livelihood, right effort, right mindfulness, and right concentration.[101]

There are two major divisions of Buddhism called Hinayana (the "Lesser Vehicle") and Mahayana (the "Great Vehicle").[102] Hinayana Buddhism (widespread in Thailand and Cambodia, and called "Southern Buddhism") is considered the lesser vehicle because it focuses on achieving personal wisdom and peace as the pathway toward Nirvana. Although stabilizing the mind and achieving wisdom are considered necessary for liberation from the *false self*, those in the Mahayana tradition would argue that these are only the first steps in preparing to take the "Great Journey." If the focus remains on the peace of the individual practitioner, then this is considered an escape and is ultimately self-defeating. Mahayana Buddhism (widespread in China, Korea, Japan, and Tibet, and called "Northern Buddhism"), because it focuses outside of the self and is more universalizing, seeks to cultivate generosity and kindness (compassion) toward others as key to achieving Nirvana.

Although neither Hinayana nor Mahayana Buddhism believes in a Creator or ruler God, deity belief is present in the Mahayana tradition. This is contained in the doctrine of the three forms of Buddha: "(1) Body of Essence—the indescribable, impersonal Absolute Reality, or Ultimate Truth that is Nirvana (Infinite Bliss); (2) Body of Bliss or Enjoyment—Buddha as divine, deity, formless, celestial spirit with saving power of grace, omnipotence, omniscience; and (3) Body of Transformation or Emanation—an illusion or emanation in human form provided by the divine Buddha to guide humans to Enlightenment."[103] Thus, although Buddhism denies a personal God, it does acknowledge a variety of concepts that could be understood as God.

In first-century CE China, Mahayana Buddhism blended easily with Chinese traditional medicine. Because of the Buddhist emphasis on compassion, welfare regulations were put into place from early on. A Buddhist prince is said to have established the first Chinese hospital in the fifth century.[104] Nevertheless, the primary way that many people in China treated illness and suffering was by praying to Kuan-yen, the Chinese Buddhist goddess. The more scientific influences from Indian medicine did not take hold in China. This was because the Buddhist attitude towards illness and disease did not focus on specific methods. Buddhism mixed together with Chinese traditional medicine promoted the idea that a vast spiritual world was responsible for illness and disease, including mental illness. Because mental illness was often thought to be due to demonic possession (particularly in Japan), any help from medicine was felt to be futile and therefore patients were referred to the priests for treatment.[105] Zen monasteries often invited persons with severe mental illness to live at least temporarily within them, as Christian monasteries in Europe did.

In Japan, unlike in other Buddhist countries, a specific treatment developed for neurosis. Called Morita therapy, this involved a Zen ritual combined with bed rest, isolation, outside work, and eventual integration back into the society.[106] Rather than allow or encourage patients to discuss problems, they were re-educated to help free them from focusing on themselves or on their personal needs and desires (in keeping with Buddhist religious philosophy of nonattachment). According to psychiatrist Bruce Scotton, what might appear to the Western therapist as passive acceptance of a painful mental state may actually be evidence that the Buddhist patient is diligently working on altering his or her consciousness and sense of desire or attachment in order to reduce suffering and treat the illness.[107]

Summary

The historical relationship between religion and mental illness—especially in Western cultures—has not always been positive. The fear that mentally ill persons were possessed by demons or evil spirits, at times accompanied by concern that such possession was infectious, led to confinement, sometimes violent attempts at exorcism, or worse, death through burning at the stake or decapitation. Nevertheless, major religious traditions throughout the world and throughout history have been at the forefront in providing humane care to the mentally ill or emotionally vulnerable. Many of the most important breakthroughs in compassionate treatment of the mentally ill were made by persons of faith crusading for those who did not have the power to speak for themselves.

In the next three chapters I examine how religious beliefs and practices are related to psychological coping and positive emotions, psychiatric disorder, and severe mental illness. What does scientific research tell us about these connections? Does religious faith represent a resource or a liability in terms of mental health?

PART II

RESEARCH ON RELIGION AND MENTAL HEALTH

CHAPTER 3

RELIGION, COPING, AND
POSITIVE EMOTIONS

Although it is clear that religious people and religious organizations have often led the way in providing compassionate care to those with mental and emotional problems, this doesn't necessarily mean that religious beliefs and practices enhance mental health, protect against mental illness, or speed recovery. In fact, as we learned in the last chapter, there are claims from both sides concerning the risks and benefits of a devout religious faith. Are religious beliefs and practices associated with worse mental health, more neurosis, and poorer adaptation to stress, as claimed by highly respected mental health professionals such as Freud, Ellis, and Watters? Is religion associated with better mental health, greater well-being, and greater family and community solidarity, as claimed by religious professionals? Or, does religion serve a selective process, including only the mentally healthy who are capable of participating in religious activities and excluding those with emotional or mental illness who cannot?

Using the methods of science, research can provide evidence to sort out which of the above views is true or whether each view has validity to some degree or another. Rather than rely on the opinions of prominent mental health professionals or on the personal testimonies of religious persons, however, let us examine over 850 studies during the twentieth century (and others conducted since then) that have objectively measured relationships between religion and mental health.[1] However, even scientific research, as objective as it attempts to be, can be influenced by biases that lead us away from the truth. Furthermore, there may be some questions related to the supernatural that the naturalistic methods of science are incapable of studying. So it is important to remember that no source of information, whether based on clinical experience, personal conviction, or scientific research, can be entirely free of error.

Before proceeding further, it is important to define terms that I will be using to describe the research. This applies especially to terms such as *religion* and *spirituality*, which are steeped in controversy and confusion.[2] I provide definitions below that describe my use of these terms in this book; however, no universally accepted definitions exist and many others can be found in the literature.

Religion is an organized system of beliefs, practices, and rituals of a community. Religion is designed to increase a sense of closeness to the sacred or transcendent (whether that be God, a higher power, or ultimate truth/reality), and to promote an understanding of one's relationship to and responsibility for others living together in a community. Religion, then, is community focused (organized into formal practices that are observable and measurable), may be authoritarian in terms of behaviors and responsibilities, and is often concerned with beliefs and doctrines that, among other goals, seek to separate good from evil.

Spirituality, on the other hand, is much broader than religion and less distinctive. Spirituality involves a more generic personal quest for understanding answers to ultimate questions about life and its meaning, and while concerned with a relationship to the sacred or transcendent, may or may not lead to religious beliefs, rituals, or the formation of a community. Spirituality is more individualistic, more focused on emotion, more inwardly directed and subjective, and has less definable boundaries, which also makes it more difficult to measure. Finally, spirituality tends to be less authoritarian and less doctrine oriented, and may even be entirely divorced from religion, without involving belief in God but rather focusing more on connections with nature, art, or other humanistic values and concerns (as in earlier pagan cultures). Because there is no agreed-upon definition and because the term has only recently come into use in the scientific literature (since the late 1980s), spirituality has been difficult to pin down and its many definitions and subjective nature make it hard to quantify.

Despite these major differences, spirituality and religion are often used interchangeably. One reason for doing so is that many people (74% to 88%) don't make distinctions between religion and spirituality, but rather report that they are both religious and spiritual.[3]

In this research review, then, I will focus primarily on religion (which is typically measured in these studies), although I will also address spirituality when possible. I will now examine the use of religion in coping and the relationship of religion to positive emotions. The next two chapters following this one will cover psychiatric disorders, substance abuse disorders, and severe, persistent mental illness.

Religion and Psychological Coping

Probability surveys of the adult population since 1940 have consistently found the United States to be a religious nation. Gallup polls of the general population between 1998 and 2003 indicated that 94–96% of the populace believes in God, over 90% pray, 65–71% are church members, 38–47% have attended church, synagogue, or temple within the past seven days, and 58–64% say that religion is very important in their lives.[4] Furthermore, many Americans turn to religion to cope when they are stressed. In December 2001, three months following the September 11, 2001 terrorist attacks, 71% of the population indicated that religion was having an increasing influence on American life, greater than at any other time since the question was first asked in 1957.[5] A study published in the *New England Journal of Medicine* found that 90% of Americans coped with the stress of 9/11 by "turning to religion."[6] During the week following the terrorist attacks, 60% of Americans attended a religious or memorial service and Bible sales rose 27%.[7]

In the United States, then, religion is often used to cope with stress (called "religious coping"). This may involve praying to God or a higher power, meditating by using a religious approach, reading religious scriptures, attending religious services, performing religious rituals, or obtaining religious counsel or direction. Many studies find that prayer and turning to religion for comfort is a common response, whether after crises (such as September 11th, the 1991 Gulf War,[8] or the 1995 Oklahoma bombing[9]), natural disasters (such as the 1993 Midwest floods[10] and 1989 Hurricane Hugo[11]), or loss of a loved one.[12] In addition, more than sixty studies have now examined the role that religion plays in coping with conditions as diverse as arthritis,[13] diabetes,[14] kidney transplant,[15] hemodialysis,[16] cancer,[17] coronary artery disease and bypass surgery,[18] heart transplant,[19] lung transplant,[20] HIV/AIDS,[21] cystic fibrosis,[22] sickle cell disease,[23] amyotrophic lateral sclerosis,[24] chronic pain,[25] and severe illness during adolescence.[26] Virtually all studies find high rates of religious coping in these stressful conditions.

Although most religious coping is positive, it can also be negative. When illness strikes, it is not uncommon to feel punished by God, angry at God, abandoned by God, abandoned by one's faith community, uncertain about God's love, or have questions about whether God has the power to make a difference. One systematic study of fifty-eight breast cancer patients found that when talking about the role that religion played in their coping with illness, 83% used positive emotion words, but 17% used negative emotion words.[27] Thus, negative religious coping is not rare. However, the frequency of negative expressions of religious coping is not nearly as common as positive expressions. This is consistent with findings from larger samples of medically ill patients and healthy persons living in the community.

For example, in a study of 577 medically ill hospitalized persons, investigators asked patients to what extent they felt punished by God, abandoned or unloved by God, abandoned by their church, or questioned God's power.[28] Patients were asked to rate to what extent they had been feeling each of these ways. The possible scores for each ranged from 0 to 9, from a low to high frequency. The average score for the sample on these expressions of negative religious coping was 1. Compare this to average scores of 7 on the same scale for positive expressions of religious coping (i.e., collaborating with God, seeking spiritual support, helping others deepen their religious faith, surrendering to the will of God). The findings are similar for healthy individuals. In a random national survey (General Social Survey, 1998) of 1,445 persons over age 18 in the United States, the average score for feeling punished by God on a 0 to 3 scale was 0.3; for wondering if abandoned by God, it was 0.2.[29] Even though it is relatively negative religious coping predicts poorer mental and physical health when studied over time and is generally associated with infrequent religious practices and low religious commitment.[30]

Religious coping is prevalent in other countries besides the United States, especially India and the Arab nations. For example, studying a sample of sixty Hindu caregivers of schizophrenic patients in India, Rammohan and colleagues found that religion was frequently used to cope with the stress of caring for a loved one with this illness.[31] The most common types of religious coping involved praying to God (90%) and lighting a lamp (83%). These religious coping behaviors increased as the loved one's severity of illness worsened. Overall, 97% of caregivers believed in God, 58% considered their religious beliefs an integral part of life, and 50% viewed religion as a source of solace, strength, and guidance.

The extent to which religion is used to cope varies depending on the seriousness of the stressor, regardless of culture. I have already described the large increase in religious behavior in the United States following the 9/11 terrorist attacks and the increase in religious coping among Hindu family members caring for loved ones with severe mental illness. This also seems true for other stressful situations such as undergoing surgery. Shrimali and Broota compared coping strategies to major and minor surgery among three groups of Hindus in India.[32] One group of 30 patients was scheduled for minor surgery, a second group of 30 was scheduled for major surgery, and 30 subjects were recruited as a matched control group. Belief in God was highest among subjects scheduled for major surgery. Post-operatively, however, level of belief in God decreased in the major surgery group, while no change occurred in the other two groups.

Use of religion as a coping behavior, however, is not universal. Northern Europe, for example, became highly secularized during the twentieth century. Although the well-developed social services system in these countries is based on strong religious values passed down from preceding more religious generations, institutionalized religion has begun to lose its influence in this region. Weekly church attendance in Sweden is only about 2–4%,[33] and the use of religion to cope during stress is about 1%.[34] In the Netherlands, only 50% indicate some degree of religiousness,[35] 43% are church members, and less than 30% say that a strong faith is important,[36] compared with 90% of Americans who say religion is somewhat or very important.[37] In Norway, a significant proportion of sick patients with severe illnesses such as cancer do not believe in God (43%) and indicate that religious beliefs provide no comfort whatsoever (45%).[38]

Directly comparing Europeans with Egyptians, Kesselring and colleagues[39] studied the meaning of illness and coping responses mobilized by 45 Swiss and 40 Egyptian cancer patients. Among Swiss patients, 38% indicated that faith in God and prayer were important sources of support, whereas 92% of Egyptian patients indicated that God or Allah was a significant factor in their ability to cope. The role that social desirability may have played in these responses (i.e., people answering the way they thought they should answer or the way they thought the interviewer wanted them to answer) is unknown.

Besides type of religion and geographic location, age may also influence the likelihood that a person will turn to religion when encountering stress. In a study of 282 European college students, Loewenthal and colleagues at the Royal Holloway University of London examined the extent to which the students used religion when coping with depression. This English sample consisted of students from Christian (n=130), Hindu (n=18), Jewish (n=35), Muslim (n=33), other religious (n=15), and no religious (n=56) backgrounds.[40] Among 26 different coping behaviors, faith in God, prayer, and religious practice were rated eighteenth, nineteenth, and twentieth, respectively, in coping effectiveness (i.e., not very effective). Even when the 56 persons with no religious backgrounds were excluded, faith in God, prayer, and religious practice still ranked only sixteenth, seventeenth, and eighteenth most helpful. When students from different religious groups were compared, Muslims rated faith in God significantly higher than other religious groups; Muslims and Christians rated prayer significantly higher than others; and Muslims and Jews rated religious practices significantly higher than others. With regard to seeking professional help, Jews were significantly more likely to do so than other religious groups, whereas Muslims and Christians were more likely to seek religious help.

Thus, older age, type of religion, ethnic background, geographic location, and severity of the stressor help to predict whether or not a person will use religion as a coping strategy. Let us now turn to the effect that religion has on mental health outcomes and coping effectiveness.

Religion and Mental Health Outcomes

Many people, whether mentally ill or healthy, report that religion helps them to cope with stress. This does not mean, however, that religious beliefs and practices are necessarily more effective than other coping strategies in relieving stress. The only way to determine this is to measure and compare the mental health of religious persons with the mental health of less religious persons, especially when they are experiencing stressful circumstances that challenge their coping abilities. Numerous studies over the past fifty years have sought to determine whether religion is more effective compared to other forms of coping. I will review some of the findings here based on a systematic review of studies conducted prior to the year 2000[41] and then discuss studies published after 2000.

EARLY VS. LATER STUDIES

Many of the early studies that examined the relationship between religion and mental health were conducted in college classrooms, where professors had ready access to eager research subjects—students. In the 1960s and 1970s, large grants were not typically available to study the effects of religion on mental health in the general population. Studies in students during that period often found that religious beliefs were associated with worse mental health—more perfectionism, withdrawal, insecurity, depression, and worry.[42] Studying associations between mental health and religious beliefs of adolescents and teenagers, however, is different than examining the effects of religion in mature adults facing major life stressors. Nevertheless, early studies in students should not be entirely disregarded. Instead, they need to be weighed in light of their limitations and the fact that almost all were cross-sectional (telling us nothing about whether religion was the cause of poor mental health or whether poor mental health preceded religious involvement and motivated them to turn to religion for cope purposes). These studies do show that at least in some populations and time periods, religious beliefs and practices were associated with worse mental health and more negative personality traits.

Recent studies have sought to correct some of the deficiencies of earlier research. Instead of using convenience samples of readily available students, later studies in the 1980s and 1990s were more likely to assess mature adults, use random or systematic sampling methods, control for confounding variables, and study subjects over time. Because confounding can be a serious problem, it is important to control analyses for covariates such as race, gender, and socioeconomic status, which was seldom done in earlier studies of college students. Recent studies also include those that are longitudinal or prospective in design. Following subjects over time can provide information about the order of effects and thus contribute evidence (if only indirectly) for making causal inferences. A few randomized clinical trials using religious interventions have also been completed, and by their design are capable of establishing causality.

What, then, is the connection between religious involvement, positive emotions, and mental disorder in these more recent studies? In the remainder of this chapter, I will review research that has examined the relationship between religion and positive emotions, and then in the next chapter, I will review studies that have explored connections between religion and psychiatric disorder.

Positive Emotions

Positive emotions are what make life worth living. American psychologist William James wrote that "how to gain, how to keep, how to recover happiness is in fact for most men at all times the secret motive of all they do."[43] The mentally healthy individual is not defined just by the absence of mental disorder, but also by the presence of positive emotions that lift their spirits above the humdrum of ordinary existence. Even persons with mental disorder can experience positive emotions, whether they are cured from their primary psychiatric disorder or not. A person with schizophrenia can still experience purpose and meaning in life, periods of joy, and spiritual well-being when, for example, he or she performs altruistic acts of love and kindness toward others.

WELL-BEING, HAPPINESS, AND LIFE SATISFACTION

Many studies have explored the relationship between religious practices and positive emotions such as well-being, happiness, hope, meaning, purpose, and optimism. Of 100 studies that examined religion and well-being prior to the year 2000, nearly 80% found a statistically significant relationship between greater religious involvement and greater life satisfaction, happiness, better mood, or higher morale.[44] The best studies methodologically were those conducted over time (i.e., prospective studies). Of the 100 studies on religion and well-being noted above, 10 were prospective cohort studies. Of these 10 studies, 8 found that greater religiousness predicted greater well-being. Relationships between well-being and religious involvement were similar in magnitude to those typically found between well-being and social support, marital status, and income.

Latest Studies

Since 2000, several studies have confirmed the association between religion and well-being in the United States, the United Kingdom, and Australia,[45] although a few have found a weak[46] or nonexistent relationship.[47] Of note is that none have reported a negative association. The connections with psychological well-being appear to be particularly strong later in life when experiencing psychosocial stressors such as ill health or loss of loved ones. For example, Fry examined the relationship between existential factors and psychological well-being in 188 persons age 65 to 87 following the loss of a spouse.[48] Using hierarchical regression, Fry found that importance of religion and spiritual beliefs/practices were strong predictors of psychological well-being, independent of social support and physical health factors. Bear in mind, however, that this study was cross-sectional, making it impossible to tell whether religious involvement preceded or followed elders' experience of well-being.

Religious support may be particularly important for older African Americans who may have few other resources to depend on. For example, Joan Cook and her colleagues at Johns Hopkins University examined predictors of life satisfaction in a sample of 831 older African Americans living in urban public housing projects in Baltimore, Maryland.[49] Although neither lifetime alcohol-related problems nor cognitive impairment were significant predictors of life satisfaction, those who indicated they depended on religious support "a great deal" experienced significantly higher life satisfaction than those who indicated less religious support. Again, this finding was independent of physical health, level of social support, or depressive symptoms.

Different expressions of religiousness (religious attendance vs. prayer vs. intrinsic religious motivation) may not all be related to mental health in the same way or may be related to different aspects of mental health. For example, the Detroit Area Study involved a probability sample of over 1,100 adults (with over-sampling for African Americans).[50] Investigators found that religious attendance and belief in an afterlife were related to greater well-being, even after psychosocial stressors and social support were taken into account. Personal prayer, on the other hand, had a weak inverse relationship to well-being. Examining another mental health measure, psychological distress, investigators again found an inverse relationship with religious attendance, but no relationship with belief in an afterlife, and a positive relationship with prayer (perhaps reflecting the increased use of prayer among those with higher distress).

In another recent study of 210 adults (whose mean age was 29), investigators found that participants with strong religious faith experienced significantly lower anxiety and lower depression scores, as well as higher ego strength and less personality psychopathology. Only modest correlations, however, were found between religiousness and well-being, suggesting again that religiousness may correlate differently with different measures of mental health in different populations.[51]

Even in areas of the world where religion plays a less significant role than in the United States, religious activity still often correlates with greater well-being. For example, in the Australian Community Survey of 989 adults, 67% did not believe in a personal God, 52% never attended religious services, and 32% never prayed.[52] Nevertheless, belief in God and frequency of personal prayer were associated with greater psychological well-being, a finding that was independent of age and gender. Likewise, a study of religious attendance and life satisfaction in Finland that involved a nationwide sample of 869 women and 773 men (where 38% of women and 50% of men never attended religious services), found that those who attended religious services at least once a month were significantly more likely to report being satisfied with life.[53]

In another European study, religiousness and life satisfaction were examined in a study of 250 adults in Greece.[54] Religiousness (church attendance and participation in religious activities, which only 32% of the sample were engaged in) was significantly associated with life satisfaction after multiple sociodemographic and physical health variables were controlled in multivariate analyses. In that study, religiousness was also associated with greater relaxation, better nutrition, and better personal hygiene.

Research from the Middle East has recently appeared in the literature, providing evidence for how relationships found in largely Christian populations might generalize to Jewish, Muslim, and Hindu samples. For example, one study examined 464 Israeli women age 75 or older from 48 old-age homes in Israel (34% indicating they were not religious).[55] Investigators found that while there was no direct association between religiousness and well-being, there was a positive correlation between religiousness and perceived health status. Similarly, in a study of 60 Israeli males ages 68 to 75 years old (37% of whom were not traditionally religious), the strongest and most powerful predictors of life satisfaction were religiosity and physical functioning.[56] Religiosity was defined as praying every day, studying the Torah, and performing religious rituals.

These same relationships have been examined among Muslims in Turkey, at least qualitatively. Thomas conducted interviews with 32 older subjects (aged 69–87 years) in Ankara and Istanbul.[57] Approximately half the subjects were religious and the other half were not. He discovered that elders who transcended problems of aging through faith experienced high levels of life satisfaction, and that no one who demonstrated such transcendence experienced low life satisfaction. According to Thomas, "These individuals had come to know God, or the transcendent, from first-hand experience, and this change in their view of ultimate reality was reflected in their personal lives in important ways and were experiencing a high level of contentment and satisfaction in their later years" (207).

Similar associations are found among Hindus in India. Anjana and Raju from the Department of Psychology at the University of Kerala, Thiruvananthapuram, India, compared the mental health of 31 reciters and 31 non-reciters of the *Bhagavad Gita*.[58] Uncontrolled analyses revealed that reciters of *Bhagavad Gita* scored significantly better on adjustment as measured by symptoms of anxiety, depression, mania, inferiority, and paranoia. They concluded that those who recited the *Bhagavad Gita* were more successful in managing adjustment problems.

Studies in the Far East likewise discover connections between well-being and religious faith. Swinyard and colleagues examined the association between happiness, materialism, and religious experience in a sample of 425 adults in the United States and 293 adults in Singapore (a largely Buddhist or Hindu nation).[59] Religiousness was operationalized as extrinsic religiosity, intrinsic religiosity, and religion as a quest. Intrinsic religiosity (religiousness as the person's ultimate concern in life) was a significant predictor of greater life satisfaction in both the United Sates and Singapore.

HOPE AND OPTIMISM

The religious worldview is generally a hopeful and optimistic one (with some notable exceptions, i.e., Branch Davidians). Rather than seeing human life as little different from other animals, here today and gone tomorrow, many world religions view men and women as special, created with a divine purpose and having a future beyond the grave. Death is not seen as the end of all existence, but as a transition to a much better place where there is no pain or suffering. The Christian tradition, for example, sees humans as eternal creatures, never truly separated from each other or from deceased loved ones with whom some day they will be reunited. Even difficult life circumstances are viewed as potentially positive and growth producing, in light of the Creator's love and desire for good in each person's life. One would hypothesize, then, that religious persons would feel more optimistic and hopeful about the future.

At least 15 studies examined associations between religion, hope, and optimism prior to the year 2000. Of those, 11 reported statistically significant positive associations between religion and greater hope or optimism. Of the remaining four studies, one found a trend in that direction and three found no association.[60] Studies using the best scientific methodology (in terms of sampling method and statistical handling of the data) all found that greater religiousness predicted greater hope or optimism. In two studies that looked at religious denomination, the results were surprising. When compared with Catholics, liberal or moderate Protestants, and Jews, investigators found that persons from Christian fundamentalist groups—those with the most rigid and constricting doctrines—experienced the highest level of optimism.[61] This could be explained by the emphasis these groups placed on hope, salvation, and successful overcoming of adversity that permeated their hymns, prayers, and sermons. As long as adherents "played by the rules" that the church laid down for them, then there was every reason to be optimistic and hopeful.

Since 2000, several other studies have examined connections between religion, hope, and optimism. For example, Sherman and colleagues at the University of Santa Clara in California conducted interviews with 95 breast cancer patients.[62] Using the Santa Clara Strength of Religious Faith Questionnaire, they found that religiousness was associated with greater optimism about the future. Likewise, Amy Ai and colleagues at the University of Michigan reported similar findings in their study of 246 adult patients awaiting cardiac surgery. They interviewed subjects two weeks prior to surgery and then measured levels of optimism the day before surgery.[63] Private prayer was assessed by examining the importance of prayer, faith in the efficacy of prayer, and intention to use prayer to cope with surgery. General measures of religiosity and type of prayers were also assessed. Only private prayer (as described above), not other measures of religiosity, predicted greater optimism prior to surgery. In a second study by this group, Ai and colleagues collected information about religiosity, war-related trauma, religious-spiritual coping, optimism and hope in 138 Muslim refugees from Kosovo and Bosnia who had recently settled in the United States. They found positive religious coping was associated with greater optimism, and negative religious coping (feeling punished or deserted by God) with less hope and more severe trauma.

Little work has yet examined the role that religious beliefs play in providing hope to patients who are experiencing the anguish of depression. Pat Murphy and colleagues at Rush-Presbyterian Medical Center in Chicago examined relationships between religious beliefs and hope in 271 persons diagnosed with clinical depression.[64] They found that religious belief, but not religious behavior, predicted greater hope in this population. Through this relationship, religious belief also had an indirect effect on the severity of depression.

In one of the few recent studies to examine religious involvement and positive emotions in teenagers, Carol Markstrom administered questionnaires to 62 African American and 63 white eleventh graders from rural areas of West Virginia.[65] Ego strengths such as hope, will, purpose, fidelity, love, and care were all associated with greater religious involvement. Unlike most previous studies, associations were particularly strong in whites.

Studying persons at the other end of the age spectrum, Neal Krause examined relationships between optimism, health, and religious attendance, congregational cohesiveness, spiritual support, and connectedness to God in a national sample of 748 white and 752 African Americans over age 65.[66] He found that older persons who had a close relationship with God were more optimistic, and those who were more optimistic had better health. In this study, however, relationships were stronger in African Americans than in whites. In his most recent study, Krause confirmed the association in older African Americans between well-being and both common (i.e., religious attendance) and unique facets of religion (i.e., the belief that religion sustains black people in the face of racial adversity).[67]

Finally, Jacqueline Mattis and colleagues in the department of applied psychology at New York University examined religiosity, spirituality, racism, and optimism in a sample of 149 African Americans of all ages.[68] Levels of self-assessed spirituality and having a personal relationship with God were associated with greater optimism, but church attendance, early religious involvement, church involvement, and self-rated religiosity were not. When other variables were taken into account in the analysis, only having a supportive and loving relationship with God was a significant predictor of optimism. Having a personalized view of God, especially for African Americans, then, appears to be an important predictor of optimism.

MEANING AND PURPOSE

Just as hope and optimism are necessary for a satisfying and fulfilling life, having purpose and meaning is also essential for good mental health. Religious beliefs provide answers to the "Where" and "Why" questions (where did I come from, why am I here, where am I going), while science and medicine answer the "How" questions. Because they address the "Why" questions, religious beliefs provide meaning, especially during times of adversity and suffering. Even religion's archenemy Sigmund Freud admitted, ". . . only religion can answer the question of the purpose of life. One can hardly be wrong in concluding that the idea of life having a purpose stands and falls with the religious system."[69] It is not surprising, then, that of the 16 studies during the twentieth century that examined the relationship between religion and purpose or meaning in life, 15 found significantly greater purpose and meaning among those who were more religious.[70] The extraordinary success of Rick Warren's book *The Purpose-Driven Life* (15 million copies sold during its first 17 months of publication) is a testament to the role that religious belief plays in finding purpose.[71]

Recent work suggests that religious and spiritual beliefs are particularly important for older adults in their search for meaning and purpose. One reason may be that religion helps to resolve the "integrity vs. despair" crisis that represents the final stage of life described by Erikson.[72] It is common for older adults to conduct a life review, where they look back over the years and determine whether life was meaningful and had purpose or not. If the conclusion is negative, then the older person will struggle with maintaining self-esteem and may cycle downward in despair, increasing the risk for depression and stagnation. This is particularly true when older adults must struggle with disabling medical illness.[73] There is recent evidence that meaning and purpose derived through religion (i.e., religious meaning) is particularly important in this regard. In a nationwide sample of black and white elders, Neal Krause found that older adults who derived a sense of meaning in life from religion tended to have higher levels of life satisfaction, self-esteem, and optimism.[74]

Religion and spirituality may be particularly important for generating purpose and meaning among minority groups. In the Krause study above, older black adults were more likely to find meaning in religion than were older white adults. This is also true for ethnic minorities during times of physical illness. Alynson Moadel and colleagues examined the spiritual and existential needs of 248 ethnically diverse patients with cancer.[75] These patients, aged 18 to 85 years, were anxious to find help to overcome their fears, find hope and peace of mind, and acquire meaning and purpose in life, death, and spiritual areas. Hispanic patients (particularly those with lower levels of education) experienced the greatest need for spiritual support, compared to white patients who reported the least need for such support.

Spiritual beliefs may also help to buffer against poverty, crime, bereavement, and other losses common among minority groups that challenge their sense of purpose and meaning in life. For example, after conducting a series of qualitative interviews with African American women, Jacqueline Mattis concluded that religion/spirituality served many purposes for these women. Religion helped them to integrate negative life events, accept reality, gain insight and courage, confront and transcend limitations, identify and grapple with existential questions, recognize their purpose and destiny, define their character, live their lives within meaningful moral principles, and achieve psychological growth despite difficult circumstances.[76]

Religious and spiritual beliefs not only protect against a sense of boredom and existential despair among older adults, the medically ill, and minorities, but also in teenagers and younger adults who have their own unique stressors to deal with. Francis examined the relationship between Bible reading and purpose in life among a sample of 25,888 teenagers (ages 13 to 15) in England and Wales.[77] After taking into account gender, age, personality, belief in God, and church attendance, Francis concluded that Bible reading had a small but important effect on these young persons' sense of purpose in life. Likewise, in a study of 296 university undergraduate students (ages 17 to 48), MacDonald and Holland found a significant inverse correlation between spiritual factors and boredom-proneness (an indicator of loss of purpose and meaning in life).[78]

QUALITY OF LIFE

Quality of life (QOL) is defined as a person's overall level of functioning, including psychological well-being, social relationships, and ability to independently care for physical needs. QOL is most often measured in people with chronic illness or terminal conditions such as cancer, HIV/AIDS, and congestive heart failure that seriously challenge them in each of these areas. QOL is usually measured using a multidimensional scale such as the Medical Outcomes Study 36-item or 12-item Short Form Health Survey (SF-36 or SF-12), depending on how much detail is sought. For cancer patients in particular, the Functional Assessment of Cancer Therapy Scale (FACIT) assesses quality of life specific to several different malignancies including breast cancer (FACIT-B), prostate cancer (FACIT-P), and mixed cancer populations (FACIT-G). This QOL instrument also has a version that assesses spirituality (FACIT-Sp). That scale includes peace, meaning, and religious faith subscales. Several recent studies have examined the connections between spirituality and QOL.

Richard Sowell and colleagues at the University of South Carolina in Columbia examined the role that spiritual activities played as a QOL resource for 184 HIV-positive women.[79] QOL was assessed using the SF-36. Spiritual activities such as praying, taking problems to God, and so on, were associated with higher QOL and less emotional distress in this population. Similarly, Sian Cotton and colleagues from California Pacific Medical Center in San Francisco examined the relationship between QOL, religious or spiritual beliefs, and spiritual well-being in 142 women diagnosed with breast cancer.[80] They found significant positive correlations between QOL (measured by FACIT-B), spiritual well-being (measured by the

FACIT-Sp), and religious or spiritual beliefs. Spiritual variables were also related to having a fighting spirit and lower levels of hopelessness, fatalism, and anxious preoccupation.

Michael Fisch and colleagues from the M.D. Anderson Cancer Center in Houston assessed the relationship between QOL (FACIT-G) and spiritual well-being (FACIT-Sp) in 163 patients with advanced cancers. They also compared self-rated QOL as judged by patients with observer-rated QOL as judged by physicians and nurses, doing so at different levels of SWB.[81] Investigators found a strong correlation between SWB and QOL. Comparison between patient and physician judgments of QOL was particularly revealing. Overall, clinician-estimated QOL matched patient-estimated QOL correctly in about 60% of cases. However, there was also an association between lower SWB and clinician underestimation of QOL. This could be attributed to patients with low SWB *overestimating their impairments* compared to more objective assessments by clinicians. This observation is consistent with other research reporting that patients' assessment of their health status is closely linked with their nonphysical sense of self, which can be heavily influenced by religious or spiritual factors.[82]

Evidence also exists for a connection between having religious faith and experiencing higher QOL in patients with heart disease, although the evidence is indirect. This study (published in *JAMA*) did not measure religiosity or spirituality. However, its findings on depression and QOL are relevant to this discussion. Ruo and colleagues at the San Francisco Veterans Administration Medical Center examined the relationship between health-related QOL and symptoms of depression in a sample of 1024 adults with coronary artery disease.[83] The primary outcome of interest, health-related QOL, was measured by frequency of chest pain, ability to perform several different physical activities, and self-assessed severity of heart disease. A fourth component of QOL included the patients' overall sense of their health status, with responses ranging from poor to excellent. In addition to depressive symptoms, other characteristics thought to be related to QOL included biological measures of cardiac function (left ventricular ejection fraction, exercise treadmill testing, and stress echocardiogram results). Age, ethnicity, education, income, marital status, medical history, smoking, alcohol use, medication use, and perceived stress were all measured and controlled for in the statistical analysis.

The strongest predictor of QOL—patients' perceptions of their overall physical health, symptom severity, and ability to function physically—was not left ventricular ejection fraction, echocardiogram-determined wall motion score, or exercise capacity determined by exercise treadmill testing. To the investigators' amazement, the best predictor of QOL was depressive symptoms. Investigators concluded that depressive symptoms were a stronger determinant of health-related QOL than any of the traditional biological measures of cardiac function. If religious or spiritual factors help to prevent or decrease depressive symptoms (see chapter 4), then it is reasonable to expect them to influence health-related QOL in patients with heart problems.

Issues of QOL may be particularly important in later life as people experience disability and pain from chronic illnesses. For example, Susan Bartlett and colleagues at Johns Hopkins University studied the relationship between spirituality, well-being, and quality of life (QOL) in a sample of middle-aged and older persons with rheumatoid arthritis (RA).[84] More advanced disease was associated with more depression, greater pain, poorer self-ratings of health, and greater physical role limitations. Spirituality, however, was associated with greater well-being and better health perceptions, even after controlling for other predicts of well-being, such as disease activity, functional disability, and age.

Other Positive Emotional States

GRATEFULNESS

Research suggests that a sense of gratitude is associated with positive emotions in general and with psychological well-being, pro-social behaviors, extraversion, and agreeableness in particular.[85] For example, Michael McCullough and colleagues developed a six-item gratefulness scale that they administered along with other measures of positive mental health to 238 psychology students.[86] Gratefulness was significantly correlated with life satisfaction, vitality, happiness, optimism, hope, and pro-social constructs such as empathy and providing emotional and tangible support to others. Gratitude was also positively correlated with a host of religious and spirituality variables, including importance of religion, frequency of religious service attendance, reading scripture, frequency of prayer, having a personal relationship with God, union with God, and spiritual transcendence.

Thankfulness has also been correlated with a lower risk of psychiatric disorder. Kenneth Kendler and colleagues at the Virginia Institute for Psychiatry and Behavioral Genetics recently examined correlations between being thankful and the presence of "internalizing" disorders such as major depression, panic disorder, generalized anxiety disorder, eating disorder, and substance abuse in 2,616 male and female twins in Virginia, finding that being thankful significantly reduced the risk of having these disorders.[87] Further research is needed on this positive emotional state and its link to religiousness, given the preliminary findings above. Unfortunately, most federal grant funding goes toward the study of mental disorders, not of positive states such as gratitude.

FORGIVENESS

Forgiveness is linked to a host of positive (well-being) and negative emotions (anger).[88] Several studies have demonstrated correlations between forgiveness and better physical health, including reduced heart rate, lower blood pressure,[89] slowed skin conductance and greater muscle relaxation,[90] lower cortisol levels,[91] and better immune function.[92] Kendler and colleagues also found forgiveness predicted less frequent substance abuse and adult antisocial personality disorder in their sample of Virginia twins.[93]

Forgiveness, in turn, has been linked to religion, which may increase the capacity to forgive.[94] Gorsuch and Hao analyzed data from a national random sample of 1,030 Americans aged 18 or older (part of a 1988 Gallup survey)[95] that measured several dimensions of forgiveness and religiosity. Although "religious conformity" was unrelated to forgiveness, "personal religiousness" was significantly related to a general forgiveness factor and to a set of primary forgiveness factors (after general forgiveness was controlled for). Protestants, Catholics, and evangelicals generally reported more forgiving responses than Jews, those with no/other religious preference, or non-evangelicals. Investigators concluded, "the more overall religious one is, the more forgiving one reports." A lack of correlation between forgiveness and religious conformity also suggested that religious persons did not answer questions in a forgiving manner just because they were conforming to how they thought they should answer (i.e., social desirability), which is a common criticism of these kinds of studies.

Research outside the United States has reported similar findings, although moderated by age. Mullet and colleagues[96] examined the relationship between religious involvement and forgiveness in a largely Catholic sample of Western Europeans: 474 adults in France, 300 adults in Italy, and 338 young adults in Portugal. Age and religious involvement influenced the willingness to forgive in an interactive fashion. Both forgiveness and religious involvement increased with age. The effect of religious involvement (especially attending religious services and taking religious vows) on forgiveness was stronger in older than in younger adults.

Mark Rye and colleagues at the University of Dayton, Ohio, examined the role of forgiveness in healing the wounds of broken romantic relationships in college.[97] Studying 58 women ages 18 to 23 who had been deeply hurt in a romantic relationship, they found that religion-based forgiveness strategies were among the most common ones used. Investigators concluded that for at least some individuals "forgiveness is tied intricately to religion/spirituality."

ALTRUISM

Altruism, the self-less caring for others, is a virtue endorsed by all major world religions. While there is still debate about whether true altruism really exists,[98] or how it affects mental health,[99] the majority of research suggests positive influences on mental health for people of all ages.[100] Whether good mental health leads to greater caring and generosity, or greater caring and generosity lead to better mental health, is still hotly debated.[101] Nevertheless, helping behaviors are generally known to produce positive moods, and prospective studies indicate that volunteering and helping others may influence a person's physical as well as mental health over time.[102] For example, Harvard psychiatrist George Vaillant directs a study of adult development that has followed over 800 men and women since the 1930s and has become known as the longest, most comprehensive examination of aging ever conducted. The study sought to identify clues to the behaviors that translate into happy and healthy longevity. In his book *Aging Well* (2002), Vaillant reports that helping behaviors focused on other people (i.e., volunteering) are among the strongest predictors of health and longevity.[103]

Even the popular media has studied the benefits of helping others. In February 1987, for example, *Better Homes and Gardens* included an article about helping others. The magazine asked readers to write in on how helping others made them feel.[104] Although hardly a scientific study, the results were intriguing. A total of 246 readers sent back responses. Seven out of 10 (68%) indicated they experienced a distinct physical sensation while helping. About 50% reported they experienced a "high" feeling, 43% felt stronger and more energetic, 28% felt warm, 22% felt calmer and less depressed, 21% experienced greater self-worth, and 13% had fewer aches and pains. These findings provide several hypotheses worth further testing.

Skeptics have challenged the idea that religious persons are more altruistic. Batson at the Department of Psychology, University of Kansas, has questioned whether religious persons are truly more altruistic than others. He bases this concern on a series of experiments he conducted with college students placed in various helping situations.[105] He argues that helping behaviors by religious persons are motivated more by egoism than by altruism. Rather than giving for the other person's benefit (altruism), Batson claims that religious persons help in order to (1) avoid social and self-punishment in the form of shame or guilt and (2) acquire social and self-rewards in the form of praise or esteem (egoism). Thus, helping behaviors by religious persons may not always be sensitive to the needs as expressed by the person being helped. What is unclear from these studies is whether helping for secular humanistic reasons is driven by any higher motives than religious helping is.

Regardless of why they help others, it appears that religious persons do so more often. This is especially true when religiousness is measured in terms of intrinsic religiosity,[106] and studied in certain subgroups of the population such as African Americans and men.[107] If financial giving is considered an indicator of altruism, then religion is certainly a major factor. In fact, of all determinants of financial giving that have been studied, frequency of attendance at religious services is the most powerful predictor.[108] According to reports by the Independent Sector, a group that monitors patterns of financial giving in the United States, regular church attenders account for 80% of all giving. For example, weekly attenders gave 2.8% of their incomes in 1998, whereas those attending less than weekly gave 1.6% and non-attenders gave only 1.1%. The same is true for volunteering. About 33% of non-church members volunteer compared to greater than 60% of church members.[109] Similarly, nearly 50% of those who attend religious services do volunteer work, compared to 33% of those who do not. Most of this volunteering and giving, however, involves meeting needs within the religious community and only about 10% to 12% extends outward to the general community.

As we have seen, generosity with finances, time, and talents predicts better mental and even better physical health, particularly if done with religious intentions.[110] Even praying for others seems to have health benefits for those who are praying. Praying for the benefit of others could be considered a form of altruism and has been shown to increase mental health and well-being, an effect that may be partly mediated by an increased sense of meaning in life.[111]

SOCIAL SUPPORT

As with forgiveness and altruism, all major world religions encourage members to support and care for one another. It is the one teaching that all can agree on.[112] Religious involvement, whether it consists of private religious activities or attendance at religious services, is consistently related to greater social support in terms of number of contacts, complexity of social network, and quality of support.[113] This is important because social support is a strong predictor of mental health and of speedy recovery from mental disorder,[114] and has been shown to buffer the adverse effects of negative life events and stress.[115]

At least 20 studies during the twentieth century examined the relationship between religion and social support. Of those, 19 found a statistically significant positive correlation between the two.[116] Several of the studies involved large random samples, ranging from 2,956 to 4,522 participants.[117] This association was again especially true for studies of minority communities and older adults. Indeed, the majority of close friendships that older Americans report (whether African American or Caucasian) are found among persons in their church, synagogue, or mosque.[118]

Given that religious communities provide social and emotional support to large segments of the population, faith-based organizations end up serving the mental health needs of millions of Americans outside of the formal mental health care system. They are particularly key to the stability of minority communities and families. For example, Ortega and colleagues surveyed a random sample of 4,522 persons in urban, rural, and isolated rural communities in northern Alabama, over-sampling for older adults, women, and African Americans.[119] Of all the variables measured, informal interpersonal contact was the strongest predictor of life satisfaction. Interpersonal contact, however, produced this effect only if friendships were church based. Researchers concluded that the greater life satisfaction of African American elderly in this study was due almost entirely to greater contact with church-related friends.

Social support received from religious sources may have a different quality than that acquired in nonreligious settings (bridge club, senior center, etc.). For example, Ellison and George in the department of sociology at Duke University analyzed data from a random sample of 2,956 community dwelling persons over 18 years of age as part of the National Institute of Mental Health Epidemiologic Catchment Area project, North Carolina site. Using multivariate analyses to control for other covariates, they found that church attendance significantly predicted number of non-kin ties, in-person contacts, and telephone calls, as well as amount of instrumental support received. There was a significant relationship between church attendance and the quality of social support even after controlling for other measures of social support.

Fiala and colleagues at Fuller Theological Seminary in Pasedena reported similar findings. They developed a scale measuring three types of religious support—support from God, the congregation, and church leadership.[120] All three types of religious support were related to greater life satisfaction in two studies involving 249 and 93 subjects after controlling for other measures of social support. Investigators concluded that religious support provides unique resources above and beyond secular types of social interaction.

Personality

The relationship between religiosity and personality is not a straightforward one. There is evidence that personality or temperament can influence the likelihood of becoming religious, and that religion itself can affect personality. The most common example of the latter is religious conversion that leads to lasting and sometimes dramatic personality change.

PERSONALITY CAN AFFECT RELIGIOSITY

First, personality can influence religiosity. Robert Cloninger has described personality along three dimensions that are biologically determined: (1) novelty seeking—a tendency to crave new experiences and excitement that is likely mediated by brain dopamine, (2) reward dependent —a tendency to be motivated by social support and positive reinforcement that is likely mediated by norepinephrine, and (3) harm avoidance—a tendency to be anxious and crave safety that may be mediated by serotonin.[121] A person who is low in novelty seeking (more conservative and less likely to take risks), high in reward dependence (socially oriented and dependent on others for approval), and high in harm avoidance (anxious, fearful, and needing reassurance) may gravitate toward religion because it meets some of those psychological needs. The person who has a tendency to be high on novelty seeking (willing to take risks, desiring new experiences, dissatisfied with tradition), who has low reward dependence (doesn't need or want support or validation from others), and low harm avoidance (experiences pleasure and excitement in dangerous situations) may shy away from religion because it does not meet the needs of his or her temperament.

These tendencies could be inherited, at least in part. A recent cover story of *Time Magazine* focused on a book titled *The God Gene* written by Dean Hamer.[122] Hamer, chief of gene structure at the National Cancer Institute, claims that human spirituality is not only an adaptive trait, but that he has located the gene responsible for spirituality and it is located on or near the gene that codes for neurotransmitters. If this is so, then some of Cloninger's ideas above begin to make sense. Of course, spirituality—or as defined in *The God Gene*, spiritual feeling—is not the same as religious belief and practice, and it is well known that drugs such as LSD or heroin elicit ecstatic experiences similar to those reported during "spiritual" states. Thus, it may be that we are talking about something very different than what most persons understand religion to be (devout commitment to revealed truth that helps to form people's lives and relationships). However, this new information is provocative and deserves further study.

GENETIC EEFFECTS

The idea of religiosity or spirituality having a genetic basis has received further support by a number of recent studies. In the past five years, at least four studies have addressed this issue. Kendler and colleagues performed genetic analyses on three dimensions of religiosity in 1,902 female twins from Virginia.[123] Correlations were higher in monozygotic (identical) than in dizygotic (fraternal) twins for some of the three measures of religiosity (personal religious conservatism, institutional conservatism, and personal devotion). When correlations are higher in identical twins compared to fraternal twins, then genetic influences are thought to play a role. For personal conservatism, no evidence (0% of variance) was found for the impact of any genetic factors (45% of the variance was explained by family factors and 55% by individual or nonspecific environmental factors). For institutional conservatism, genetic factors appeared to play a minor role (12%) (vs. 51% for family and 37% for individual/environment). Over a quarter (29%) of the variance of personal devotion, however, was due to the influence of genetic factors (vs. 24% for family and 47% for individual).

In this study, personal conservatism was measured using two items: (1) "Do you believe that God or a universal spirit observes your actions and rewards or punishes you for them?" and (2) "Do you agree with the following statement: 'The Bible is the actual word of God and is to be taken literally, word for word'?" Institutional conservatism was measured by an ordering of religious affiliation: (1) fundamentalist Protestant, (2) Baptist, (3) Catholic, (4) mainline Protestant, and (5) other or unaffiliated. Personal devotion was assessed by three questions: (1) "How important are your religious and spiritual beliefs in your daily life?" (2) "When you have problems or difficulties in your family, work, or personal life, how often do you seek spiritual comfort?" and (3) "Other than at meal time, how often do you pray to God privately?" Thus, importance of religious belief, use of religious coping, and frequency of prayer had the most genetic basis (although genetics could explain less than one-third of the variance in responses).

As noted above, work has also been done on isolating specific genes that could influence the tendency toward or away from spiritual activity. Comings and colleagues studied 81 college students and 119 patients from an addiction treatment unit.[124] They administered a survey that included three self-transcendence measures, and genotyped subjects for the dopamine D-sub-4 receptor (DRD4) gene. The three self-transcendence subscores were significantly correlated with the DRD4 gene, and the "spiritual acceptance" subscore had the highest correlation. Based on these results, the investigators concluded that "the DRD4 gene may play a role in the personality trait of spiritual acceptance."

The actual biochemical pathway by which such genetic influences could have an effect has also been examined. Kurup and Kurup studied the isoprenoid pathway in atheistic-oriented and spiritually inclined individuals to determine whether left or right hemispheric dominance correlated with these tendencies.[125] HMG CoA reductase activity, serum digoxin, RBC membrane Na(+)-K(+) ATPase activity, serum magnesium, and tyrosine/tryptophan catabolic patterns were analyzed. Spiritually inclined individuals tended to show right hemispheric chemical dominance, whereas atheistic individuals tended to show left hemispheric dominance. Investigators concluded that chemical dominance and hypothalamic digoxin might help to regulate the predisposition to spirituality or atheism.

Finally, Abrahamson and colleagues investigated genetic and environmental influences on social attitudes among 654 adopted and non-adopted children and their biological and adoptive relatives as part of the Colorado Adoption Project.[126] General tendencies toward having conservative beliefs and values were assessed, as well as religious attitudes. Multivariate genetic analyses discovered that both conservatism and religious attitudes were strongly influenced by family environmental factors throughout adolescence. However, while they found a significant genetic influence on conservatism, no evidence for such an influence on religious attitudes was found.

Thus, all studies agree that family and other environmental or individual factors predominate in their influences on religious or spiritual tendencies. Three out of four also agree that there is some genetic influence, although how much and which aspect of religiosity is most affected remains uncertain. Also controversial is the specific neurotransmitter or other chemical likely involved in determining whether a person's tendency is toward or away from spirituality. The question is whether or not this kind of biologically/genetically determined spirituality or capacity for spiritual experience has anything to do with devout religious belief or commitment that is not based entirely on feelings/emotions.[127]

RELIGION-PERSONALITY RESEARCH

A number of studies have examined the relationship between religiosity and various personality traits. In general, religious involvement tends to be associated with greater cooperativeness,[128] less hostility,[129] lower sense of alienation,[130] more altruism and concern for others,[131] greater capacity to forgive,[132] and a greater sense of internal control.[133] In other studies, religion has been associated with greater authoritarianism,[134] guilt,[135] dogmatism,[136] and social desirability.[137] More recently, Ramanaiah and colleagues tested the hypothesis that college students who are high and low on spiritual well-being have different personality profiles.[138] They administered the Revised NEO Personality Inventory and the Spiritual Well-being Scale to 319 psychology undergraduates. Investigators found that students with high spiritual well-being scored lower on neuroticism and higher on extraversion, agreeableness, and conscientiousness, compared to low spiritual well-being subjects.

In one of the few longitudinal studies of personality, investigators followed 100 adults ages 55 to 80 over six years (Duke Longitudinal II Study of Aging).[139] Religious coping was examined as a predictor of 16 personality traits measured with the Catell 16-PF at the beginning and at the end of the study period. After controlling for age, sex, social class, health, and stressful life events, researchers found that persons who used religion to cope scored lower on factor E (dominance, aggressiveness, hostility, rebelliousness) and higher on factor G (responsibility, strong superego, concern over moral standards, and strength of character). Over time, male religious copers showed a decline in factor Q3 (controlling or compulsive) and female religious copers experienced a decline in factor Q4, suggesting an increase in relaxation, tranquility, and composure over time.

Thus, the relationship between religion and personality is a complex one. On the one hand, temperament (biologically driven and genetically determined) may influence tendencies toward or away from religion. On the other hand, religiosity may itself influence personality in several positive (or negative) ways as described above.

Religion and Poor Mental Health

Not all studies find that religion is linked to better coping, greater well-being, or positive emotions and personality traits. In our review of the literature on religion and mental health prior to the year 2000, we discovered that approximately 6% of studies (43 of 724) reported worse mental health among those who were more religious.[140] Conventional wisdom and modern research suggests that religion can be used to justify hatred and aggression,[141] prejudice and discrimination,[142] physical abuse,[143] and control or domination over others.[144] Religion has been correlated with dogmatic thinking,[145] obsessive traits,[146] and perfectionism.[147] It may be used to deny the facts and encourage magical, unrealistic thinking[148] or inappropriate pacifism or dependency.[149] Religion can promote negative attitudes toward psychiatric care,[150] replace psychiatric care,[151] delay diagnosis and impede effective treatment,[152] and justify non-compliance[153] (a particular problem in minority populations[154]). I summarize a few of these studies below.

HATRED AND AGGRESSION

Although not a scientific study, in his book *Holy Hatred,* newspaper editor James Haught compiled hundreds of newspaper articles detailing atrocities committed in the name of religion, including events in Yugoslavia, Northern Ireland, Sudan, Egypt, New York City, Sri Lanka, Iran, Algeria, and Russia.[155] He pays special attention to activities by extremist Muslims and other fringe groups such as the Branch Davidians in Waco, Texas. Although I could not locate any systematic studies of the relationship between hatred, aggression, and religious involvement, it is not surprising that intensely held religious beliefs can be destructive at times.

PREJUDICE AND DISCRIMINATION

Nearly forty years ago, Weima administered a 25-item Dutch version of the California F scale (authoritarianism), the Anti-Semitism scale, Anti-Protestantism scale, and Religious Conservatism scale to a sample of 67 male members of Ecclesia Circles (Catholics who met monthly to discuss subjects of interest in the field of religion) and 101 Catholic students at the

State University in Utrecht, Holland.[156] Authoritarianism was significantly and positively related to religious conservatism in both groups. Religious conservatism was also related to anti-Semitism in both groups, although the relationship was stronger in the Ecclesia Circles.

Allport and Ross surveyed 309 members of church groups in Massachusetts (94 Catholics and 28 Baptists), New York (55 Lutherans), South Carolina (44 Nazarenes), Pennsylvania (53 Presbyterians), and Tennessee (55 Methodists).[157] Using an intrinsic-extrinsic religiosity measure, they divided subjects into intrinsic (n=108), extrinsic (n=106), and indiscriminate (n=95) types, comparing them on measures of prejudice that assessed anti-black, anti-Jewish, and anti-other attitudes. They found that churchgoers were more prejudiced than non-churchgoers in the sample, although the relationship depended on religious orientation. Those with an extrinsic religious orientation (religion as a means to some other end, such as social status) were significantly more prejudiced than those with an intrinsic religious orientation (religion as an end in itself). Church members who were the most prejudiced were those in the indiscriminately pro-religious group (i.e., scored high on both intrinsic and extrinsic items). Researchers concluded that certain religious motivations (extrinsically and indiscriminately pro-religious) might foster greater prejudice against those who are different.

PHYSICAL ABUSE

Bottoms and colleagues examined how some religious beliefs can foster, encourage, and justify child abuse.[158] These investigators reviewed cases of religion-related child abuse, withholding medical care for religious reasons, abuse related to attempts to rid a child of evil, and child abuse perpetrated by clergy. Researchers also reported results from a national survey of almost 20,000 mental health professionals that asked about any experiences with religion-related abuse that they had during their time in practice. Based on this exhaustive survey, investigators identified 417 cases of alleged abuse. Of those, 271 were considered "pure" cases (rather than having mixed etiology). Of those 271 (of which 177 were clergy abuse), corroborative evidence was present in about half (26–57%). The evidence was strong enough to lead to a conviction, however, in less than 10%. Although the rate of such abuses appeared rather low, investigators concluded that society should protect the rights and welfare of children when they are threatened by religious beliefs and practices.

Ellison and colleagues examined whether there was any connection between religion and domestic violence using a national sample of 2,242 men and 2,420 women ages 19 or older (National Survey of Families and Households).[159] They reported that denominational monogamy (both parents having the some denomination) was unrelated to domestic violence in men. However, men who held much more conservative theological views than their partners were at slightly increased risk for domestic violence (an effect that reached statistical significance). Women, on the other hand, were less likely to perpetrate domestic violence if they attended religious services one or more times per month and if both spouses were either conservative Protestant or both Catholic.

Bowker reports two studies involving battered women. In the first study, she surveyed 146 battered wives from southeastern Wisconsin.[160] Approximately 40% sought help from clergy after 132 incidents of wife abuse. Counseling sessions averaged 11 in number and extended over an average of four months. The study was covered in *Women's Day* magazine. As part of that story, the magazine invited readers to join the research effort by writing to Dr. Bowker and completing a 6-page questionnaire. A total of 854 questionnaires were completed, bringing the combined sample for the two studies to over 1,000 battered women from all over the United States. The religious affiliations of battered women were 49% Protestant, 31% Catholic, 15% other religions, and 5% none. The religious affiliations of husbands were 39% Protestant, 29% Catholic, 12% other, and 20% none. Forty-eight percent of husbands never attended church and only 10% attended church weekly. Wives were more likely to attended services, with only 23% never attending services and 26% attending weekly. Overall, approximately one-third of the women received help from clergy, and of those, 34% rated help from clergy as somewhat or very effective (vs. 38% for district attorneys, 39% for police, 47% for social service or counseling agencies, 50% for lawyers, 56% for battered women's shelters, and 60% for women's groups). Thus, help from clergy was rated among the lowest of all helping professionals in terms of effectiveness. The authors concluded that while a significant proportion of battered women sought clergy for help, they on the whole perceived clergy to be relatively ineffective in helping them.

DOMINATION OVER OTHERS

Although not a research study, Hochman discusses the role that miracles and mystery can play in establishing power and control over others.[161] He notes that the suspension of natural and ordinary routines by the occurrence of miracles has the capacity to produce an atmosphere of awe, and is often the basis for development of strong authoritative leadership in religious cults (and to a lesser extent, perhaps, to religious authority in more traditional settings). Hochman notes that cults typically have many secrets that keep both potential recruits—and sometimes members—unaware of offensive aspects of the cult. By emphasizing their intellectual and spiritual powers, cult leaders can often control the lives of their followers. Members may spend much time living and working together, but know relatively little about each other's thoughts and feelings. Hochman concludes that an emphasis on miracles, mystery, and authority could explain, for example, the mass suicide at Jonestown, Guyana, by members of the People's Temple cult.

DOGMATIC THINKING

Dogmatism involves the arrogant, stubborn assertion of an opinion or belief. Strickland and Weddell surveyed regular attenders at a Southern Baptist and Unitarian church (a senior high and adult group in each church).[162] A total of 93 completed questionnaires (26 Baptist youth, 21 Baptist adults, 31 Unitarian youth, 15 Unitarian adults); 93% were white. The survey included measures of intrinsic-extrinsic (I-E) religious motivation, dogmatism, and racial prejudice. Investigators found no association between I-E score and prejudice (except in Baptists, where intrinsic religiosity was associated with less prejudice). However, they found a statistically significant relationship between I-E score and dogmatism (i.e., greater intrinsic religiosity was associated with being more dogmatic).

OBSESSIVE THINKING

Several studies report that religious persons have a tendency toward obsessive thinking. For example, Raphael and colleagues examined three groups of 50 psychiatric patients: 50 with obsessive-compulsive disorder

(OCD), 48 consecutive referrals to a psychotherapy group, and 51 consecutive referrals to general adult psychiatric services.[163] Although religious affiliation was the only religious characteristic measured, the percentage of subjects with a religious affiliation was highest in the OCD group (24.5% vs. 18.8% vs. 16.3%, respectively). Investigators concluded that religious affiliation may be a factor in the development or maintenance of OCD. In fact, a faith-based cognitive therapy to help treat religious persons with obsessive thoughts has been developed.[164] See part IV for a broader discussion of this issue.

PERFECTIONISM

Perfectionism involves the personality trait where people want everything in their lives to be perfect or exact. If things don't turn out the way they expect them (best grades, highest performance), then they become anxious. Richards and colleagues at Brigham Young University (BYU) conducted a study of 15 Mormon BYU students struggling with perfectionism.[165] Students attended eight group counseling sessions that focused on teaching clients about perfectionism and relied heavily on cognitive therapy methods to help clients overcome perfectionism. Investigators used Propst's (1980) *Cognitive Therapy-Meditation Manual* and discussed Mormon sermons with themes of accepting oneself despite imperfections, forgiveness, grace, Christ's atonement, and spiritual growth as a lifelong process. Religious imagery was also used. At the conclusion of treatment, students showed significant improvements on depressive symptoms, perfectionism, self-esteem, and spiritual well-being. Although this study doesn't prove that religious persons have more problems with perfectionism than nonreligious persons, it does establish that perfectionism can be a problem for some religious persons and that there are faith-based psychological approaches that may help.

DEPENDENCY

Dreger examined personality differences between 30 religious "conservatives" and 30 "liberals" (based on their responses to a Salvation Opinion questionnaire) in this 1952 study. Subjects were church members in their mid-thirties who were selected from a wide range of congregations in the United States (from Pentecostals and Baptists to Presbyterians and Unitarians). Projective tests (Rorschach and others) were used to determine personality traits. Dreger reported that religious conservatives showed significantly greater dependency on projective tests than did religious liberals.[166]

Thus, we find that in some studies and case reports religion is not associated with better mental health. Studies that document a negative relationship between religion and mental health can be difficult to interpret since they are almost always cross-sectional and thus plagued by "the chicken or egg" dilemma. Is religion the cause or the result of poor mental health in these studies?

If one considers that many persons will use religious beliefs in order to cope with distress, what is surprising is that so few of these cross-sectional studies find negative associations between religious coping and mental health. We would expect cross-sectional associations between emotional distress and religious coping to be *positive* because people "turn to religion" as their distress increases (i.e., the fox-hole effect, discussed in chapter 4). Positive associations in such studies, however, are not, surprisingly, very common. For example, of 62 studies that quantitatively looked at the correlation between religious coping and mental health, we found only 3 studies where religious coping was associated with greater distress or worse mental health (all were cross-sectional).[167] This low frequency of positive correlations suggests that religious coping may in fact be benefiting individuals.

Nevertheless, the studies discussed in this section suggest that for some people and in some circumstances, religion may actually impair mental health. More research is clearly needed to better understand such phenomena.

Social and Psychological Strain

Religion can also, in subtle ways, have negative effects on social relationships and at times can cause sadness, stress, and confusion. Such "psychological strains" can interfere with happiness and may even precipitate episodes of psychiatric disorder in vulnerable individuals. Although little systematic research documents such effects, conventional wisdom and clinical experience argue that psychosocial strains caused by strongly held religious beliefs are not uncommon. Julie Exline, an assistant professor in the Department of Psychology at Case Western Reserve University, divides sources of psychological and social strain into four areas: interpersonal strain, negative attitudes toward God, inner struggles to believe, and difficulties related to virtuous strivings.[168]

INTERPERSONAL STRAIN

Under this topic fall two common areas where religious beliefs cause psychological distress and social conflict: religious disagreements and negative attitudes towards other religious groups. If a person converts to a particular religious belief system, this may cause great strain in relationships with family members or close friends. For example, the person from a devout Christian family who converts to Buddhism, or a Buddhist from a traditional Buddhist family who converts to Christianity, will likely encounter much resistance. Family members are often upset by such decisions and may completely ostracize the person from any relationship with the family at all. Even in the best of circumstances, religious arguments with family and friends can create disharmony, anger, and pain. Another example may be a person who converts to evangelical Christianity and then distances himself or herself from close friends, or attempts to convert those friends to his or her way of thinking. Again, this may cause strife and disrupt the person's social network.

These issues can become particularly distressing when one spouse is from a different religious background (over half of couples today[169]), or when one spouse is more religious than the other (as Ellison found for cases of abuse). Disagreements over leadership roles, the raising of children, ways of spending time together, establishment of family traditions, and financial decisions can all arise over differing religious views. This creates stress in the relationship, and helps to explain why the divorce rate is so much higher among couples with different religious affiliations.[170]

Even among persons from the same religious background, intensely held beliefs that differ may cause strife in the relationship. For example, certain doctrines regarding the existence of hell or the devil may create anxiety in a person, or may cause that person to try to convince family or friends to believe in a certain way to avoid eternal damnation. Such conversations may become quite heated given the high stakes involved (i.e., fearing that a loved one is going to hell and will be eternally separated from them). Such conflicts may become particularly intense when loved ones are dying, creating stress for both the dying person and for the family member who is unable to convince the loved one to believe in a way that will prevent their feared demise.

Distress may also result when persons who are not particularly religious, or hold to more personal self-constructed spiritual views, experience resentment or anger toward religious persons who don't practice what they preach. They may read about religious leaders who become involved in affairs, financially manipulate followers, or sexually abuse children, and react with disgust and anger toward those who are religious. This may adversely affect interpersonal relationships, given the great numbers of religious people in this country, as well as cut them off from potential sources of psychological and social support. Exline notes that this disgust may evolve from disapproval of religious persons as hypocrites to seeing them as morally wrong or even evil, justifying strong negative attitudes toward such persons and their religious traditions.[171] Such negative feelings may also go the other way. In other words, devoutly religious people may see the nonreligious as morally inferior or evil, causing them to separate from such persons or even possibly persecute them. All of this disrupts interpersonal relationships and creates stress, divisions, and, sometimes, physical harm.

NEGATIVE ATTITUDES TOWARD GOD

When people experience emotional pain or difficult life circumstances, they often call out to God for comfort and help. As pain and distress go on and on, however, it is easy to become frustrated. While many experience comfort and a strengthening in their relationship with God when suffering, others experience a growing distance from God as their prayers for help seemingly go unanswered. There is the sense that God is not listening, doesn't care, or perhaps may even be punishing them. This can give rise to anger and resentment toward God, and lead to an avoidance or separation from anyone connected with God (other church members or pastoral staff). The result may be chronic anger, isolation, loneliness, and loss of meaning and purpose in life. Research shows that the loss of spiritual well-being and religious struggles that result from such feelings predict worse mental and physical health, and may even lead to a desire to end life.[172] On the other hand, those who are able to express and resolve their anger at God experience better mental health.[173]

People can also develop strained relationships with God, just as they would develop conflict with a parent or other authority figure. God as a father figure, for example, may evoke a similar relationship as with one's own father, and if that relationship was not a good one, then the relationship with God may not be either. Religious doctrines or religious figures may also be used to threaten and cajole children into obeying.[174] This can leave the child with a sense that God is a punishing or ruling figure, and if the parent-child relationship is not close, then God can be seen as distant and uncaring. Rather than seeing God as merciful, loving, and forgiving, the child may grow up seeing God as a ruthless judge who gives out rewards and punishments for good or bad behavior.

Even if a person does not feel angry or resentful toward God, he or she may have difficulty trusting and relying on God. Exline notes, for example, that some conservative Christian groups require a confessing of sins, giving up control, turning one's life over to God, and then depending on God to direct and lead them.[175] This may be quite difficult for someone who puts great importance on self-reliance, self-determination, and sense of autonomy—values highly esteemed in today's culture. Considerable psychological conflict may result as the person wrestles with relying on self vs. relying on God.

INNER STRUGGLES TO BELIEVE

Nonbelievers may not be able to logically and rationally endorse a belief system due to lack of scientific support or to apparent inconsistencies and contradictions. Given the dominant religious culture in which they live, however, this can precipitate inner struggles. These struggles over belief may result from a desire for life to have greater meaning, for a belief system to instill moral values in children, or for the support offered by a faith community, and may create distress for the spiritual seeker. Research suggests that those who are not raised in a religious home tend not to become religious later in life unless they do so through powerful emotional or social experiences.[176] These personal experiences enable nonbelievers to bypass their intellect or have less confidence in their intellect as the only road to truth so that they can embrace a faith. The whole process, though, can be quite disturbing.

Believers, on the other hand, may not agree with their own religious tradition's position on all subjects. For example, a Catholic woman may disagree with her church's position on birth control or abortion; an Episcopalian man may disagree with his church's stance toward homosexuality; or a Pentecostal teenager may disagree with her church's doctrines against alcohol use or smoking. These disagreements about belief can create internal conflict as well as social conflict with other family members or close friends within religious organizations. Some persons solve this problem, according to Exline, by choosing a "cafeteria-style religion" or "do-it-yourself spirituality" where they pick and choose only those doctrines from different religious faiths that agree with their own personal beliefs.[177] Whether this is an expression of individual freedom and choice—or self-deception—is debatable.[178] Regardless, such struggles with religious doctrine invariably cause strain within the individual and their social group.

PROBLEMS WITH VIRTUOUS STRIVINGS

Many religious people strive to better themselves in ways endorsed by their religious group. Such strivings often involve self-sacrifice, nonparticipation in certain kinds of activities, or avoidance of certain kinds of people, any of which may run counter to their social group or to the culture at large. Others may not understand why religious people are behaving this way and may exclude them or make fun of them because of their choices. This may cause the religious person to feel torn between a desire to serve God and a need to be approved and included by others.

Even more common is failure to live up to the values espoused and strived toward. Such values may include honesty, generosity, forgiveness, humility, or kindness. People may easily fall short of attaining these virtues because of their limited capacity for self-control or discipline,[179] and the result may be self-condemnation, hopelessness, or excessive guilt. This can cause them to give up entirely and reject these values as unobtainable, precipitating a downward spiral in the opposite direction. As the religious person becomes more and more deeply committed, he or she may become more and more sensitive to these failures, giving rise to other negative emotions and a drop in self-esteem.

Thus, devout religious belief, strivings toward religious belief, or sudden changes in religious belief can all create intrapsychic stress and social tension that lead to mental distress or worsen a preexisting psychiatric disorder. The person with mental disorder may be particularly sensitive to these stresses and strains due to an already low self-esteem, exaggerated sense of guilt, or compulsive and perfectionist nature. As important as they are, areas of religious stress and strain remain largely unexplored today.[180]

Religion as a Selective Process

Another possible explanation for the frequently reported positive relationships between religion and mental health is that religion serves as a selective factor. Persons disabled by negative emotions, especially at the level of a mental disorder (as explored in the next chapter), may be unable to engage in religious activities. Similarly, the negative, socially withdrawn person may not fit in very well in a faith community, where positive attitudes and social extroversion are highly valued and expected. Persons with such negative dispositions, then, may shy away from attending religious services. This is likely to be especially true for persons with psychiatric disorders such as depression or schizophrenia, whose symptoms can interfere with their ability to pray, read the Bible, or to engage in other religious activities. If true, this could help to explain associations between religious involvement, positive emotions, and pro-social traits.

Prospective vs. Cross-sectional Studies

Longitudinal or prospective research provides more information regarding causal relationships than cross-sectional studies; however, such studies still cannot establish whether religious beliefs and activities lead to better or worse mental health. When subjects are followed over time, everything else being equal, those at the start of the study who are more likely to pray or depend on religion to cope often end up experiencing better mental health down the road. The same phenomenon occurs for those experiencing physical pain. Although praying is usually associated with greater pain in the short run, it tends to predict a greater reduction in pain over the long term than experienced by those who do not pray. This is because increased pain causes people to initially turn to religion to cope (as discussed above), but as they engage in religious activities like prayer, this helps to reduce their experience of pain over time.[181] Such results from longitudinal research on religion and mental health are consistent with findings from randomized clinical trials that I will discuss in chapters 4 and 6.

Summary

A number of early studies, often in college students, found that religious beliefs were correlated with negative emotions or unfavorable character traits. There is evidence that religion may foster depression, worry, prejudice, physical abuse, dogmatic thinking, dependency, and obsessive traits. Religious beliefs likely cause considerable psychological and social strain for both religious and nonreligious persons alike, although the area has not been studied very well. Finally, religious communities may selectively exclude persons with emotional or social problems from religious activities, or these persons may be less able to engage in religious practices, creating a false positive association between religious activities and better mental health, especially in cross-sectional studies.

Nevertheless, when problems with health or situations arise that are out of a person's control, people often turn to religious beliefs or to a faith community for support. This is especially true in areas of the world such as the United States, India, Hispanic nations, some African nations, and Arab countries, although it is not as common in mainland northern European countries. In the United States, religious coping is most prevalent among ethnic minorities, women, the elderly, and those with chronic illness. Furthermore, such religious beliefs and practices are usually associated with greater well-being, hope, and optimism; more purpose and meaning in life; greater quality of life; and more pro-social traits in terms of forgiveness, sociability, and altruism. These positive findings are particularly notable when studies are conducted in adult community-based samples or medically ill populations. Finally, religious involvement is consistently related to both a higher level and a higher quality of social support, particularly among older adults and African Americans. In the next chapter, we look at the connections between religion and mental disorders.

CHAPTER 4

RELIGION, PSYCHIATRIC
SYMPTOMS, AND DISORDERS

In the last chapter, I focused on relationships between religiosity, positive emotions, virtuous character traits, personality, and social support. In this chapter, I examine psychiatric symptoms and psychiatric diagnoses such as anxiety disorders, depressive disorders, eating disorders, personality disorders, and substance abuse disorders. I will discuss severe persistent mental illness (schizophrenia, bipolar disorder, and other chronic psychotic disorders) in chapter 5. Here I will explore whether religious beliefs are associated with fewer (or more) symptoms of nonpsychotic psychiatric disorder, and whether religious involvement predicts faster (or slower) resolution of psychiatric symptoms.

First, however, it is necessary to explain how having psychiatric symptoms may be different from having a psychiatric disorder. Psychiatric symptoms are common in the general population and usually exist on a continuum from very mild to very severe. Many people without psychiatric disorder or mental illness experience such symptoms, but they never reach the threshold necessary to cause trouble with functioning or persist for prolonged periods as mental disorders do. Who doesn't experience periods of anxiety or sadness? These emotions are a normal part of life—where things go wrong, failures happen, and disappointments occur all the time in relationships, jobs, and goals.

However, this is completely different from the experience of anxiety that paralyzes people's actions or confines them to home or makes them repeatedly check locks or wash their hands. It is completely different from depressive symptoms that make persons feel worthless, drain hope, and drive them to kill themselves rather than endure continual and seemingly unending pain and suffering. In anxiety or depressive disorders, these feelings don't just pass away after a few hours or days, but last for weeks, months, sometimes years. Having a disorder is totally different from the fluctuating moods that most of us have.

A psychiatric disorder is said to exist when mental or emotional symptoms become so severe that they interfere with a person's ability to function at work, at home, or in social relationships. Interference with psychological, social, or occupational functioning, then, is the hallmark of psychiatric disorder and is required for it to exist. I will discuss religion's relationship to both psychiatric symptoms and psychiatric disorder in this chapter.

Anxiety

Anxiety is a normal emotion experienced when we anticipate something threatening in the future. Whether the event is a physical threat to our bodies or a psychological threat to our self-esteem really doesn't matter. Anxiety is useful because it alerts us to prepare ourselves to handle the potentially negative experience. However, anxiety can become continuous even in the absence of threatening circumstances and may interfere with a person's ability to function at his or her highest level.

Many studies have examined the connections between religion and anxiety. There is an old saying that refers to this relationship: "Religion comforts the afflicted and afflicts the comfortable." It suggests that religion can be a two-edged sword when it comes to anxiety, increasing it in some circumstances and decreasing it in others. At least 76 studies prior to the year 2000 examined the relationship between anxiety and religion.[1] Of these, 69 were observational studies (either cross-sectional or prospective cohort studies) and 7 were randomized clinical trials. A majority of the observational studies (35 of 69) found lower anxiety or less fear among those who were more religious, 24 found no association, and 10 studies found greater anxiety.

The 10 studies that found greater anxiety among the more religious deserve further explanation. Bear in mind that all of these studies were cross-sectional. On the one hand, religion may cause or arouse anxiety. Religious persons can feel anxious or guilty over real or imagined "sins" and may fear retribution either in this present life or in the hereafter. Doctrines that emphasize the devil, hell, and eternal damnation can instill fear in children or adults in order to constrain behavior. Religious doctrines may cause internal conflicts as people strive to live according to religious ideals, but are drawn by human desires toward other paths. On the other hand, anxiety can also be a strong motivator of religious belief because of the comfort and sense of control that it offers. Again, consider how Americans coped with September 11th—90% turning to religion and increasing religious activity following the event. "Fox hole" religion involves a turning to religion during times of greater danger or anxiety, such as during war or other desperate situations. When do people pray the most? When they are anxious or worried about a situation over which they have little or no control.

Recall that longitudinal studies are those that assess the relationship between two variables over time providing information about the order of effects (i.e., whether religion came first and is causing the emotional problem, or whether the emotional problem came first and is motivating the religious behavior). Even if one variable can predict changes in another variable over time, however, it is still possible that both variables are associated with some third underlying characteristic that is really the cause of the connection between the two. Thus, as discussed earlier, the evidence for causality provided by longitudinal studies is indirect and only a randomized clinical trial can provide direct evidence for causality.

To help us sort out whether religion is causing or being caused by anxiety, let us examine the results of studies that observe people over time (longitudinal) and of clinical trials that test religious interventions to determine whether the overall effect of religion is to increase or decrease anxiety. Of the five longitudinal studies that examined the relationship between religion and anxiety prior to the year 2000, four found that people who were more religious at the beginning of the study were less likely to experience fear or anxiety when surveyed months or years later.[2] Of the seven clinical trials that tested a religious treatment for anxiety, six found that the religious intervention reduced anxiety levels.[3] These studies included religious treatments from Christian, Islamic, Hindu, and Buddhist orientations, and often involved meditation. These studies will be described further in chapter 6.

TYPE OF RELIGIOSITY

The reason for being religious (i.e., religious motivation) may also influence the relationship with anxiety. What is driving or motivating a person's religious activities? Is it just to impress people? Is it for financial or economic gain? Is it only to make social contacts? Or is the person religious for religion's sake alone, regardless of whether any material or social gain results? Research has found that having an *intrinsic* religious orientation (i.e., being religious for religion's sake) rather than an *extrinsic* religious orientation (i.e., being religious in order to acquire something more highly valued than religion) may influence the religion-anxiety relationship. In a study conducted 20 years ago, Baker and Gorsuch administered measures of intrinsic religiosity, extrinsic religiosity, and anxiety to 52 persons in a religious wilderness camp in Southern California.[4] They found that anxiety level was negatively correlated with intrinsic religiosity, but was positively correlated with extrinsic religiosity.

Other negative psychological constructs, such as poor social integration, ego weakness, and suspiciousness have all been positively correlated with extrinsic religiosity but negatively correlated with intrinsic religiosity. Recent investigations have replicated these findings in Christians, Buddhists, and Muslims.[5]

One of the most interesting examinations of the religion-anxiety relationship was a study of Buddhists from Thailand and Christians in Canada. Overall anxiety and worry were significantly lower among both Buddhists and Christians who scored high on intrinsic religiosity.[6] Buddhists who were more extrinsic in their religious orientation, however, experienced more worry and anxiety than did extrinsic Christians. The researchers suggested that differences in belief system could have accounted for these findings. Most Christian groups emphasize mercy and redemption from a forgiving God at any time during life, including old age. In Buddhism, there is no help from a personal savior but rather the promise of enlightenment. If enlightenment is not achieved before death, however, the Buddhist will not be liberated from the cycle of death and rebirth. As a result, study authors concluded, "Therefore, for Buddhists higher levels of worry might be associated to a greater extent with the realization that their extrinsic religious behavior does not help in alleviating individual responsibility or guilt."[7]

More recent studies conducted since the year 2000 also suggest an association between greater religiousness and less anxiety in both U.S. and non-U.S. samples, from Muslim adolescents to Lithuanian adult service professionals, from Mexican migrants in the United States to South African sawmill workers.[8] An example of one of these studies involved 2,453 Kuwaiti adolescents ages 14 to 18.[9] Anxiety and self-rated religiosity were inversely related for both boys and girls, effects that achieved a high level of statistical significance. Investigators explained the results as due to the fact that Islamic teachings help to reduce anxiety through encouragement of religious practices.

Overall, then, there is little evidence to suggest that religion is a primary cause for persistent anxiety in most people, even though this may occur in some individuals. Instead, the research indicates that anxiety is a powerful motivator of religious activity, which may result over time in the lowering of anxiety (that may then be followed by a reduction in religious activity, as evident in the months following 9/11). Let us now examine the relationship between religion and specific anxiety disorders.

POST-TRAUMATIC STRESS DISORDER (PTSD)

Bei-Hung Chang and colleagues at Boston University's school of public health and Bedford Veterans Administration hospital conducted two studies on religion and sexual assault trauma using representative national samples of female and male veterans. In the first study of 3,543 women who used Veterans Administration ambulatory care services, investigators found that higher religious service attendance predicted better mental health and fewer depressive symptoms in women with sexual assault (using standard measures of mental health and depression).[10] In that study, religious coping (personal religiousness) was also associated with better mental health and less depression whether or not women had a history of sexual assault. In a second study of 2,427 males receiving Veterans Administration ambulatory care services (a 2-year prospective study), Chang and associates again found that religious attendance and religious coping attenuated the association between sexual trauma and the development of depression or poor mental health.[11] Both of these recent studies document the role that religion can play in buffering the adverse mental health effects of traumatic events that otherwise could lead to PTSD.

We have been discussing how religion affects anxiety symptoms following trauma. What about the reverse? How does experiencing a severe trauma affect a person's religious beliefs? Religious beliefs may weaken or decline in importance if the person feels punished by God or abandoned by God, whereas beliefs might strengthen as the person turns to God for comfort and hope. The effect probably varies depending on the person's particular beliefs and level of commitment to those beliefs prior to the trauma.

For example, Falsetti and colleagues examined relationships between religious belief, experiencing a negative trauma, and having post-traumatic stress disorder (PTSD) in a sample of 120 adults from the St. Louis area participating in a DSM-IV Field Trial Study on PTSD.[12] Subjects in the PTSD group were composed of individuals seeking psychiatric care (n=56). They were compared to a community sample of people who had experienced a negative trauma but did not have PTSD (n=64). The types of traumatic stress among those with PTSD included sexual assault (32%), undergoing a natural disaster (14%), and witnessing someone being seriously injured (8%). Two-thirds of the PTSD sample indicated multiple traumas. Intrinsic religiosity was measured using a validated 10-item scale, and changes in religious beliefs were assessed after the first/single trauma and after the most recent trauma. Information about change in religious beliefs was obtained retrospectively. Persons in the PTSD group were more likely to report changes in religious beliefs than those in the non-PTSD group. For the overall sample, 17% experienced a decline in beliefs after the trauma whereas 14% experienced an increase or strengthening of religious belief. For the PTSD sample, 30% experienced a decline in belief, whereas 20% reported a strengthening of belief.

Although the above study found that more persons turned away from religion than toward it following a traumatic event, these findings conflict to some degree with the study referred to earlier on religiosity after September 11th, showing that 9 out of 10 Americans turned toward religion.[13] The latter study, however, asked a somewhat different question and did not specifically target persons with PTSD. Severe psychological trauma, such as that seen in PTSD, may shake a person's religious worldview so seriously that it becomes inaccessible as a source of comfort and hope. How could a loving God who is in control allow such a horrible thing happen? This may precipitate a lifelong search for an answer.

Consider the findings of a recent study of 1,385 veterans from Vietnam (95%), World War II, and/or Korea (5%) involved in outpatient or inpatient PTSD programs.[14] Alan Fontana and Robert Rosenheck, from the division of the VA National Center for PTSD and Yale University School of Medicine, examined the interrelationships between veterans' exposure to traumatic stress, PTSD, change in religious faith, and use of mental health services. They used structural equation modeling to show that veterans' traumatic experiences during war weakened their religious faith. Weakened religious faith, in turn, was an independent predictor of use of VA mental health services—independent of severity of PTSD symptoms and level of social functioning. Investigators concluded that the use of mental health services was driven more by weakened religious faith than by clinical symptoms or social factors. This remarkable study, then, found that changes in religious faith was one of the strongest predictor of veterans seeking mental health services over the years, even stronger than the severity of the clinical symptoms themselves. They concluded that pastoral counseling to address spiritual issues may need to become a more central part of the treatment of PTSD patients.

OBSESSIVE-COMPULSIVE DISORDER (OCD)

Freud's first paper on religiosity pointed out the similarity between religious practices and obsessive-compulsive neurosis.[15] Even a special term *(scrupulosity)* has been used to describe obsessions and compulsions associated with religion.[16] Nearly a decade ago, Steketee and colleagues found in a sample of OCD patients that religiosity was significantly correlated with severity of OCD symptoms, but not with measures of general anxiety, social anxiety, or depression.[17] This suggested some degree of specificity in the religion-OCD symptom relationship. They did not, however, find a difference in degree of religiosity between the 33 patients with OCD and 24 patients with other anxiety disorders, meaning that religiosity per se probably did not lead to OCD. Rather, the evidence favored an influence for religion on the manifestation of the disorder (50% of the sample was Catholic).

Also studying a largely Catholic sample, Sica and colleagues compared OCD symptoms between three groups: (1) members of convents and nunneries, (2) members of Catholic associations, and (3) college students in northern Italy.[18] Members of convents and nunneries were categorized as "high religiosity" (n=54). Members of well-known Catholic associations who regularly attended church activities, were well grounded in religious practices, and spent most of their spare time participating in religious activities were categorized as "medium religiosity" (n=47). The college student group consisted of those who indicated no interest in religious matters ("low religiosity") (n=64). OCD symptoms were assessed using three validated measures of OCD symptoms. Scales measuring depressive symptoms and anxiety symptoms were also administered. Age (mean age 22), gender, and years of education were comparable across the three groups.

Results indicated that members of convents and nunneries (high religiosity) scored significantly higher on anxiety and depressive symptoms than either the actively religious group (medium religiosity) or the low religiosity group. The medium religiosity group (religiously devout lay Catholics), however, tended to score lower on both measures of anxiety and depression compared to the low religiosity group. The high religiosity group scored significantly higher than low religiosity subjects on only 1 of 5 OCD subscales (impaired mental control) of the first measure. On the second OCD measure, high and medium religiosity subjects scored significantly higher than low religiosity subjects on 4 of 6 subscales (control of thoughts, importance of thoughts, responsibility, and perfectionism). On the third OCD measure, however, it was low religiosity subjects who scored significantly higher than high religiosity subjects on importance of thoughts (the opposite of that found on the second OCD measure), and there was no difference between groups on the other two subscales. Based on these findings, investigators concluded, "religion might play a role in obsessive-compulsive disorder phenomenology" (813). It should not be surprising, though, that religious subjects score higher than nonreligious subjects on subscales measuring a sense of responsibility or degree of perfectionism, since these are values endorsed by many religious groups (being responsible and paying attention to detail are considered positive traits). This illustrates a problem with some OCD scales. They often include questions that assess traditional religious values. How such bias may have contributed to other findings above is not clear.

Other recent research examining OCD patients has not found evidence that links religiousness to this disorder. In a study conducted in Tel Aviv, Israel, investigators compared religiosity between 22 adult patients with

OCD, 22 patients with panic disorder (PD), and 22 normal controls (age- and sex-matched patients undergoing minor surgery).[19] Five Jewish religiosity scales were administered across the three groups. No differences were found on any of the measures, except that PD patients scored significantly lower on religiosity than controls. Likewise, other recent studies of OCD patients from Christian, Jewish, and Islamic religious backgrounds report little evidence for a link between religiousness and OCD.[20] These studies, however, did not examine religiousness and severity of symptoms within OCD patients, as Steketee had done.

There is also evidence that obsessive and compulsive symptoms are more likely to be picked up in very religious persons, more likely than in nonreligious persons who have the same level of OCD symptoms.[21] This means that there may be a bias in the detection of OCD symptoms in religious people. Contaminated OCD symptoms scales and bias in the detection of OCD symptoms may help to explain why religiosity and severity of symptoms are associated in OCD patients. Alternatively, certain types of religiosity may either foster or support OCD-like traits or OCD itself.

When religious obsessions and compulsions are present, however, at least two studies suggest a worse prognosis. The first study involved 60 outpatients in Spain with OCD followed for 1 to 5 years. Obsessions with sexual or religious content were unique in predicting poor long-term outcomes despite pharmacological and behavioral treatment.[22] The second study involved 153 outpatients with OCD in London enrolled in a randomized clinical trial examining the effects of behavioral therapy.[23] Higher scores on sexual/religious obsessions again predicted poorer outcomes after controlling for initial symptom severity. Further research is clearly needed in both clinical and nonclinical samples to help sort out whether religiousness or type of religion makes a difference in the etiology, course, or detection of OCD.

Depression

Because religion is a source of hope, optimism, and well-being, one would expect lower rates of depression and suicide among those who are more religious. Clinical experience and common sense, though, argue that religion may foster guilt and remorse over sin that could worsen depression or complicate recovery. Although there is evidence supporting both viewpoints, most of it favors a role for religion in preventing depression or facilitating its resolution.

At least 101 studies prior to the year 2000 examined the relationship between religion and depression, and 68 examined the relationship between religion and suicide.[24] Eight of the 101 depression studies were randomized clinical trials. The majority of the 101 depression studies found less depression among those who were more religious. Of the 93 cross-sectional or longitudinal studies, 60 found significantly lower rates of depressive disorder or fewer depressive symptoms among the more religious. Of the 22 longitudinal studies, 15 found that greater religiousness at baseline predicted lower depression scores when subjects were followed up later.

Three longitudinal studies have examined the effects of religiousness on the outcome of depressive symptoms or depressive disorder. These studies enrolled depressed patients and followed them over time, examining whether baseline religiousness increased or decreased the speed of remission during a 6 to 12 month follow-up period. All three studies found that greater religiousness predicted faster recovery from depression over time. In the first study, Braam and colleagues followed 177 older adults in the Netherlands for over 12 months to identify factors influencing change in depressive symptoms.[25] Subjects who indicated religion was not very important were almost six times more likely to remain chronically depressed. This was especially true for older women. Among depressed women who indicated that religion was not important, none (0%) recovered from depression; among women who indicated religion was very important, 50% recovered (p<0.01).

The second study was the first to examine the effect of religiosity on the course of depressive disorders. The NIMH Diagnostic Interview Schedule was used to identify depressive disorders in medical patients admitted to general medicine, cardiology, and neurology services of Duke University hospital.[26] Depressed patients (n=87) were then followed for an average 47 weeks after discharge, during which time weekly change in depressive symptoms was measured to determine the time it took for patients to fully remit from their depressions. Of nearly 30 baseline characteristics, level of intrinsic religious (IR) motivation was one of five characteristics of patients at baseline that predicted the speed at which their depressions got better. For every 10-point increase on the IR scale, whose scores ranged from 10 to 50, there was a 70% increase in speed of depression remission, after controlling for the effects of other predictors. In patients whose physical functioning did not improve during the course of the study, i.e., the chronically disabled, the effect was even stronger (over a 100% faster speed of remission for every 10-point increase on the IR scale).

In the third study, investigators sought to clarify the role that social support and other clinical factors played in the relationship between religiousness and depression among persons with severe depression.[27] Investigators followed 114 elderly patients for 6 months to assess factors that might influence response to treatment following hospitalization. All patients were so depressed at the start of the study that they required acute psychiatric hospitalization, and were treated using a standard medication regimen. At baseline, subjects completed measures of public and private religious practice, a measure of positive and negative religious coping, and two scales assessing subjective and instrumental social support. A geriatric psychiatrist completed an observer-rated depression scale at baseline and 6 months later. Public religious practices and positive and negative religious coping were related to depression scores at baseline (all in the expected directions). Positive religious coping (seeing God as a partner, seeking God's love and care, focusing on religion to stop worrying) measured at baseline also predicted lower depression scores 6 months later, independent of social support, demographic, and clinical factors such as use of electroconvulsive therapy and prior episodes of depression. Although religious coping was positively related to social support, it was inversely related to depression on follow-up after controlling for social support. Researchers concluded, "Clinicians caring for older depressives should consider inquiring about spirituality and religious coping as a way of improving depression outcomes" (905).

At least 8 clinical trials have now examined the effects of religious interventions on the course of depression.[28] Five of the 8 clinical trials found that depressed patients receiving religious interventions recovered more quickly than patients receiving secular interventions or no treatment at all.[29] These studies were all performed in religious patients and included treatments from Muslim, Christian, and Buddhist perspectives (and will be discussed in greater detail in chapter 6). Thus, the majority of cross-

cross-sectional research, prospective cohort studies, and clinical trials all indicate that religion helps to prevent the onset of the depression and, when depression does occur, facilitates recovery.

The effects of religion on buffering against depression or improving recovery appear to be strongest during times of stress, especially poor health, financial difficulties, severe trauma, or difficulties involved in caring for loved ones. Numerous studies demonstrate stronger inverse relationship between religious involvement and depression among those struggling with chronic physical disability,[30] persons in the general population coping with stress,[31] those experiencing the traumatic stress of sexual assault,[32] partners of patients with AIDS,[33] family members caring for a loved one with Alzheimer's or end-stage cancer,[34] and those coping with the loss of loved ones,[35] suffering through natural disasters,[36] or dealing with the economic stresses.[37] Interestingly, during the most difficult times in life it seems that religious beliefs and practices make the most difference.

I will now review a few recent studies on the religion-depression relationship, discussing them by the age group of participants studied: children and adolescents, young and middle-aged adults, and older adults. Most of these reports have appeared since the year 2000.

CHILDREN AND ADOLESCENTS

Interpersonal religious experiences

Given the influence of peers, interpersonal religious experiences may be particularly important in protecting adolescents and teenagers from depression. Michelle Pearce and colleagues in the Department of Psychology at Yale University examined the relationship between depressive symptoms and religiosity in 744 adolescents (mean age 13 years).[38] They found that several measures of religiousness were associated with lower levels of depressive symptoms, including religious attendance and self-rated religiosity. Especially important, however, was having positive interpersonal religious experiences (positive interactions with those in the faith community). Negative interpersonal religious experiences (conflict with clergy or church members) were associated with significantly higher levels of depression. Investigators emphasized how religious-based social support during adolescence may foster positive interpersonal religious experiences.

Schapman and Inderbitzen-Nolan at the University of Nebraska also found that religious activity was associated with less depression in 261 teenagers ages 13 to 18.[39] Thus, involving teenagers in religious activities with one another to build positive relationships within a faith-based setting may help to shield them from the development of depression as they struggle with other changes and stresses of this stage.

Mother and child depression

Religious beliefs of parents may influence both their own risk of depression, as well as the risk that their children face. Lisa Miller and colleagues at Columbia University in New York City conducted a prospective study of 60 depressed mothers and 151 offspring assessed once a year for 10 years.[40] Investigators found that among mothers, religious importance and Catholicism (assessed during the final interview, assessment 10) was related to fewer episodes of major depression during the previous 10 years. These same religious measures in mothers (importance and Catholicism) were also related to fewer episodes of major depression in their offspring during the previous 10 years (although the relationship was only marginally significant). Among offspring, however, their own religiosity was not associated with a lower risk of major depression. Finally, mother-offspring concordance for denomination (again, measured at the final assessment) was associated with a lower prevalence of major depression in offspring during the previous 10 years. Researchers concluded that maternal religiosity influences the character of child rearing, shapes the home environment, and therefore may influence the likelihood that offspring will experience depression.

In a similar study, Varon and Riley from the division of child and adolescent psychiatry at Sinai Hospital in Baltimore examined the relationship between maternal church attendance and adolescent mental health and social functioning in 143 youth.[41] Two-thirds were at risk for developing a psychiatric disorder (i.e., scored one standard deviation above the median on one of two mental health measures). Investigators found that youth whose mothers attended religious services at least once a week experienced greater overall satisfaction with their lives, more involvement with their families, better skills in solving health-related problems, and felt greater support from friends.

In another study involving mothers and adolescents, Horowitz and Garber in the department of psychology at Vanderbilt University examined the relationship between religiosity and depressive disorder over time in 240 adolescents based on maternal depression history.[42] Adolescents were first evaluated in sixth grade and then every year for 6 years. Adolescent religiosity (frequency of praying in a house of worship and importance of religion) did *not* moderate the relation between chronic maternal depression and adolescent depressive disorder. Both maternal and adolescent depression during grades 7 through 11 predicted lower religious attendance during the twelfth grade (controlling for prior religious attendance), suggesting that depression was having an adverse effect on church attendance. Religious attendance in sixth grade tended to predict a lower likelihood of developing depression during grades 7 through 12 (p<0.07), although this effect was weaker than the effect of depression on attendance. Thus, depression and religious activity may have a bi-directional effect on each other over time in adolescence.

Physical maturation

Studying religiosity and depression in adolescents from a different perspective, Miller and colleagues from Columbia University examined the impact of physical maturation on the relationship between religiosity and depression in a random sample of 3,356 adolescent girls in North Carolina.[43] They assessed physical maturation based on self-reported secondary sexual characteristics and age menstruation onset. Religiosity, in turn, was assessed using measures of personal devotion, personal conservatism (based on religious beliefs), institutional conservatism (based on denominational affiliation), and religious attendance. Controlling for age and ethnicity, they found that personal devotion and religious attendance were associated with a 19% to 26% decrease in the prevalence of depression among immature girls and a 32% to 43% decrease in highly mature girls. Personal and institutional conservatism, however, were associated with a 17% to 24% decrease in depression among immature girls but no decrease in highly mature girls. Investigators concluded that the protective effects of religiosity among adolescent girls depend on both physical maturation level and type of religiosity.

History of childhood depression

Miller and colleagues at Columbia also recently reported the results of an 11-year follow-up study of 146 children with a history of childhood depression and 123 control children with no such history.[44] This is one of the few studies that followed children for over a considerable period examining how religiousness in childhood and adulthood influenced the development of depression over time. Depression in childhood and during the 11-year follow-up was assessed using a structured diagnostic interview. Religious attendance and denomination were assessed in children at baseline and then at the end of the follow-up period (when they were adults). In addition to frequency of attendance at religious services and denomination, they were also asked about importance of religion during the adult evaluation.

Investigators found that importance of religion at the adult evaluation tended to predict a decreased risk of depression in female children during follow-up (51% lower), but only in those who had not been depressed as children. Among female children depressed in childhood, greater religious importance at the adult evaluation tended to predict a 2.4 times *greater* risk of developing depression during follow-up. Frequency of religious attendance in childhood predicted an 84% lower likelihood of developing depression during follow-up for female children without a history of depression and there was as similar trend for attendance measured at the adult evaluation as well (65% lower). No such effects, however, were seen in females who were depressed as children. With regard to male children, there was no association between religious attendance in childhood or adulthood and depression during follow-up in those with or without a history of depression. However, male children with a depression history had a 78% lower risk of developing depression if they indicated a Catholic affiliation at the adult evaluation and a similar trend was present for Catholic affiliation in childhood. These effects were not present in male children without a history of depression.

Of particular interest was the greater likelihood of developing depression in female children with a history of childhood depression and strong adult religiousness. Investigators hypothesized that childhood religiousness may have caused girls to gravitate toward religion as a source of comfort (depression leading to religion). Alternatively, depressed girls may

have integrated their depressed cognitive style into personal religious beliefs, possibly developing punitive or guilt-inducing forms of adult religiousness that could foster the development of depression (religion leading
to depression). Investigators also explained that Catholic rituals or Catholic promotion of social cohesion in childhood could help to prevent the
later development of depression in vulnerable young males.

Teenage pregnancy

The particular kind of stress that a teenager encounters may also influence the likelihood that religion will have positive or negative effects on
mood. For example, Sorenson and colleagues assessed the relationship between religion and depression in a group of 261 teenage mothers identified before delivery and followed for 4 weeks after delivery, most of who
were unmarried.[45] They found that Catholics, those affiliated with more
conservative religious groups, and those who attended religious services
more frequently all had higher depression scores. The highest depression
scores were found among girls who cohabitated with someone while continuing to attend religious services. The authors concluded that religion
fosters feelings of guilt or shame, eroding feelings of competence, self-
worth, and hopefulness, and encourages withdrawal of community support from those who do not conform to social norms. The finding of
greater depression in actively religious teenagers who act contrary to the
teachings of their religion (i.e., live with a partner and bear children out of
wedlock), however, is not terribly surprising.

In summary, recent research in children and adolescents confirms earlier research suggesting that religious involvement reduces the likelihood of
depression. However, the particular stressor and whether or not the
teenager has a history of depression may influence the kind of effect that
religion has.

YOUNG AND MIDDLE-AGED ADULTS

Social support

Interpersonal religious relationships may also play a role in protecting
adults from depression, just as it does in adolescence. Jan Nooney and Eric
Woodrum at North Carolina State University analyzed data on a national-

ly representative sample of 1,445 adults from the 1998 General Social Survey. Using structural equation modeling, they found an inverse relationship between religious attendance, prayer, and depressive symptoms.[46] In that model, religious attendance predicted increased church-based social support, which in turn predicted fewer depressive symptoms. Prayer predicted positive religious coping (as defined earlier), and positive religious coping, in turn, predicted less depression. Note that church-based social support was not "simply" social support, such as the same kind of support that one gets by attending a bridge club or community center. Rather it was support derived through relationships developed within a faith community, and was measured using a standardized scale developed for this purpose.[47]

Bereavement

Death of a loved one, particularly when it involves a child, is a major stressor that often results in depression. Maura Higgins at the Graduate School of Social Work, Boston College, examined associations between religious characteristics and depressive symptoms in a national sample of 621 adults aged 24 to 65 years who had experienced the death of a child.[48] Religious measures included belief in an afterlife and frequency of attendance at religious services. Higgins found only weak support for an inverse relationship between religion and depression. Other variables, including gender, marital status, ethnicity, age, family income, and education all appeared to have a stronger relationship with depression than religious variables. Marital status had the strongest inverse relationship to depression for women, and education had the strongest inverse relationship with depression for men. As noted for PTSD, severe psychological trauma may challenge a person's religious worldview, making it difficult to rely on religion for comfort.

Psychiatric inpatients

In one of the first studies to examine the relationship between religious commitment and depressive symptoms among hospitalized psychiatric patients in Canada, Baetz and colleagues in the Department of Psychiatry at the University of Saskatchewan surveyed 88 consecutive adult patients admitted to their psychiatric service (two-thirds with major depression).[49] Approximately two-thirds of patients believed in a God who rewards and punishes, 27% attended religious services at least weekly, and 35% prayed once or more daily.

After controlling for age, sex, education, marital status, and social support, investigators found that frequent church attendance was associated with less severe depressive symptoms, shorter current lengths of stay, higher satisfaction with life, and lower rates of current and lifetime alcohol abuse (all statistically significant relationships). Higher intrinsic religiosity was also associated with fewer depressive symptoms and less current alcohol use. Religious coping was associated with shorter lengths of hospital stay. Prayer frequency was weakly associated with less depression, although the finding did not reach statistical significance. Researchers concluded that certain religious practices may protect against severe depressive symptoms, shorten hospital stay, and enhance life satisfaction in this patient population. Given the cross-sectional nature of their data, however, it is just as likely that these inverse relationships were due to severe depression preventing the religious activities assessed (such as religious attendance, for example).

Social support and religion

Does greater social support by itself explain why those who frequently attend religious services experience less depression? In the United States, where religion and social activity are both common and strongly correlated, this may be difficult to tease out. Studies in less religious parts of the world, however, may shed light on this question. For example, Hintikka and colleagues in the Department of Psychiatry of Kuopio University Hospital in Kuopio, Finland, examined the effect that social support had in mediating the relationship between religious attendance and low levels of depression.[50] Their sample consisted of 1,179 patients receiving community mental health services. Only 20% of women and 11% of men attended religious services regularly. Using logistic regression, they found an inverse relationship between depression and regular religious attendance in females, but not in males. Increased social support among those who attended religious services regularly did not account for the negative association between attendance and depression in women. Investigators concluded that while religious attendance may be important in preventing depression in Finish women receiving mental health services, increased social support was not the reason. Although social support may be important, the effects of religious attendance likely involve psychological factors as well (optimism, hope, meaning and purpose, better health behaviors).

Thus, recent cross-sectional studies in young and middle-aged adults report an inverse correlation between religious involvement and depressive symptoms, similar to that reported in earlier research. Questions of causality remain, however, and the effects appear weaker among those suffering from severe psychological trauma secondary to loss of a child.

OLDER ADULTS

Type of stressor

Recent research in older adults suggests, as in teenagers, that the particular type of stress people experience may determine whether religion protects against depression or worsens it. Studying a random sample of 2,537 older adults living in California (average age 65 years, mostly Caucasian),[51] Strawbridge and colleagues found that religious attendance and private religious activity were associated with fewer depressive symptoms among persons experiencing health-related or financial stressors. However, for those experiencing family stressors or problems with children, increased religiousness was associated with more depressive symptoms. Investigators explained the findings as follows. When people experience stressors that conflict with expectations that they have of themselves (based on religious beliefs), then this may foster the development of depression. Religious beliefs may be more helpful in coping with problems originating outside the individual, such as physical illness or financial stressors, than with problems due to personal failures or relationship struggles. In other words, because religion emphasizes the importance of harmonious family relationships, religious people who are having difficulties in this area may be more upset by them. Although the findings make sense, causal inferences should be made carefully since this was a cross-sectional study.

Similar findings, however, were reported by Ken Branco, who examined the effects of religiosity on depression in response to health, non-family, and family relationship stressors.[52] His sample consisted of 1,449 nursing home patients (mean age 83 years) from 10 different states. Evidence that religiosity prevented the development of distress was found in white men only. Prior church attendance moderated the effects of nonfamily relationship stressors in white women only. Among blacks, religiosity moderated the effects of both health stressors and nonfamily relationship stressors (but not family stressors). Among whites, in fact, religiosity appeared to exacerbate the effects of family conflict on depression, as Strawbridge had found in his largely white sample. This study suggests that in addition to type of stressor, both gender and ethnic background may need to be taken into account.

European studies

Does the relationship with depression depend on the part of the world where such studies are done? A recent investigation in highly secular Western Europe suggests that it does not (confirming earlier reports[53]). Braam and colleagues examined the relationship between religious activity and depression in older Europeans as part of the EURODEP study.[54] First, associations were studied between church attendance, religious denomination, and depression in six EURODEP study centers located in five countries and involving a sample of 8,398 persons. Second, the relationship between "religious climate" and depressive symptoms was determined based on data from the European Values Survey administered to 17,739 persons from 11 European countries. Investigators found a lower prevalence of depressive symptoms among regular church attenders, an effect that was most evident among Roman Catholics. In addition, fewer depressive symptoms were found among older women in countries with high rates of regular church attendance (generally, Roman Catholic countries). Levels of depressive symptoms were significantly higher among older men living in Protestant countries. Researchers concluded that religious practices were associated with less depression in elderly Europeans and may help to facilitate coping with negative stressors in later life.

Dying patients

Although many studies find an inverse relationship between religiousness and depression in persons with serious physical health problems, there are exceptions. In a study of 162 terminally ill patients with a life expectancy of less than 6 months, investigators examined the relationship between spirituality, religiosity, and observer-rated depressive symptoms.[55] Of the 162 patients, 78 were dying with AIDS and the remainder with cancer. The FACIT-Sp scale measured spirituality in these patients (using a meaning/peace and faith subscales). After controlling for other relevant variables, patients who scored high on the meaning/peace subscale (not surprisingly) were less likely to experience depressive symptoms. The faith subscale, however, was unrelated to depression and a 2-item religiosity index (self-rated religiousness and religious attendance) was positively related to depression. Thus, those persons who scored higher on religiosity were more likely to be depressed.

This finding, however, may have resulted from a statistical artifact. In the uncontrolled analysis, religiosity was unrelated to depression; only after controlling for meaning, peace, spiritual faith, and social support did the positive relationship between depressive symptoms and religiosity emerge. Thus, it is likely that the "effective ingredients" of religion had already been explained away by these other variables, leaving perhaps only the negative aspects. Negative aspects may have involved religious turmoil that led to greater distress in persons who were more religious, particularly those dying with AIDS.[56] Studies in patients with HIV/AIDS, however, have not typically found a positive relationship between religiousness and depression. Instead, religiousness has usually predicted fewer depressive symptoms, greater mastery, higher self-esteem, better quality of life, and more satisfying adjustment to the illness.[57] While important, a single study with an unusual finding must be interpreted in light of what other investigators have found.

Relationship with God

Rather than religion per se, it may be the type of relationship one has with God (particularly if medically ill) that influences whether religion leads to or protects from depression. Levin examined the association between a "loving relationship with God" and depressive symptoms in a sample of 205 medical outpatients.[58] An 8-item scale was used to measure the extent to which patients felt they loved God and were loved by God. After controlling for measures of religious involvement, social resources, psychological resources, physical health status, social and demographic variables, he found a statistically significant inverse correlation between a loving relationship with God and feelings of depression. Levin concluded, "One's relationship with God thus may represent an important personal resource for mitigating the emotional consequences of poor health and other deleterious life circumstances, as well as a marker for successful religious coping" (379).

In summary, the majority of both earlier and more recent studies in children and adolescents, young and middle-aged adults, and the elderly document a role for religion in protecting against depression. Not all studies report this finding, however, and it may only be true for certain kinds of religiosity, for certain kinds of stressors, and for certain kinds of people.

SUICIDE

The idea that religion protects against depression is further supported by research on suicide, the ultimate adverse consequence of severe depression. Research indicates that persons with strong religious beliefs, and especially those who are involved in a supportive religious community, consistently have more negative attitudes toward suicide, fewer suicidal thoughts, and are at lower risk for committing suicide. Of 68 studies that examined the relationship between suicide and religiousness prior to the year 2000, 57 found lower rates of suicide or more negative attitudes toward suicide among those who were more religious. This is true even when religiousness was assessed as crudely as national rates of religious book production. Countries that publish and sell the most religious books (Ireland, Italy, etc.) consistently have the lowest national suicide rates.[59] This may partly result from the culture's effect on suicide reporting (i.e., in religious countries, people may be more reluctant to report suicide as the cause of death because it is frowned on by society), although it is doubtful that this is the entire explanation. Muslim, Christian, and Jewish religious traditions (in that order) are particularly strong in condemning suicide as a response to personal problems or suffering,[60] whereas Buddhist, Tao, and Hindu traditions, while opposed to suicide, are not as strongly so.[61] More recent studies confirm the protection that religion may levy against suicide.

Young persons

Studying a community sample of 1,098 African American and white adolescents, Greening and Stoppelbein asked subjects to rate the likelihood that they would die by suicide.[62] They also assessed levels of depression, hopelessness, intrinsic and extrinsic religiosity, orthodoxy, social support, and style of causal attribution. After controlling for other predictors, religious orthodoxy—defined as a commitment to core beliefs—was the single strongest predictor of negative attitudes toward suicide. In addition, the adolescents' degree of orthodoxy moderated the effect that depression had on perceived suicide risk. The authors concluded, "Commitment to core, life-saving beliefs may help explain the religion-suicide link for adolescents."

Older persons

Religion also "works" at the other end of the age spectrum in helping to prevent suicide. In a study conducted by investigators at Johns Hopkins, the University of Pennsylvania, and the National Institute of Mental Health, a sample of 835 African American older adults (average age 73 years) from six urban public housing developments were assessed for active and passive suicidal ideation.[63] Characteristics of subjects with suicidal ideation included elevated anxiety, social dysfunction, somatic symptoms, low social support, absence of a confidante, older age, lower education, more depressive symptoms, and poorer cognitive functioning. However, multivariate analyses demonstrated that only two variables uniquely predicted suicidal ideation: depressive symptoms and low religiosity were associated with passive suicidal ideation, and only low life satisfaction and low religiosity were predictive of active suicidal ideation. Religiosity in this study was measured using a single question: "Are religious or spiritual beliefs a source of support and comfort?"

Dying persons

Finally, in a study recently published in one of the world's most prestigious medical journals, *The Lancet*, Colleen McClain and colleagues at Fordham University and Sloan Kettering Cancer Center in New York City assessed the relationship between spiritual well-being, depression, and desire for death in a sample of 160 terminally ill cancer patients with less than 3 months to live.[64] An observer-rated depression scale, a hopelessness scale, and a scale measuring attitudes toward a hastened death were administered, along with the FACIT-Sp spiritual well-being (SWB) scale. Assessment of suicidal ideation was based on a single item that measured recurrent thoughts of death or suicide (rated from "absent" to "high risk for suicide requiring suicide precautions"). Investigators found large, significant negative correlations between SWB and desire for hastened death, hopelessness, and suicidal thoughts. When other relevant characteristics were controlled in the analysis, SWB was the strongest predictor of each of the three outcomes above (stronger even than depression scores), and there was a strong inverse relationship between SWB and depression. Although depression was strongly correlated with desire for a hastened death in participants with low SWB, depression was not correlated at all with desire for death in those with high SWB. The strongest effect was seen for the peace and meaning subscale of the FACIT-Sp, although the religious faith subscale was also inversely related to hopelessness. Investigators concluded that spiritual well-being may provide substantial protection against end-of-life despair in dying patients.

Eating Disorders

Theoretical reasons exist why eating disorders ought to be *more common* among those who are devoutly religious. Sarah Huline-Dikens discusses this in terms of concepts of asceticism, ethical codes of sacrifice, loyalty, sexual denial, original sin, and self-punishment as understood in the Judeo-Christian tradition.[65] She argues that there are many connections between the religious ascetic and the anorexic. Similarly, Griffin and Berry reviewed historically the concept of holy anorexia and analyzed the pictorial and language content of advertisements displayed in the media and on the Internet.[66] They concluded that religious messages identifying eating with guilt or reward could lead to "atypical" eating disorders in certain vulnerable religious persons. The evidence from systematic research, however, does *not* support these speculations.

In one of the few objective studies of this relationship, Larry Forthun and colleagues at Penn State University examined associations between intrinsic religiousness, family risk of eating disorder, and disordered eating in a sample of 876 college women between the ages of 18 and 29.[67] They found that when intrinsic religiousness was higher, there was no relationship between family risk and disordered eating. At low levels of intrinsic religiousness, however, family risk and disordered eating were significantly and positively correlated. The opposite pattern was true for extrinsic religiousness. Investigators concluded that intrinsic religiousness served to protect women against developing an eating disorder even in family situations where the risk was high.

Similarly, Faune Taylor Smith and colleagues at the Center for Change (Orem, Utah) and Brigham Young University investigated the effects of religious orientation, religious affiliation, and spiritual well-being on treatment outcome in 251 patients ages 12 to 56 years with eating disorders (anorexia nervosa, bulimia nervosa, or other eating disorder).[68] Analyses revealed that neither intrinsic religiousness nor religious affiliation improved or worsened treatment outcomes. However, improvements in spiritual well-being during treatment were significantly correlated with positive gains in eating attitudes, body shape concerns, and other indicators of better psychological and social functioning.

Personality Disorder

The relationships between personality disorder and religiosity are complex. As noted in the last chapter, personality or temperament can affect the likelihood of becoming religious, reflecting genetic or hereditary influences. Religious conversion, however, can also lead to dramatic and lasting personality change.

Although personality disorders have been considered relatively resistant to change, religious experience may be one of the few factors powerful enough to initiate and sustain such change. Consider the alcoholic, drug addict, delinquent, or prodigal son who "finds God" and is "born again." Such persons are known to change their lifestyles and social relationships because of newly found religious beliefs that are no longer compatible with previous ways of living. In many of these cases, religion may not change personality completely, but rather moderate or suppress certain traits or characteristics and promote the development of others. This may be especially true for persons with severe personality disorder like antisocial or borderline personality disorders, for which psychological treatments have been notoriously ineffective. Frequently underestimated, religious conversion can bring power for change that rivals that brought about by traditional mental health treatments.

Consider what Harvard psychiatrist George Vaillant wrote in the *Archives of General Psychiatry* as he describes the role that religious organizations can play in helping to transform the lives of those with personality disorder:

Finally, one-to-one therapeutic relationships are rarely adequate to change the sociopath. A therapist even five times a week—is not enough to satisfy an orphan. At the start of the recovery process, only the church, self-help residential treatment, and addicting drugs provide relief for a sociopath's pain; they all work 24 hours a day. . . . Only group membership or caring for others, or both, can eventually provide adults with parenting that they never received. . . . The psychopath needs to absorb more of other people than one person, no matter how loving, can ever provide. The sociopath needs to find groups to which they can belong with pride.[69]

ANTISOCIAL BEHAVIORS

The vast majority of studies prior to the year 2000 found that antisocial activities such as delinquency and crime were much less common among the religious. At least 36 studies examined this relationship, most of them conducted among young people.[70] Nearly 80% (28 of 36) found significantly lower rates of delinquency or crime among persons who were more religious. In one of the best and most definitive reports, sociologist Rodney Stark analyzed data from a national random sample of 11,995 high school seniors.[71] He found that those who attended religious services regularly were significantly less likely to get into trouble with the law. Correlations were robust in all areas of the country except the Pacific Northwest. Wallace and Forman reported similar findings in their analysis of data from a national random sample of 5,000 high school students. This study was part of the Monitoring the Future Project conducted by the University of Michigan. Importance of religion was inversely related to carrying a weapon to school, interpersonal violence, and driving while drinking.[72] Frequency of religious attendance was also related to fewer intentional and unintentional injury behaviors.

Sociologist Byron Johnson has emerged as one of the leading investigators in the area of religion, delinquency, and crime. A recent report from the Center for Research on Religion and Urban Civil Society (CRRUCS) described results from a study of non-drug crimes, using drugs, and dealing drugs in 2,300 black males ages 16 to 24 living in Boston, Chicago, and Philadelphia.[73] The probability of committing a non-drug crime decreased from 31% for church nonattenders to 19% for those who attended church more than once a week (frequent attenders); the probability of using drugs decreased from 48% for nonattenders to 26% for frequent attenders; and the probability of drug dealing fell from 33% for nonattenders to 14% for frequent attenders. This study confirmed earlier findings suggesting that religiosity exerted a direct effect on delinquency that could not be explained by secular pathways such as social control or socialization.[74]

In another recent CRRUCS report, Johnson examined the effects on recidivism (return to prison for crimes after release from prison) for inmates who attended a faith-based rehabilitation program.[75] The program involved Bible teaching, life-skills education, and group accountability. A total of 177 prisoners released from the Texas state prison system were involved in this 2-year prospective study. The recidivism rate for those in the program was compared to that of 1,754 inmate controls matched to study prisoners by race, age, offense type, and a risk factor score for reincarceration. Of the 177 prisoners, 75 completed all phases of the program (called graduates), 51 were paroled early, 24 voluntarily quit the program, and 27 were removed for disciplinary reasons or at the request of the staff. Johnson found that 17.3% of the 75 program graduates were arrested during the 2-year post-release period, compared to 35% of the matched control group. Only 8% of program graduates were re-incarcerated, compared to 20% of matched controls. Although this study has been criticized[76] and needs replication, these results support the introduction of faith-based rehabilitation programs into prisons to help reduce the high recidivism rates among the growing population of U.S. prison inmates, 15% of whom have chronic mental illness.[77]

Substance Abuse

This topic has been dealt with thoroughly in a white paper prepared for the Center for Substance Abuse Treatment (CSAT), which documented a huge literature base on religion and substance abuse.[78] Nearly 140 studies have examined the religion-substance abuse relationship, 90% of which find less substance abuse among the more religious. Since that report, however, the National Center on Addiction and Substance Abuse (CASA) at Columbia University released a 52-page, two-year study entitled, "So Help Me God: Substance Abuse, Religion and Spirituality."[79] The study found that adults and teens who indicated religion was very important in their lives or who attended religious services weekly or more were far less likely to smoke, drink, or use illegal drugs. In addition, they reported that individuals who both received professional treatment and attended spirituality-based support programs (such as Alcoholics Anonymous or Narcotics Anonymous) were far more likely to remain sober than if they received professional treatment alone. These results were based on analysis of data from three major national surveys: the 1998 National Household Survey, CASA's National Survey of American Attitudes on Substance Abuse, and the General Social Survey.

More specifically, the CASA study found that adults who did not consider religion very important were at least 50% more likely to use alcohol and cigarettes, three times more likely to binge drink, four times more likely to use illicit drugs other than marijuana, and at least six times more likely to use marijuana, compared to adults who strongly believed that religion is important. Compared to those who attended religious services at least weekly, adults who never attended religious services were almost twice as likely to drink, three times more likely to smoke, five times more likely to abuse illicit drugs other than marijuana, seven times more likely to binge drink, and almost eight times more likely to use marijuana.

With regard to teens, those who did not consider religious beliefs important were almost three times more likely to drink, binge drink, or smoke, four times more likely to use marijuana, and seven times more likely to use illicit drugs, compared with teens who strongly believed that religion is important. Compared to teens who attended religious services at least weekly, those who never attended services were twice as likely to drink, more than twice as likely to smoke, more than three times as likely to use marijuana or binge drink, and four times more likely to use illicit drugs. Director of the study was Joseph A. Califano Jr., former U.S. Secretary of Health, Education and Welfare in the Clinton administration. These findings accurately reflect those of 86 studies conducted prior to the year 2000 that examined the religion-alcohol relationship, 76 of which reported significantly lower alcohol use and abuse among those who were more religious (including 8 of 9 prospective studies).[80] This was also true for the 52 studies that examined the relationship between religiousness and illicit drug use and abuse, 48 of which found significantly less drug use among the more religious.[81]

Recent research both in the United States[82] and Europe[83] since the year 2000 confirms these findings. I focus in this section on the European studies. A recent study that analyzed data from a random sample of 1,526 adults in Poland (Polish General Social Survey) found that in both men and women, frequency of religious attendance and prayer predicted less smoking and lower rates of excessive drinking.[84] Likewise, Winter and colleagues from the Department of Public Health at the University of Helsinki examined factors affecting adolescent alcohol use in rural and urban regions of Finland in a sample of 1,904 adolescents and 989 mothers.[85] They found that alcohol use was lowest in rural areas where religiousness was highest. There was also a correlation between religiousness and alcohol use in urban regions, although it was much weaker than in rural areas. Overall, highly religious adolescents were 47% less likely to use alcohol. Investigators also found that high religiousness among mothers was more protective against adolescent alcohol use in rural regions than in urban areas. Among adolescents whose mothers were low on religiousness, 14% abstained from alcohol use; among those whose mothers were highly religious, 24% in urban regions and 53% in rural regions did not drink.

Recent work has focused on identifying aspects of Christian practice in England that are most effective in preventing substance abuse. Hope and Cook from the University of Kent at Canterbury compared the following four statements as predictors of never having smoked, drunk alcohol, or tried drugs: "usually go to church on Sunday," "have given my life to Jesus," "read the Bible every week," and "pray most days."[86] The sample consisted of 7,661 church-affiliated persons aged 12 to 30 years living in England. Analyses were stratified by age (12 to 16 years and 17 to 30 years). All four statements were associated with a lower likelihood of substance abuse. However, the strength of the association varied depending on age group. Church attendance was the primary factor that predicted less substance abuse in adolescents ages 12 to 16. For older subjects ages 17 to 30, however, "have given my life to Jesus" and "read the Bible every week" were more predictive of abstinence. The authors concluded that socialization through involvement in a church among young teenagers protects them against substance use, whereas when youth grow older, the internalization of Christian commitment becomes more important as a protective mechanism.

Alcohol use and depression are frequently linked.[87] There is evidence that the level of religious involvement can influence that relationship. Musick and colleagues at Duke University analyzed data from a 3-year prospective study of 1,897 Baptists aged 65 or older living in central North Carolina.[88] Religious attendance was inversely correlated with alcohol use, as expected, and this effect was stronger in rural than in urban areas (as reported in other studies). Researchers hypothesized that persons living in rural areas were more likely than those living in urban areas to be surrounded by friends and families from the same religion and would therefore be more likely to conform to the norms of that group.

Investigators then assessed the use of alcohol and depressive symptoms at different levels of religious activity, thinking that the effects of alcohol use on depression would be strongest among respondents who attended religious services more frequently (given a stronger internal conflict about alcohol use). This hypothesis, however, was not supported. Instead, they found a stronger relationship between alcohol use and depression among rural Baptists who attended religious services *less frequently*. In fact, rural Baptists who used alcohol and did not attend church regularly had higher levels of depressive symptoms than any other urban or rural group. This unexpected finding, investigators explained, may have resulted from the fact that drinking alcohol exacerbated the guilt and stigma associated with lower levels of religious attendance. An alternative explanation is that older rural Baptists using alcohol may not have had the church-related social support necessary to buffer the adverse effects of drinking on their mood. A final possibility is that depressed rural Baptists who start drinking may stop going to church because they feel too guilty to go (because of their drinking).

In summary, although there is still some question about how religion impacts substance abuse and in what settings, active religious involvement appears to be a powerful deterrent to drug and alcohol use and abuse in both the young and the old, in both men and women, in both the United States and Europe (and no doubt, in Arab countries as well).

Summary

It is not true that religious beliefs and involvement never cause mental health problems or adversely affect the course of a psychiatric disorder. Despite this, however, greater religiousness appears to be associated with a lower prevalence of mental disorder and fewer self-destructive behaviors, consistent with the findings reported for positive emotions in chapter 3. Religious beliefs and practices are inversely associated with anxiety and depression in the majority of cross-sectional studies, usually predict less depression and faster recovery from depression in prospective studies, and, when examined in randomized clinical trials, religious interventions cause a faster reduction in clinical symptoms than secular therapies alone or no treatment. This is also true, in general, for negative character and personality traits, antisocial activities that involve crime or delinquency, and use of drugs or alcohol.

Thus, while not all studies report mental health benefits for religion, the vast majority of both qualitative and quantitative studies do. As a result, it is no longer possible to argue that religious involvement is usually neurotic, harmful, or incompatible with mental health, as once claimed. Furthermore, clinicians should view patients' religious beliefs as not only having negative effects on the psyche, but also as a resource, especially when dealing with situational life stressors, health problems, severe loss, or trauma. In the next chapter, we will find out if this is also true for those who grapple with severe and persistent mental illness.

CHAPTER 5

RELIGION AND SEVERE, PERSISTENT MENTAL ILLNESS

Although the use of religion to help cope with stress is well established, less is known about how religious belief and activity are related to severe, persistent mental illness (i.e., schizophrenia, recurrent mania, psychosis, or severe personality disorder). For centuries, it was thought that a person with severe mental illness was possessed by demons and should be treated by expelling the demons through a process called *exorcism*. This was/is true for almost every major religious group around the world.[1] Mental health professionals have been concerned that religious beliefs and practices, and religious interventions in particular, may worsen psychosis in patients with schizophrenia or other psychotic disorders, especially those already having difficulty separating fantasy from reality. What, then, is the relationship between religious beliefs, activity, and severe mental illness?

Challenges of Mental Illness

Living day in and day out with recurrent, severe mental illness is not easy. It is often a life filled with fear, paranoia, uncertainty, and perhaps more than anything else, loneliness. Other than family members, who wants to associate with a person with severe and persistent mental illness? Emotions and behavior may be unpredictable. Taunted by strange hallucinations, unable to distinguish reality from fantasy, cast into a pit of deep despair or transported to the heights of manic elation, they may for long periods of time be unable to communicate with others. This makes the establishment and maintenance of relationships very difficult. Drugs or alcohol may lure them with the false promise of relief, yet ease the pain only momentarily and make them even less attractive as social partners. Unable to depend on the mentally ill persons' mood or cognitive state, employers often shun them. Unable to hold down a job, they often struggle with financial problems and sometimes even have difficulty finding a safe and warm place to sleep at night. The treatments are not easy either. Required medications have side effects that drain energy, cause fatigue and sluggishness during waking hours, disrupt sexual function, cause weight gain or loss of hair, and may interfere with driving safety. The bottom line: persons with long-term mental illness have a lot to cope with. Yes, and often they turn to religion.

Religious Coping

Religious coping is common among those with severe mental illness in religious areas of the world. In a small study of 28 patients with chronic mental disorders (mostly schizophrenia), Karen Lindgren and colleagues from the University of Maryland found that 47% indicated that spirituality/religion had helped "a great deal," 57% prayed every day, and 76% thought about God or spiritual/religious matters on a daily basis.[2] More recently, psychologist Leslie Tepper and colleagues at UCLA and Fuller Theological Seminary surveyed 406 patients with persistent mental illness at a Los Angeles County mental health facility.[3] More than 80% of patients indicated they used religion to help them to cope. In fact, the majority of patients spent as much as half of their total coping time in religious practices, with the most common practice being prayer. Investigators concluded that religious beliefs and activities are particularly important for those experiencing more severe mental symptoms, and that religion serves as a "pervasive and potentially effective method of coping for persons with mental illness, thus warranting its integration into psychiatric and psychological practice" (660).

Studies in other areas of the United States support these findings. William Sullivan at Southwest Missouri State University in Springfield collected data from 40 psychiatric patients, discussing various sources of strength.[4] Nearly half of the patients he interviewed (48%) indicated that spiritual beliefs and practices were essential to coping with their illness. In another study, Ziatka Russinova and colleagues at the Center for Psychiatric Rehabilitation at Boston University conducted an Internet survey of adults with severe mental illness who used alternative health care practices (nutritional supplements, chiropractic, herbs, guided imagery, yoga, massage, religious/spiritual activities).[5] A total of 157 individuals responded: 40 persons with schizophrenia, 70 with bipolar disorder, and 39 with major depression. For persons with schizophrenia and major depression, the most common alternative health practice they reported benefit from was religious/spiritual activity (57.5% and 56.4%, respectively). For persons with bipolar disorder, only "meditation" surpassed religious/spiritual activity in frequency of use (54.3% vs. 41.4%).

Although such findings underscore the importance that religion plays in coping with mental illness, not all studies are positive—particularly with regard to help from the faith community. For example, in a small qualitative study conducted in Sioux Center, Iowa, investigators from Dordt College did not find that the faith community played much of a role in the coping of 17 people with serious mental illness.[6] The majority of participants indicated that although their personal religious beliefs were vital in providing a sense of meaning and hope in the face of their illness, they felt estranged from their religious communities (as some of the stories in chapter 1 also illustrate).

The way religion is used to cope may also determine whether it has a positive or negative effect on adjustment to severe mental illness. Natalia Yangarber-Hicks at the University of Cincinnati examined relationships between religious coping styles, empowerment, level of adaptive functioning, and recovery activities in persons with severe and persistent mental illness.[7] She discovered that the "collaborative/deferring" approach to religious coping (i.e., seeking control through a partnership with God in problem solving and deferring to God in certain matters) predicted higher quality of life and greater involvement in recovery-enhancing activities. A self-directing coping style (i.e., coping without God's help) and a pleading style (i.e., pleading to God for direct intercession), however, were associated with more negative psychosocial outcomes.

Whether or not persons turn to religion for help coping with mental illness may depend on the part of the world they live in and their ethnic or religious background. For example, Wahass and colleagues examined ways of coping with auditory hallucinations by Western and non-Western patients with schizophrenia.[8] The sample included 33 persons from Great Britain and 37 from Saudi Arabia. Researchers found that Saudi patients were more likely than British patients to use religion to cope with hallucinations (43% vs. 3%, respectively). Saudi patients commonly used prayer, reading the Qur'an/Bible, or listening to religious cassettes to help them cope. British patients, on the other hand, were more likely to use distraction or other approaches.

The religiousness of an area of the world, however, does not always affect the likelihood that those with mental illness will use religion to cope. For example, recent surveys of the Australian population indicate that only 60% consistently believe in God (vs. 95% in the United States) and 25% attend church monthly or more often (vs. 60% in the United States).[9] However, a study of 79 psychiatric patients at Broken Hill Base Hospital in New South Wales found that 79% rated spirituality as very important, 82% thought their therapist should be aware of their spiritual beliefs and needs, and 67% indicated that their spirituality helped them to cope with psychological pain.[10]

Type of psychiatric disorder may also influence the likelihood of religious or spiritual coping. Reger and Rogers examined the differences in religious coping between 356 persons with persistent mental illness, comparing individuals with schizophrenia, schizoaffective, bipolar, and depressive disorders.[11] They discovered that patients with chronic schizophrenia or schizoaffective disorder were more likely to find religion helpful in coping compared to those diagnosed with depressive disorders. Because this is one of the few reports comparing religious coping across different disorders, future studies are needed to replicate these findings.

CAUSE OR COINCIDENCE

Again, we struggle with the chicken or egg phenomenon that has come up over and over again in this book. Is religion more common in persons with severe mental illnesses because it is used to cope with symptoms? Is it more common because religion somehow causes or contributes to the development of severe mental disorder (due to parental influences during childhood,[12] religious strains during adulthood, or perhaps, as some believe, to demonic possession)? Or is religion's presence in such disorders simply a coincidence, given the religious nature of the society or culture? Let us explore these questions in light of what is known about possession and exorcism, religious conversion, religious delusions, and associations between religiousness and psychotic symptoms or psychotic disorders.

Demonic Possession and Exorcism

There was a widespread belief in Europe during the fifteenth through seventeenth centuries (brought to the New England colonies) that demons or evil spirits were the cause of symptoms in some persons with mental illness. This belief has been common within many different cultures around the world at different times throughout most of recorded history. However, in Europe and later in the American colonies, the belief in demonic possession became so strong that violent actions were taken to rid the population of such persons, with many burned at the stake as witches or sorcerers (see chapter 2).

Even today many people in underdeveloped countries (and developed ones, too) persist with such beliefs (although seldom persecute the mentally ill as they did during the late Middle Ages). This is particularly true in countries where the causes and treatments for mental illness are not well understood, and is reflected perhaps best in the beliefs of family members. For example, Vlachos and colleagues surveyed 80 mothers of psychotic patients from southwestern Greece, asking them what they thought caused the psychosis in their children. Researchers found that 85% of mothers reported magico-religious beliefs concerning the cause.[13] Interestingly, the frequency of such beliefs did not depend on whether the family was religious or not. The likelihood of such magico-religious beliefs increased as education level decreased.

Parmanand Kulhara and colleagues from the Department of Psychiatry at the Postgraduate Institute of Medical Education and Research in Chandigarh, India, report similar findings.[14] They examined the magico-religious beliefs that family caregivers held concerning the causes of illness in 40 patients with schizophrenia in northern India. The effects of these beliefs on treatment-seeking behavior were also explored. Beliefs were assessed using a Supernatural Attitude Questionnaire. Results indicated that the majority of patients had sought treatment related to magico-religious beliefs, particularly when relatives thought that psychotic symptoms were due to spiritual factors (74% of this group sought such treatments). Investigators concluded that belief in supernatural influences is common in patients' relatives and treatment is often based upon such beliefs.

Reports on beliefs that attribute psychosis to supernatural causes have apparently fallen off in recent years, at least in some areas. In a study of relatives of 254 patients with chronic schizophrenia conducted by the Schizophrenia Research Foundation in India, family members were given a list of possible causes of the illness.[15] Despite their general lack of education about schizophrenia, they only rarely indicated that demons, spirits, or evil forces were the primary causes for the illness.

Al-Faraj and Al-Ansari, working at the Manama Psychiatric Hospital in the Middle Eastern country of Bahrain, asked 50 family caregivers of schizophrenic inpatients and 50 caregivers of nonpsychotic inpatients about the nature and cause of mental disorder in their loved ones.[16] Only 20% of caregivers believed that patients were suffering from a specific mental disorder and only 8% of the caregivers of psychotic patients thought they had psychosis. The cause of the condition was most often attributed to psychosocial factors. However, nearly 60% of patients had consulted religious or traditional healers, even though only 5% of family caregivers would admit that they thought the cause was religious or spiritual.

Although beliefs concerning spiritual factors in mental illness may be less common than in earlier times, they nevertheless persist in some pockets of the population—even in developed countries. For example, research indicates that a substantial number of psychiatric patients in the United States attribute their illness to religious factors. In a survey of 52 patients on the psychiatry service at the University of Minnesota hospital in Minneapolis, William Sheehan and Jerome Kroll reported that 23% of patients thought their illness resulted from sinful acts, 10% thought they were in the hospital because they had sinned, and 19% thought they needed penance before they could improve.[17] Diagnosis (schizophrenia vs. depression) was unrelated to thoughts about religion being the cause of illness.

Many fundamentalist religious groups around the world today (including the United States) continue to consider exorcism a valid method of treating a mentally ill person to rid them of their demons, although this is becoming less common. Even some mental health professionals, however, report a high prevalence of "possession states" among patients with schizophrenia.[18] If demonic possession is responsible for the development of chronic mental illnesses such as schizophrenia, then exorcism should be an effective treatment. Is there any evidence of this? The answer is no.

No systematic research shows that exorcism is a successful treatment for patients with schizophrenia or any other severe and persistent mental illness. Although some patients may exhibit less dramatic and violent manifestations of their illness following exorcism, they continue to remain schizophrenic and require biological treatments for their illness.[19] William P. Wilson, professor emeritus of psychiatry at Duke University and former head of biological psychiatry at that institution, acknowledges that while possession states may occur, the possessed person does not have the blunting of affect, disturbances of thought, or ambivalence that typifies the condition of schizophrenia.[20] Furthermore, possession states are thought to be associated with evil, which seldom characterizes the person with schizophrenia.[21] By evil, I mean the willful desire to hurt or destroy another person in the absence of revenge, fear, or other provoking cause.

Mental health professionals disagree on the role that exorcism plays in the treatment of other severe mental illnesses. Dennis Bull at Dallas Theological Seminary discusses therapeutic exorcism for dissociative identity disorder (multiple personality disorder).[22] Approaching the issue from the patient's view that he or she is possessed by demons, Bull describes how patients can be empowered to use their own spirituality to expel these perceived entities and thereby help to resolve the illness. He also reviews the history of exorcism and the literature that deals with both the negative and positive aspects of the practice. Bull concludes that positive outcomes can result in some cases if the therapist avoids coercive methods, utilizes knowledge about the psychodynamics of dissociative disorder, and enters into the patient's worldview. Illustrative cases are presented and both legal and ethical concerns are discussed.

Elizabeth Bowman from the Department of Psychiatry at Indiana University, however, argues against exorcism as a treatment for this condition.[23] Referring specifically to persons with severe dissociative disorders, Bowman discusses the adverse psychological consequences of mistaking "alter" personalities for demons and subjecting such persons to exorcism.

She also discusses the positive and negative aspects of membership in a conservative religious group, in light of the fact that most persons with dissociative disorders are female and have a history of child abuse. The major positives of belonging to a "healthy" conservative religion are establishing a connection with a benevolent, powerful God, developing healthy relationships with others in the congregation, having a reliable source of social support, helping with behavioral control, deterring suicide, enhancing self-esteem as a child of God, fostering hope, and providing meaning and purpose for suffering. The major negatives of membership in a conservative religion might include the institutionalization of male dominance, the confusion of human male images with God, the cultural value placed on silent, submissive women, the absence of a nurturing female God image, the discouragement of anger over abuse, and the encouragement of premature forgiveness.

In modern psychiatry today, then, demonic possession is not thought to play a significant role in any severe and persistent psychiatric disorder, nor is exorcism recommended as a form of treatment. Given the lack of research on such phenomena, however, this conclusion—as reasonable as it may seem—remains tentative until more systematic investigations are done. In any case, religious and spiritual beliefs of patients and family members clearly influence their understanding of mental disorder and the treatments they seek for themselves and loved ones.

Religious Conversion

Although demons are unlikely to be a major cause of severe mental illness, intense religious experiences may play a role in precipitating an episode of such illness. There is some evidence that the emotional energy released during sudden religious conversion may destabilize a person who is vulnerable to psychiatric illness, or may even precipitate acute psychosis in normal persons.[24] John of God (patron saint of psychiatric nurses) and Anton Boisen (founder of Clinical Pastoral Education) are examples of persons whose intense religious experiences were followed by a psychotic breakdown and acute hospitalization (see chapter 1). In a review of this topic, Wootton and Allen report that the *speed* at which religious conversion occurs may influence its impact on mental health.[25] Conversion experiences may be gradual and slow, or sudden and dramatic. When religious conversion is sudden, there is a greater likelihood that it may be associated with psychotic decompensation. This is contrasted with religious conversion that occurs more gradually, "in the course of real maturing . . . after a reasoned, thoughtful search," says Georgetown University psychoanalyst Leon Salzman.[26] William James also wrote that sudden conversion is more likely to occur in the "sick soul" than in the "healthy minded,"[27] suggesting that mental illness itself may predispose to sudden religious conversion—rather than vice versa.

Wootton and Allen's review was based on the expert opinions of mental health professionals and isolated case reports. In one of the first systematic studies of religious conversion and mental illness, Wilson and colleagues compared the religious histories of 72 people with schizophrenia from the inpatient services at two psychiatric hospitals in North Carolina with those of 109 persons from the same area without mental health problems.[28] Researchers found that people with schizophrenia were actually *less* likely than people without it to have religious conversion experiences, especially before their twenty-first birthday when initial psychotic breaks tend to occur. Religious conversion can mark a time of personality integration and improvement in mental health, including increased ability to communicate with others, decreased use of alcohol, and decreased symptoms of depression, anxiety, confusion, and anger, as Wilson demonstrated in another study of 63 persons with conversion experiences.[29] Furthermore, there is evidence from a study of 330 medically ill persons aged 70 or older that religious conversion can have a profound effect on the way that persons deal with crisis later on in life and their ability to successfully overcome those crises.[30]

Although religious conversion often occurs in the setting of stress or mental instability, it doesn't have to. In one of the largest studies to date, Max Heirich at the University of Michigan examined the settings in which conversion occurred among 152 recently converted Catholic Pentecostals in Ann Arbor.[31] He compared these converts to 158 controls from similar backgrounds who had not experienced a conversion. When examining the characteristics of converts, he found that life stress and emotional upheaval appeared unusually common in this group. However, when compared to the 158 controls, life stress and emotional problems were virtually the same. The most important factor precipitating conversion was interpersonal influence—discussions with friends, relatives, or religious professionals. Thus, psychological or situational life stress and social influences play important roles in religious conversion.

Several studies have found an increase in religiousness (spending more time in religious places) as a symptom in schizophrenic patients experiencing their first psychotic break. This is especially true in studies of patients from India, where between 22% and 27% of such patients experience increased religiousness.[32] Given the high prevalence and importance of religion in India, however, this is not entirely unexpected, since religion would likely be used to cope with disruptive or strange experiences resulting from a first episode of schizophrenia. Studies have found that increased religiousness is more common in Indian patients with first-time schizophrenic breakdowns than in European white patients.[33] Even in Europe, however, religious delusions are still more common in initial presentations of schizophrenia than are found in patients with other psychiatric disorders. For example, Gutierrez-Lobos and colleagues at the University of Vienna studied 639 first-ever admitted patients presenting with delusions in Austria.[34] They found that religious or metaphysical contents occurred significantly more frequently among patients with schizophrenia than in those with delusions from other disorders. None of these studies examined religious conversion specifically or its relationship to initial psychotic decompensation.

Thus, there is no convincing evidence from systematic studies that religious conversion per se "results in" or causes persistent, lasting mental illness in a person not otherwise predisposed.

Religious Delusions

Religious delusions are not infrequent among persons with severe mental illnesses such as schizophrenia or other chronic and acute psychoses.[35] Religious delusions are particularly important because they have been associated with a greater risk of self-harm and poor outcome. There are numerous dramatic cases that illustrate such negative consequences, some based on Jesus' Sermon on the Mount: "If your right eye causes you to sin, gouge it out and throw it away. It is better for you to lose one part of your body than your whole body to be thrown into hell. And if your right hand causes you to sin, cut it off and throw it away."[36] For example, Erol and Kaptanoglu report a case of a thirty-nine-year-old male with schizophrenia who gouged out both of his eyes, driven by guilty feelings resulting from religious delusions.[37] Other cases include castration[38] and limb amputations during the midst of psychosis.[39] Most recently, a mother in McKinney, Texas, killed her baby daughter by cutting off both her arms, following the biblical passage above.[40] Individual cases, however, provide less information than systematic research that allows results to be generalized.

In 1986, Cothran and Harvey from the University of South Florida assessed the religiousness of consecutively admitted patients (18 with mania and 23 with schizophrenia) to a state psychiatric facility in New York, and compared them to 53 normal controls selected from the general population.[41] Of the patients with psychotic illness, 17 were not delusional, 11 had delusions without religious content, and 13 had delusions with religious content (31.7% of total). Four of 18 patients with mania (22%) and 9 of 23 patients with schizophrenia (39%) had religious delusions. Although patients with religious delusions reported higher religiosity, they were less likely to admit to fundamentalist beliefs and were less involved in organized religion than were non-delusional patients and normal controls. Furthermore, the religiosity of psychotic patients appeared to be of a different nature than that of nonpsychotic patients or normal controls.

In a more recent study, Ronald Siddle and colleagues from the Department of Psychology at North Manchester General Hospital (United Kingdom) investigated the prevalence of religious delusions in a sample of 193 inpatients admitted with schizophrenia.[42] There was no correlation between psychotic symptoms in general (measured using a standardized scale) and self-assessed degree of religiosity. Among all patients studied, 24% had religious delusions. Not surprisingly, those with religious delusions were more likely to describe themselves as religious than patients with other delusions, but the difference wasn't as great as might be expected (80% vs. 64%). Subjects with religious delusions, however, were much sicker: they had more severe symptoms (hallucinations and bizarre delusions, in particular), poorer functioning, and were on more antipsychotic medication than patients with schizophrenia who had other delusions.

When patients were examined longitudinally, however, investigators found evidence that religiosity varied depending on the severity of psychotic symptoms.[43] In a reduced sample of 155 psychotic patients with schizophrenia, they measured religiosity during the time when symptoms were more active and again after treatment. As psychotic symptoms diminished, investigators reported a reduced need for religion in these subjects. This is not surprising, though, since the psychological distress related to psychosis could have caused many patients to initially turn to religion for comfort. As both psychotic symptoms and psychological distress became less severe with ongoing treatment, the need for religion to cope also became less acute.

There is other evidence that the severity of religious delusions may be associated with the general religious activity of patients. Glen Getz and colleagues from the Department of Psychiatry at the University of Cincinnati compared Catholic and Protestant patients with religiously unaffiliated patients.[44] They found that while there was no difference in the severity of religious delusions between the three groups, Protestant patients were more likely to experience religious delusions than either Catholics or nonaffiliated patients. The severity of religious delusions was significantly related to overall frequency of religious activity.

Religious delusions appear to be specific to the patient's religious background and cultural environment. For example, Kam-shing Yip in the Department of Applied Social Studies at Hong Kong Polytechnic University interviewed four adult Chinese patients with schizophrenia.[45] He found that traditional Chinese religious beliefs and superstitions, such as fortune telling, Buddhist gods, Taoist gods, historical heroic gods, and ancestor worship, influenced the content of delusions and hallucinations manifested by these patients.

Thus, religious delusions are common among psychotic patients, particularly those with severe, persistent mental illnesses such as schizophrenia, and may be associated with more severe symptoms and greater religious activity. However, the type of religious activity engaged in is not always the same kind as that practiced by patients without psychosis or persons in the general population.

In practice, clinicians often find it difficult to distinguish between "normal" religious beliefs and religious delusions, especially in patients with schizophrenia or other psychotic disorders. Pierre provides guidelines for mental health professionals to help in this regard.[46] He notes that the field of psychiatry has taken divergent approaches to this problem. Freud, on the one hand, considered all religious beliefs delusional (or illusions, at best), and *DSM-III* and prior versions followed this pattern. *DSM-IV*, on the other hand, has seriously restricted the requirements necessary for the diagnosis of religious delusions, perhaps overly so. In order to distinguish between normal and psychotic religious beliefs using a more middle-of-the-road approach, Pierre says it is necessary to consider several factors. First, since shared beliefs may become normalized, it is important to recognize that entire delusional subcultures can exist and this must be taken into consideration in the evaluation of a patient's beliefs. Second, he notes that either religious or delusional beliefs can result from neurological lesions and therefore a careful neurological workup is required when other clinical indicators are present. Third, he points out that because religious beliefs lie outside of the scientific domain, they can easily be incorrectly labeled as delusional by therapists unfamiliar with the beliefs (necessitating input from religious professionals more familiar with the belief system). Fourth, he encourages clinicians to consider what kind of impact the religious beliefs are having on a person's ability to function. Interference with social and occupational functioning, along with the likely influence of cultural factors, Pierre says, should be the primary method of determining whether or not a religious belief is delusional. To this I will add that clergy or members of the patient's faith community usually do not have a difficult time recognizing religious delusions as such. This is because of their bizarre nature, and because such delusions are also associated with other psychotic symptoms or altered thinking that give away their true nature.

Religiosity and Psychosis

Besides occasional acute psychosis following conversion and religious delusions found in persons with severe mental illness living in religious areas of the world, is there any evidence that religious beliefs actually predispose to the development of persistent mental illness? Several authors writing over twenty years ago noted that religious beliefs were unusually common among persons prior to the onset of schizophrenia.[47] Some recent evidence also suggests that bipolar manic episodes can be induced by religious practices, specifically meditation in the yoga or Zen tradition.[48] These observations, however, are based on either clinical experience or anecdotal case reports, not systematic research. I now examine systematic research conducted in both psychiatric patients and the general population on the relationship between religiosity and the tendency toward psychosis or severe mental illness.

CLINICAL SAMPLES

For reasons not clear, studies carried out in the United Kingdom consistently report a link between religiosity and schizophrenic-type symptoms that is seldom found in other countries. Jan Neeleman and Glyn Lewis at Maudsley Hospital in London compared religious beliefs and attitudes of psychiatric inpatients with those of surgical patients hospitalized on the orthopedic service.[49] Patients with schizophrenia and depression were more likely to report personal religious experiences compared to orthopedic controls (48% and 38% vs. 17%, respectively). Psychiatric patients were also more likely to be religious and report receiving comfort from religion. Investigators did not, however, distinguish healthy religious beliefs and experiences from psychotic delusions.

Joan Feldman and John Rust from the Institute of Psychiatry at the University of London also found a positive relationship between religiosity and schizotypal thinking in 67 patients with schizophrenia (although the relationship was the exact opposite in 140 normal controls).[50] Investigators hypothesized that increased intrusive schizotypal thinking in patients with schizophrenia may have become encapsulated into the rigidly held belief system of religious individuals. They concluded that their results supported a connection between religious experience and factors associated with the onset of schizophrenia.

Both of these studies, however, were cross-sectional in nature. Thus, we do not know whether (1) religiousness prior to psychiatric illness caused persons to experience mental health problems, (2) religiousness affected the expression of mental illness that resulted from other causes, or (3) religion was turned to for comfort after the psychiatric illness began. For that reason, it is important to examine results from longitudinal research (and intervention studies, see chapter 6) to determine whether religion leads to severe mental illness, is coincidental, or is a consequence of it.

In a 1-year prospective study of 128 African American schizophrenic patients consecutively admitted to seven hospitals and mental health centers in the Missouri Division of Mental Health, Chu and Klein from the Nebraska Psychiatric Institute in Omaha interviewed patients on admission, discharge, and a year after discharge (or on readmission if occurring before that time).[51] Patients from urban areas (n=65) were significantly less likely to be re-hospitalized if they said prayers once daily (vs. more often). They were also less likely to be re-hospitalized if their families encouraged them to continue religious worship during their hospital stay. Religious affiliation affected re-hospitalization rates for both urban and rural patients. Fewer re-hospitalizations occurred if the patient's family was Catholic, and more re-hospitalizations occurred if they had no religious affiliation. All findings above were statistically significant.

In one of the largest and methodologically most rigorous of all studies to examine religious influences on the course of schizophrenia,[52] Abraham Verghese and colleagues at the Christian Medical College in Vellore conducted a two-year multi-center prospective study of 386 outpatients with schizophrenia from psychiatric clinics in Lucknow, Vellore, and Madras, India. Among patients who reported a decrease in religious activities at baseline, health outcomes deteriorated over time (p<0.001). Researchers concluded, "If these associations are confirmed, it is possible to plan some intervention programs, such as changing the attitudes of others to the patient, and giving more importance to various types of religious activity. Religiosity is important in Indian culture and the increase in religiosity that was related to better outcomes in the present study could be a means of effectively handling the anxiety of the patient" (502).

Brent Brenda, a professor in the School of Social Work at the University of Arkansas in Little Rock, examined predictors of re-hospitalization in a random sample of 600 homeless Vietnam veterans aged 46 to 65 involved in a Midwestern U.S. hospital program.[53] These men had a chronic history of abusing drugs and alcohol and many also had co-morbid severe mental illness. The researcher estimated the time to re-hospitalization during the 2-year study period using Cox proportional hazards. Predictors included personal characteristics, history of drug and psychiatric treatment, social support, religiosity (5-item scale), and combat experience in Vietnam. Almost three-quarters of the sample (72%) were readmitted to the hospital during the 2-year follow-up for problems related to substance abuse or mental illness. Religiosity (prayer, Bible study, discussion of religion, church attendance, and belief in a supernatural being) predicted longer time spent in the community before readmission to the hospital. In other words, subjects scoring high on religiosity were about one-third less likely to be readmitted than others during the study period. This is the third prospective study that has reported better outcomes for patients with greater religious involvement.[54]

Thus, although cross-sectional studies from England suggest a correlation between religiousness and severe mental illness, prospective studies that follow these patients over time do not find that greater religiousness precipitates or worsens the course of illness. There is also no evidence that sensitive spiritual interventions in patients with schizophrenia or other psychotic disorders worsen the condition or exacerbate psychosis.[55] We will return to spiritual interventions for severe mental illness in chapter 6.

NONCLINICAL SAMPLES

A series of studies involving healthy nonclinical samples of teenagers and adults in England have examined the relationship between religiousness and schizotypal or psychotic personality traits. Stephen Joseph and Debbie Diduca at the University of Warwick examined the association between religiosity and schizotypy in a sample of 492 British teenagers 13 to 18 years old.[56] Stronger Christian attitudes were associated with higher scores on perceptual aberration but lower scores on impulsive nonconformity and magical ideation. When analyses were stratified by gender, the association with higher scores on magical ideation (i.e., more schizotypy) was present only in boys and the association with lower scores on impulsive nonconformity (i.e., less schizotypy) was found only in girls. Investigators concluded that while religiosity may be associated with psychosis proneness in boys of this age, it was associated with greater psychological well-being in girls.

John Maltby and colleagues from the school of psychology at University of Leicester in the United Kingdom reported a similar pattern when investigating religious orientation and schizotypal traits in 195 English university students ages 18 to 49.[57] Among men, but not women, an intrinsic orientation toward religion was associated with more borderline personality traits. A more recent study by Maltby examined this relationship again, but this time in a larger and somewhat older adult population.[58] Assessing religious experience, religious orientation, and schizotypy in a sample of 308 English people aged 20 to 59 years, they found that having an intrinsic orientation toward religion was associated with *lower* levels of schizotypy, whereas religious experience and extrinsic orientation towards religion were associated with higher levels of schizotypy.

Another study by Joseph and colleagues surveyed 180 English adults (mean age 40 years) using the Eysenck Personality Questionnaire, schizotypal trait measures, and Batson's Religious Life Inventory to obtain scores on external, internal, and quest dimensions of religiosity.[59] When they entered personality and schizotypal trait measures together to predict scores on religiosity, schizotypal traits emerged as a predictor of religious quest but not the other dimensions of religiosity.

Recall that Feldman and Rust also found significantly less schizotypal thinking among those who were more religious in their sample of 140 normal British adults. This corroborates the results from two other studies of normal populations outside of Great Britain—one involving 315 young persons in Hong Kong and another involving 608 university students in Venezuela,[60] which found less schizotypal thinking among the more religious.

Thus, the findings in healthy populations are conflicting. While some investigators report an association between schizotypal traits and religiosity in younger English males, this relationship did not hold up in younger females. Relationships between religiosity and schizotypal traits in young persons outside of Great Britain generally find less schizotypal thinking in persons who are more religious. In mature adult populations, likewise, intrinsic religiosity is either unrelated to schizotypal traits or inversely related to them, even in England. Be aware that these studies involve nonclinical samples, so "psychological traits" picked up on these psychological tests are simply tendencies, and not severe enough to warrant a formal diagnosis or treatment.

Differences among Religious Groups

The association between religiousness and psychosis or schizotypal thinking may be influenced by the particular beliefs that a person holds, particularly those involving less traditional types of religion. The emergence of psychotic symptoms themselves may also prompt a change in religious affiliation from traditional to less traditional. Renate Armstrong and colleagues at East Moline State Hospital in Illinois compared the strength of religious belief of 121 non-psychotic patients to that of 88 psychotic patients at their psychiatric facility.[61] For Catholics and Protestants, religious beliefs were stronger among non-psychotic patients than among psychotic patients; however, the opposite pattern was found for Unitarians (i.e., religious beliefs were stronger among psychotic patients).

In a small study that compared different religious groups on psychiatric outcomes following conversion, Ullman examined 40 converts to traditional (10 Jewish and 10 Catholic) and nontraditional religious groups (10 Baha'i and 10 Hare Krishna). Subjects had converted 2 months to 10 years previously. Jewish and Catholic converts were significantly more likely to have a history of seeking outpatient psychiatric help compared to Baha'i or Hare Krishna converts (32% vs. 5%). However, Baha'i and Hare Krishna converts were significantly more likely to have had a psychotic episode requiring psychiatric hospitalization (25% vs. 5%) and were more likely to have experienced a chaotic lifestyle prior to conversion (75% vs. 40%).

In a recent English study, the presence of delusional thinking was compared between persons involved in new religious movements (Hare Krishna and Druids), Christians, nonreligious persons, and psychotic inpatients with delusions.[62] A total of 142 subjects completed two delusional inventories as part of this study. Persons in new religious movements (NRM) scored significantly higher than Christians or nonreligious persons on all delusional measures. In fact, they could not be differentiated from deluded psychiatric inpatients on the number of delusional symptoms or on level of conviction. However, NRM members were considerably less distressed and preoccupied by these experiences than delusional psychiatric patients. Researchers found no difference in delusional symptoms between nonreligious persons and Christians, indicating that religious beliefs by themselves could not account for the findings in the NRM group.

Individuals with mental illness may also change their religious affiliation at the time they develop psychosis and then turn to religious groups that are more extreme. Dinesh Bhugra from the Institute of Psychiatry at the University of London conducted studies in Trinidad (an island in the Caribbean) and in London of first-onset schizophrenia among four ethnic groups: Trinidadian, London white, London Asian, and London African-

Caribbean. He found that patients with first-onset psychosis among these groups were likely to change their religion in an attempt to regain a degree of self-control as their self-concept began to change with the onset of symptoms.[63] Thus, rather than a particular religion or type of religious belief leading to psychosis, it may be more likely that psychosis-prone individuals change their affiliation to less conventional or more extreme religious groups.

Other Benefits of Religious Involvement

The majority of epidemiological studies suggest that persons with severe mental disorder do better if they are involved in or connected with a faith community, as noted in the majority of studies described above. Additional research supports this conclusion. For example, Alan Breier and Boris Astrachan in the Department of Psychiatry at Yale studied the characteristics of Connecticut Mental Health Center patients who committed suicide between 1970 and 1981, comparing them with a control group.[64] They found that 20 patients with schizophrenia who committed suicide were less often affiliated with a religion or indicated their affiliation as "other" (40%) compared to 81 non-suicidal schizophrenic controls (25%). Patients with schizophrenia who committed suicide were also less likely to be Protestant-affiliated compared to the control group (10% vs. 40%, p<0.05). This study suggests that certain types of religious affiliation may help counter the worsening of symptoms in patients with schizophrenia that eventually leads to suicide.

Kirov and colleagues in the Department of Psychological Medicine at the University of Wales at Cardiff assessed religious faith and religious coping in a sample of 52 consecutively admitted psychotic English patients.[65] Subjects ranged in age from 18 to 66 years, and were interviewed after their index admission. Nearly 70% indicated they were religious and 22% indicated that religion was the most important part of their lives. Nearly one-third of the sample (30%) reported that their religiousness had increased since the onset of illness and almost two-thirds (61%) used religion to cope with illness. Patients who used religion to cope had better insight and, interestingly, were *more* compliant with antipsychotic medication. The results from this study help to dispel the widespread belief that religious patients often discontinue their medication when they become psychotic.

Summary

Persons with severe and persistent mental illness frequently use religion to help them to cope with the stress these conditions cause. This is especially true in religious areas of the world (the United States, India, the Middle East) and for members of certain religious groups (Hindu, Christian, Muslim). Spiritual explanations (including demonic possession) for severe mental illnesses are common, especially in places where education about mental illness is limited. Even when non-spiritual explanations for illness are given, many patients and families still seek treatment from non-traditional spiritual healers rather than from mental health professionals.

Despite the high prevalence of religious delusions in psychotic patients, especially those with schizophrenia, there is no evidence that exorcism is effective in treating persons with these conditions. There is also little evidence that religious beliefs or religious conversion predispose to the development of schizophrenia or other severe mental illnesses, nor that schizotypal or psychotic traits are more common among religious persons. Increase in religious activity and changes in religious affiliation, however, are common after a first psychotic break. Several prospective studies now demonstrate that religious involvement by people with schizophrenia or other severe mental illness predicts lower rates of re-hospitalization and less health deterioration over time.

Compared to the huge number of studies in nonpsychiatric populations, there is a void in research that systematically examines the role that religion plays in the etiology, course, and treatment of persons with severe mental illness. Further research is clearly needed to better understand when religion serves as a resource and when it acts as a liability in this population.

CHAPTER 6

INTEGRATING RELIGION
INTO MENTAL HEALTH
TREATMENTS

Based on the research presented in the last four chapters, there appears to be a growing consensus that religious factors in one way or another influence the mental health and well-being of persons with mental illness. No doubt there are instances where religion is used neurotically as a psychological defense, or when help from the faith community is slow or disappointing. Much of the time, however, religious involvement has a positive effect on coping and well-being, helps to prevent depression, and buffers against stress that causes psychological deterioration in persons with mental illness. This was the conclusion of nearly 500 studies during the twentieth century that reported statistically significant associations between religion and better mental health (478 out of 724 studies),[1] and as we've seen, many of the studies published since the year 2000 have further confirmed these findings. I now examine two questions.

First, how does religion improve coping with stress, enhance well-being and quality of life, and speed recovery from depression, and does the particular religion make a difference? Second, how can this information be used to design psychological and social treatments for those with emotional problems or serious mental illness, and what are the results of studies that have evaluated such interventions?

Ways that Religion Helps

Here I discuss the pathways by which religious beliefs and practices reduce stress or improve coping. Religion both *provides things* and *expects things in return*. There is no free lunch. What religion expects from people, however, may actually be an important part of the mechanism by which it conveys its positive effects. For example, take the doctrines concerning acceptable and unacceptable behaviors and lifestyles. Although religious teachings have often been considered "prudish" and "backward" in our modern society, we are now discovering that such constrictions on lifestyle may actually promote health and enhance well-being. Below are ten ways that religion could improve mental health.

1. PROMOTES A POSITIVE WORLDVIEW

Religious beliefs provide a worldview that is positive, coherent, optimistic, and caring. Again, I will use the Judeo-Christian worldview as an example, although these likely apply to other religious worldviews as they exist within particular cultures. In Judeo-Christian belief, a forgiving, merciful, just, and all-powerful God exists who is separate from creation and controls everything that happens both on earth and throughout eternity in the life beyond. This is a personal God who experiences emotions like we do, is interested in and cares about people, recruits them to help carry out divine purposes, and responds to pleas for help and assistance. According to this worldview, the universe is a friendly place that has been designed specifically for humans.

Such a worldview is different from the secular, purely scientific understanding and explanation of life. That viewpoint sees events occurring entirely as a result of random chance. There is no greater meaning to events other than the actual event itself. The universe is viewed as impersonal, hostile, and threatening—ruled by the law of conquer or be conquered. Humans are seen as simply another species of animal that is temporary and evolving into other creatures that someday will be very different. Humans, in this worldview, are rather insignificant—here by chance and soon to be gone. From this perspective, the religious worldview is seen as pure fantasy, springing from human imagination in response to fear and uncertainty.

But is the religious worldview simply wishful thinking—a refusal to confront the cold reality of the way things are? If science alone defines reality, and reality includes only the material world that can be observed and measured, then religion is exactly that—wishful thinking. Those from a religious perspective, however, disagree with this reasoning. They say that science is not capable of defining all of reality nor is it the sole determinant of what is real or not real. Instead, they claim that there is much of reality that exists outside of the observable and the measurable. Regardless of which view is truer in the ultimate sense, the mental health consequences of one worldview compared to the other may be profound, especially for the person with severe mental illness.

The scientific worldview works wonderfully for researchers, educators, academicians, and those blessed with good health, material resources, and interesting occupations. For those who are experiencing severe stress, multiple losses, socioeconomic deprivation, or prolonged pain or suffering, however, it does not work so well. The reason is because the scientific worldview is completely devoid of meaning, and it is *meaning* that enables those who suffer to survive.[2]

Finally, the treatment of mental illness and the mentally ill person's response to that treatment may also be affected by worldview. This is especially true when the worldview of those who provide treatment is substantially different from the view of those who receive it. This idea will be explored further later.

2. HELPS TO MAKE SENSE OF DIFFICULT SITUATIONS

People need to understand why they have been singled out to have mental illness or endure severe emotional pain—why their hopes and prayers for healing have not been answered. They need to be able to integrate this event into their worldview and sense of self. People need to understand what this illness means for them, their future, and their families' future. They need to know how they are going to cope with the illness, how they will bear the burden of a changed life that may involve long-term discomfort and restriction. Religion provides answers to the why question. Those answers may not be entirely satisfactory for some, but for others, they help the person make sense of something that seems totally senseless.

3. GIVES PURPOSE AND MEANING

This is particularly true for people undergoing negative life experiences or difficult situations—and that includes those with mental or emotional problems. Meaning is important because it provides a sense of purpose and direction for life that gives hope for better times ahead and gives significance to present difficulties. People need renewed purpose and meaning in order to continue to fight the illness and make the efforts necessary to recover and rehabilitate. They need to know that they can still contribute and are still valuable, despite their illness and disability. Religious and spiritual beliefs often lie at the core of what gives life purpose and meaning in these circumstances. In the Christian tradition, all situations, no matter how difficult, can result in good things: "And we know that in all things God works for the good of those who love him, who have been called according to his purpose."[3]

4. DISCOURAGES MALADAPTIVE COPING

Religious beliefs discourage negative responses to stress such as alcohol or drug use, risky sexual behaviors, or other behaviors that worsen mental health in the long run. Rather than turning to these unhealthy sources of comfort and solace, religion encourages people to turn to God, prayer, and their community instead. It also helps people to make better decisions (i.e., don't steal, forgive, etc.) that are less likely to result in further stress or in difficult life situations that worsen or precipitate mental illness.

5. ENHANCES SOCIAL SUPPORT

Most studies (19 of 20) during the twentieth century found that religious persons have more social connections and experience a higher quality of social support. This includes family and marital bonds that tend to be stronger among the more religious. In our systematic review, 35 of 38 studies of religion and marriage found that spouses who were more religious or from similar religious backgrounds had more satisfying and durable marriages.[4] The presence of supportive relationships from family and friends at times of stress is a key factor in helping persons cope successfully and in preventing the development or worsening of mental disorder. For the person with severe and persistent mental illness, having an intact family is very important for their ongoing care. Support and understanding from another person is also the basis for the standard therapeutic modality used to treat persons experiencing stressful life circumstances (i.e., supportive psychotherapy). The religious community can also provide such support.

Emotional problems and severe mental illness cause people to feel isolated, lonely, and disconnected from others. They are often alienated from friends and family, may be living among strangers, worried about what will happen next. Spiritual beliefs and practices help people feel more connected. Phone calls or visits from a pastor or member of a congregation, or knowing that members of a faith community are praying for them—all help to re-establish connection with others. Feeling connected to, cared for, and loved by God also helps to relieve loneliness, especially when no one else is around.

6. PROMOTES OTHER-DIRECTEDNESS

Religion influences mental health by directing one's attention outside of the self. As noted earlier, every major world religious leader has instructed his followers to support and care for one another—Moses, Jesus, the Buddha, Hindu holy men, and Muhammad—all emphasized this teaching as a key to happiness and spiritual progress.[5] Such teachings promote forgiveness, mercy, kindness, compassion, and generosity toward others. Other-directed actions can themselves produce healing in those whose lives have been scarred by deprivation, neglect, loss, and struggle. Focusing attention outside the self helps to prevent brooding over personal problems, resentments, and entitlements. Well-being is enhanced as one sees others benefiting from one's actions. This helps a person feel more involved in the world and more related to others in it. The effect that such other-directed activities may have on resolving deep-seeded emotional problems in those with mental illness is only beginning to be explored. Research in the mental health fields has fallen far behind work in other medical disciplines that has examined the effect of other-directed activity on those with physical illness.

For example, 132 people with multiple sclerosis were trained to listen actively and to provide compassionate, unconditional positive regard to others with the same condition (called "peer support").[6] During this 2-year study, investigators reported improvement in confidence, self-aware-ness, self-esteem, depression, and role functioning among those who pro-vided the peer support. The same is true for those suffering with chronic arthritis. Twenty-one adults with either osteoarthritis or rheumatoid arthritis (with an average disease duration of ten years) were recruited into a study that trained people with arthritis to lead arthritis self-management courses.[7] Subjects were assessed at three points in time: before their train-ing, six weeks after training, and six months after training. By six months after training, participants reported significant increases in arthritis self-efficacy for pain, cognitive symptom management, communication with their physician, and significant decreases in depressed mood. They also re-ported having more confidence, greater happiness, even a changed out-look on life. Focusing on spiritual matters or on the needs of others around them often helps people to put their own concerns and worries in perspective. By encouraging care for others, religion provides a way for persons with mental illness to heal themselves.

7. HELPS TO RELEASE THE NEED FOR CONTROL

Emotional pain and psychiatric illness can take control away from a person, causing anxiety and a sense of helplessness. As a result, many des-perately seek to regain that control. They fight any efforts by family care-givers or health professionals that are perceived as taking away control. Religious beliefs and practices help people to regain control and mastery over their situations by empowering them with resources to do so (prayer). Religious beliefs also help people to give up control when it is ap-propriate and necessary. Belief and trust in God are often what enable them to do so. This improves their ability to cooperate with their care providers and makes life easier on everybody.

8. PROVIDES AND ENCOURAGES FORGIVENESS

As indicated in chapter 6, persons with severe mental illness sometimes interpret their illness as punishment for past sins. Religion provides ways by which people can receive forgiveness and thereby be released from the burden of guilt or shame. Religion also encourages forgiveness of others, and thereby helps to free people from bitterness and resentment that may be gnawing at their peace and well-being. We know from research presented in chapter 3 that forgiveness infuses both the receiver and the giver with positive emotions.

9. ENCOURAGES THANKFULNESS

Being thankful and grateful for their health and relationships helps persons with severe mental illness cope better with conditions and maintain a positive attitude. As Emmons and colleagues have shown, simply writing down each day a list of things to be thankful for produces positive emotions almost immediately.[8] Religious beliefs encourage an attitude-of-gratitude, and religious scriptures provide role models to help accomplish this.

10. PROVIDES HOPE

Hope is the engine of motivation. It is what keeps a person moving toward health and healing.

Emily Dickinson said it this way:

> Hope is the thing with feathers
> That perches in the soul,
> And sings the tune—without the words,
> And never stops at all,
>
> And sweetest in the gale is heard;
> And sore must be the storm
> That could abash the little bird
> That kept so many warm.
>
> I've heard it in the chillest land,
> And on the strangest sea;
> Yet, never, in extremity,
> It asked a crumb of me.[9]

Without hope, people give up, neglect themselves, and strike out at others trying to help them. Spiritual beliefs are a powerful source of hope for many patients: "With man this is impossible, but with God all things are possible."[10]

Religious Understanding of Mental Illness

A religious perspective on mental illness can lighten the burden by emphasizing that even these dreaded conditions have the possibility of good. Pain, suffering, and fear associated with mental illness are not experiences that anyone would seek after. However, what does a person do if he or she has such a condition? Assuming that everything possible has been done (psychotherapy, medication, behavioral change) to relieve the symptoms and treat the disorder, what does one do if the treatment has not been successful or has only been partially successful? Many, many persons today must live with recurrent, persistent emotional or mental illness. What about these people? Are they doomed to a life of senseless pain and suffering? Certainly, they should hope for and seek information about new treatments that may relieve their symptoms. Every effort should be made to stay alert for such future developments. However, what does the mentally ill person do in the meantime?

In order to survive and maximize quality of life, it may help to adopt a religious view that sees mental illness as having a special *meaning or purpose*—that something good may someday result from the illness. Religious faith makes it possible for people to see their illnesses as serving a higher purpose. I suggested this briefly in the introduction and I return to elaborate more on it here.

Religious faith may help to transform a person's view of his or her illness. Although not easy, it is possible to view mental illness as a gift that not only helps to deepen and sensitize the person who has it, but also can serve a key role in the "formation" of our faith communities.

From this perspective, mental illness can have at least three purposes. It can (1) sensitize the emotionally or mentally ill person to the pain and suffering of others, uniquely equipping them with the insight and ability to help; (2) draw the sufferer closer to God or deepen their spirituality; and (3) challenge those in the faith community to support and include him or her as an integral part of the congregation. I will discuss each of these below.

SENSITIZED TO THE SUFFERINGS OF OTHERS

Until one has undergone pain, discouragement, isolation, confusion, and fear, it is difficult to really understand and appreciate these experiences that people with mental illness must deal with on a day-to-day basis. Having gone through such experiences, a person is more able to empathize with and feel the suffering that others must endure. From this comes a greater desire to help and to share one's own experiences. This helps both the giver and the receiver feel less alone. The receiver now realizes that at least one other person knows what it is like to live with this condition and has survived. If that is possible, then this gives hope that he or she, too, might be able to make it. In *The Wounded Healer*,[11] Henri Nouwen discusses the role that emotional pain plays in making a person able to help others navigate through similar situations. It is that pain that often qualifies a counselor to lead others out of darkness and toward the light. Thus, having mental illness may help make a person qualified to support others who are similarly afflicted, as John of God and Anton Boisen were able to do.

DRAWN INTO A DEEPER, CLOSER RELATIONSHIP WITH GOD

C. S. Lewis said, "God whispers to us in our pleasures, speaks in our conscience, but shouts in our pain: it is his megaphone to a deaf world."[12] Indeed, it is emotional distress that gets our attention and stretches our coping abilities to their maximum. As those coping abilities are stretched, a person is more likely to call out to God for assistance or have greater interest in spiritual matters that give hope for relief. Adversity often shows that a person's own skills and resources are not sufficient to get him or her out of a situation, and that only when he or she taps into that which is beyond and outside of the self, healing is found. Of course, mental illness and emotional pain can also destroy a person's relationship with the Divine if anger and resentment set in. People may struggle with feelings that God doesn't love them, is unconcerned about their pain, or is even punishing them. Spiritual struggles like this, as we learned earlier, negatively impact both psychological and physical health, underscoring the need for pastoral counseling to help resolve such conflicts.

CHALLENGE THE FAITH COMMUNITY

Persons with mental illness challenge faith communities by providing members of those communities with an *opportunity* to live out their faith in a meaningful way. If people of faith have no opportunity to provide support to others, to show care and compassion to the needy, or to include those who are different into their social group—then how can they live out the religious beliefs and ideals that are at the core of their faith traditions? Those with mental illness remind members of the faith community who they (the faith community) are and what their purpose is here on earth. If the faith community responds by loving, supporting, and including the mentally ill, then it can say with pride that it is carrying out the great commandment. If not, then how is the faith community different from any other social group or secular organization? The very identity and uniqueness of our faith congregations hinge on their response to this challenge. If the faith community welcomes and provides a distinct place and role for those with mental illness, then at least in the Christian tradition, it is doing what its founders intended. This will require that people in the church will have to get their hands dirty. Sometimes the mentally ill are not the easiest persons to associate with or work with, but they are those whom we have been called to minister to, sacrifice for, bear the burdens of.

In this way, mental illness may be viewed as a religious calling that qualifies a person to understand and help others with similar problems, that forces him or her to grow and mature spiritually, and that presents those in religious communities with an opportunity to support, care about, and include the mentally ill as part of their religious family. Having this perspective on mental illness infuses it with meaning and instills hope that something good can come out of it—something good that otherwise might never be possible. This spiritual attitude can give meaning and purpose to mental illness and make the burden of having it a lot lighter.

When Religion Doesn't Help

As I've said repeatedly in this book, religion does not always promote better mental health and stronger social relationships. Religion may induce excessive guilt, shame, and fear with its prohibitions against unacceptable behavior. It can foster social isolation and low self-esteem in persons engaged in homosexual activity, extramarital sex, those who become pregnant out of wedlock, or others behaving in ways not sanctioned by the religious community. Religion may restrict personal growth by promoting rigid thinking or may foster an attitude of self-righteousness. Religion can be used maladaptively or neurotically to block therapeutic interventions, and may even discourage seeking professional help altogether.

Most religious beliefs and practices based within established religious traditions, however, help to maintain mental and social health. Religion may be especially helpful for persons with severe and persistent mental disorders who must cope with many stressors that threaten to destabilize their illness, although further research is clearly needed on how and when religion worsens the course of mental illness.

Differences among Religions

Are the mental health benefits of religion restricted to only certain types of religion? Is Christianity more effective in preventing mental problems or reducing their severity than, say, Judaism or Islam or Buddhism? As noted above, there are only a few studies that compare the rates of mental illness between different religious groups. The information we have suggests that devout, sensible religious practices typically encouraged within each of the major world religions usually correlate with better mental health. This does not mean that the content of belief does not matter or that all religions teach the same thing, but only that world religions lasting for thousands of years usually promote pro-social values that help to bind communities together and address the problem of suffering, even though the way they do that may be quite culture-specific.

The essential therapeutic factors are those described above: (1) promoting a positive worldview that gives meaning, (2) encouraging love of neighbor that fosters the giving and receiving of support, and (3) prohibiting unhealthy addictive behaviors or obsessive preoccupation with selfish desires and concerns. These are common to almost all major world religions, although their emphasis may vary across traditions. Most of the data from systematic research on religion and mental health come from

Christian populations (90% of studies),[13] although studies of Islamic,[14] Jewish,[15] Hindu,[16] Buddhist,[17] and Tao[18] practices seem to support generalizing the findings to these religious groups as well. Nevertheless, further research on religion and mental health is needed in non-Christian religions to see whether the vast majority of research done in Christian populations applies equally well to persons with other belief systems.

Relevant to this question is research finding that people in "Christian" nations do not appear to be that much happier than those living in non-Christian nations, especially if socioeconomic conditions are taken into account. A 1999 Roper Starch survey of a representative sample of 22,500 respondents ages 18 years or older in 22 countries examined level of happiness. Countries included in the study were: Argentina, Australia, Brazil, China, Denmark, Egypt, France, Germany, Hong Kong, Hungary, India, Italy, Kuwait, Malaysia, Mexico, Nigeria, Russia, Spain, the United Kingdom, Ukraine, the United States, and Venezuela. Among the 10 happiest countries (based on percent "very happy") were the United States (46%), Kuwait (Muslim) (41%), India (Hindu) (37%), and Malaysia (Muslim) (34%).[19] The gross domestic product (GDP) per capita of these nations, however, is quite different. GDP per capita gives an estimate of the purchasing power per person, and is computed by taking the value of all goods and services produced within a nation in a given year divided by the nation's population.[20] In Kuwait the GDP per capita is $15,000, in India it is $2,200, and in Malaysia it is $10,300, compared to $36,200 in the United States. Thus, the difference in happiness between the Christian United States and Hindu India is only 9%, when the GDP difference is 1,650%.

For Christianity, however, the personal nature of God and the emphasis on social responsibility are important elements that likely influence individual mental health and the care of those with mental illness.[21] Belief in an involved, personal, and loving God provides Christians with a divine relationship that may help to dispel loneliness, provide hope, and facilitate self-acceptance, as described above. The emphasis within Christianity on serving others as part of its social mission is relevant not only to effects on individual mental health, but underscores the role and responsibility of the Christian community in caring for those with mental illness. Again, this does not mean that other religions do not also stress these aspects or that Christian programs are more effective in delivering social or mental health services than are Jewish, Buddhist, or Islamic programs, but only that beliefs with regard to social activism are particularly strong in the Christian religion.[22]

Certainly, part of this has to do with Christianity's evangelical focus, where the drive to care for others may be related to a desire to convert them. The true test, however, is to what extent Christian motivations lead to compassionate care not only to the mentally ill among its own members, but also to needy persons outside its tradition whether they convert or not (i.e., as the good Samaritan treated the wounded Jewish traveler).

Using Religious Faith in Treatment

If religious beliefs and practices have the potential to positively impact mental health, then it would seem natural that psychiatric interventions might utilize the religious resources of religious patients to speed their recovery and healing. This does not mean that religious interventions should be used in nonreligious patients or that nonreligious patients should be encouraged to become religious. Rather, it means that psychotherapeutic interventions in religious patients might utilize the religious beliefs of these patients in treatment. Attempts have been made to integrate religion into psychotherapy, or at least take into consideration patients' religious background and strengths.

Integrating religion or addressing religious issues in mental health care is important, given the fact that studies show that the vast majority (over three-quarters) of psychiatric inpatients have religious needs,[23] many of which remain unmet during their hospital stay. As we saw above, religious beliefs and practices may help prevent the onset or facilitate the resolution of emotional problems and psychiatric disorders. Finally, a significant minority of psychiatric patients in the United States (23%) believes that religious factors are the cause of their illness.[24] Thus, ignoring the role that religion plays in mental health care is not longer tenable.

A number of randomized clinical trials have tested the effectiveness of religious interventions in religious patients with depression or anxiety. These have included Christian cognitive-behavioral therapy,[25] Christian rational emotive therapy,[26] Islamic therapy using the Qur'an and prayer,[27] and Tao cognitive therapy.[28] The majority of these clinical trials have found that religion-based psychotherapies with religious patients are more effective than secular psychotherapies or no treatment. I will now review some of these studies below.

Rebecca Propst and colleagues from the Graduate School of Professional Studies at Lewis & Clark College conducted a randomized clinical trial that compared the effectiveness of religious cognitive-behavioral therapy (religious CBT) to traditional secular cognitive-behavioral therapy (secular CBT), ordinary pastoral counseling (PCT), and no treatment (a wait-list control; WLC) (four study groups) in the treatment of depression.[29] Subjects were 59 religious patients who had experienced depression for an average of 12 months. Religious CBT was used with Christian religious rationales, religious arguments to counter irrational thoughts, and religious imagery. The intervention consisted of eighteen 50-minute sessions over 3 months. Subjects were assessed before treatment, at termination of treatment, and at 3 months and 24 months after treatment using a variety of depression, severity of illness, and social adjustment scales. Therapists delivering the intervention were divided into religious and nonreligious therapists.

The findings were as follows. Only religious CBT resulted in significantly lower immediate post-treatment, self-rated depression scores than the WLC group, although the secular CBT and PCT groups showed a non-significant trend in that direction. With regard to observer-rated depression scores, only the religious CBT and PCT groups tended to show lower post-treatment scores compared to the WLC group. The religious CBT group also scored significantly better on a severity of illness scale than did the WLC group. Finally, only the religious CBT group tended to score better in overall functioning than the WLC group.

Whether or not the therapist was religious also had an impact. When nonreligious therapists administered RCBT, the subjects scored significantly lower on post-treatment self-rated depression scores than either the WLC group or the secular CBT group. Similar findings were present for observer-rated depression and severity of illness scores. At the 3-month post-treatment assessment, subjects who received religious CBT from nonreligious therapists and subjects who received secular CBT from religious therapists were also doing significantly better.

Thus, Christian-based religious CBT achieved a faster decrease in symptoms than did either the secular therapy or the pastoral care groups, and the effect of the religious CBT was greatest when administered by nonreligious therapists. Cognitive-behavioral therapy is the most commonly used psychotherapy for the treatment of depression in the United States today, and therefore these findings have wide relevance.

MUSLIM PSYCHOTHERAPY

Azhar and Varma from the Department of Psychiatry at the School of Medical Sciences in Kelantan, Malaysia, conducted a randomized clinical trial to examine the effects of brief psychotherapy on depression using a Muslim perspective compared to secular psychotherapy.[30] Subjects were 64 Malaysians with strong Muslim backgrounds, all fulfilling criteria for depressive disorder. Both groups received weekly secular psychotherapy and low doses of antidepressant medication. The study group, however, received an additional 45-minute session of religious psychotherapy once per week. A psychiatrist blind-to-treatment group assessed patients at 1 month, 3 months, and 6 months of treatment. Subjects receiving additional Muslim-based psychotherapy that involved reading verses from the Holy Qur'an and saying Muslim prayers experienced faster relief of depressive symptoms than subjects receiving secular psychotherapy and antidepressant medication alone. The group reported similar findings when they utilized this treatment protocol for subjects with bereavement.[31]

Azhar and colleagues also examined the effects of Muslim-based psychotherapy on 62 devout Muslim subjects with generalized anxiety disorder.[32] Subjects were randomized to either traditional treatment (supportive psychotherapy and anti-anxiety drugs) or traditional treatment plus religious psychotherapy. Religious psychotherapy again used Muslim prayer and reading verses of the Holy Qur'an specific to the person's situation. Anxiety symptoms in subjects receiving religious psychotherapy improved significantly faster than in those receiving traditional therapy. Thus, Muslim-based psychotherapy, when added to traditional therapy, results in faster relief of both depression and anxiety symptoms in devoutly Muslim subjects.

TAO-BASED PSYCHOTHERAPY

Zhang and colleagues compared the effectiveness of Chinese Taoist cognitive psychotherapy (Taoist CT), tranquilizers (benzodiazepines), or a combination of both in 143 Chinese patients with generalized anxiety disorder. Taoist CT is a type of cognitive therapy based on Taoist religious philosophy.[33] Patients were randomized to receive Taoist CT only, tranquilizers only, or Taoist CT plus tranquilizers. Investigators found that while tranquilizers rapidly reduced symptoms within the first month of treatment, they lost their effects by 6 months. Taoist CT, while it reduced symptoms more slowly than tranquilizers, was still effective after 6 months of treatment. Most important, combined treatment (Taoist CT plus tranquilizers) led to both rapid relief of symptoms and long-term relief as well.

RELIGIOUS PSYCHOTHERAPY FOR
THE NONRELIGIOUS

With the exception of one study to my knowledge, religious therapies have only been tested in religious patients. Razali and colleagues in the Department of Psychiatry at the University of Sains Malaysia School of Medical Sciences conducted a clinical trial involving Muslim-based religious cognitive psychotherapy (religious CP) as a treatment for generalized anxiety disorder. Subjects were 85 religious and 80 nonreligious Muslims. Subjects were randomized depending on their religiousness to one of four groups: religious subjects who received religious CP, religious controls, nonreligious subjects who received religious CP, and nonreligious controls. All subjects received standard treatment for generalized anxiety including tranquilizers, supportive psychotherapy, and/or simple relaxation exercises. Religious CP included extensive use of the Qur'an and Hadith (sayings of Muhammad) to alter negative thoughts, change negative behaviors, and increase religiousness. The four groups were assessed at 4, 12, and 26 weeks of treatment. Religious subjects receiving religious CP improved significantly faster than religious controls. However, there was no difference between nonreligious patients receiving religious CP and nonreligious controls.

Thus, patients for whom religion is important will likely be more receptive to religious psychotherapies and other religious interventions, and these therapies may be more effective in this group than in nonreligious patients. No studies have yet examined psychiatric patients in general asking them whether they wish to have religious issues addressed in psychotherapy or receive religious psychotherapy. It is safe to say, however, that all patients wish to have their religious beliefs (or lack of religious beliefs) respected, valued, and understood by their therapists.

SPECIAL POPULATIONS

Including religious considerations into psychotherapy may be particularly important for certain subgroups in the population such as African Americans and Hispanics. Cooper and colleagues in the Department of Medicine at Johns Hopkins compared the views of 76 African American and white primary care patients on how important they viewed different aspects of depression care.[34] Subjects rated the importance of 126 aspects of care. From the 30 aspects rated highest by patients, nine domains were created: (1) health professionals' interpersonal skills, (2) primary care provider recognition of depression, (3) treatment effectiveness, (4) treatment problems, (5) patient understanding about treatment, (6) intrinsic spirituality, (7) financial access, (8) life experiences, and (9) social support. The biggest difference between African American and white patients' ratings was the likelihood of rating spirituality as extremely important for depression care. African Americans were three times more likely to rate it as important than whites.

Because the population of the United States is a melting pot of people from different ethnic backgrounds, cultures, and religions, this challenges mental health professionals to be knowledgeable about religious beliefs and practices from many different perspectives and to understand their role in the etiology and the treatment of mental disorder. Minority and immigrant populations may deal with psychiatric issues almost exclusively from a religious perspective. The *Handbook of Religion and Mental Health* discusses how different religious belief systems influence psychotherapy and medical treatments, including Catholic, Protestant, Mormon, Unity, Jewish, Buddhist, Hindu, and Muslim perspectives, written by mental health professionals with these religious backgrounds.[35]

Interventions in Those with Severe Mental Illness

Roger Fallot at Community Connections in Washington, D.C., describes several ways in which spiritual and religious concerns can be addressed as part of rehabilitation services for those with severe and persistent mental illness.[36] These include taking a spiritual history, incorporating spiritual resources into psychotherapy, linking the mentally ill person to faith communities and spiritual resources, and offering spiritually oriented group therapy. I will focus on the last of these, spiritually based group therapy, given the increased amount of attention that this approach is now getting.

A number of mental health professionals have described group therapy for the treatment of persons with severe and persistent mental illness. One model described by Phillips and colleagues at Bowling Green State University involves a 7-week semi-structured psychoeducational program. During this time participants discuss religious resources, spiritual struggles, forgiveness, and hope.[37] Another model is described by therapist Nancy Kehoe who bases her treatment on experiences gained during 18 years of conducting spiritually based group therapy for chronically ill psychiatric patients.[38] Kehoe's group is for adults and is usually held in a day treatment center. She has found that psychodynamic-oriented groups foster tolerance, self-awareness, and positive exploration of value systems. The groups are bound by rules that promote the toleration of diversity, respect for other members' beliefs, and ban proselytizing. Although many staff were first concerned that discussing spiritual issues might worsen delusions or strengthen unhealthy religious defenses, these concerns have not proven true (for either Kehoe's or Phillips's groups).

Others using group therapy have also reported positive results, including an increased understanding of feelings, problems, and questions related to spiritual aspects of their lives, an increased sense of spiritual support, and a greater sense of connection with group members and facilitators.[39] These groups are often held at day treatment programs in psychiatric outpatient settings and include anywhere from 6 to 12 members. Spirituality-based group therapies have yet to be subject to rigorous evaluation using a randomized clinical trial format.

In fact, there is some evidence that benefits do not always accrue from spiritual approaches. For example, Salib and Yoakim at Hollins Park Hospital in Warrington, United Kingdom, reported an association between the experience of spiritual healing and the occurrence of schizophrenic relapses in a sample of 40 older Egyptian patients.[40] This was a case-control study that compared schizophrenic subjects who had received some type of spiritual healing with those who had not. They compared 20 patients who reported having received spiritual healing with 20 patients, matched for age, gender, and duration of illness, who did not report such experiences. Relapses over an 18-month period were examined. "Spiritual healing" was defined as excessive use of prayers, reading verses of the Qur'an or Bible for at least 1 hour each day, excessive attendance at mosques or churches (more than 5 times per week), and attending sessions that involved the use of witchcraft or exorcism. More subjects who received spiritual healing relapsed than did those who had not (17/20 vs. 12/20, p=0.03).

Relapse was particularly common among patients receiving exorcism or witchcraft (4.3 times more likely to relapse, p=0.01). Unrelated to relapse were intensity of religious beliefs or frequency of prayer/meditation. The authors concluded that spiritual healing could have contributed to relapse in these patients with chronic schizophrenia. However, this was not a clinical trial nor was it a prospective study of a spiritual intervention, and investigators could not determine whether relapses occurred immediately after the attempts at spiritual healing or long afterwards. Furthermore, investigators' definition of spiritual healing was quite atypical and involved primarily "excesses" of spiritual activity or atypical types of spiritual healing. Finally, the study was unable to determine whether frequent relapse may have in fact increased the likelihood of turning to spiritual forms of healing after more traditional treatments had failed to prevent relapse.

OTHER RELIGIOUS OR SPIRITUAL INTERVENTIONS

Lindgren and colleagues at the University of Maryland administered an individual spiritual intervention to 28 patients with serious mental illness (over two-thirds with schizophrenia).[41] This was an open trial and there was no control group. The spiritual intervention consisted of four $1^{1}/_{2}$-hour sessions designed to help subjects utilize spiritual beliefs to improve their self-esteem. Subjects that received the intervention experienced significant increases in perceived spiritual support, but there was no effect on depression, hopelessness, self-esteem, or purpose in life. Of particular note is that the intervention did not cause a worsening of symptoms in any domain.

Carson and Huss at the University of Maryland School of Nursing conducted a spiritual intervention in 20 Christian patients with schizophrenia hospitalized in a state mental institution.[42] The 10-week intervention, implemented by student nurses, involved spending one-on-one time with patients. During this time, nurses focused on prayer and scripture reading, emphasized God's love and concern, and communicated to the patient their worth and value to God. Outcomes were assessed at the beginning and at the end of the intervention, and results were compared to patients in a control group. Investigators reported that patients receiving the intervention became more verbal about concerns, expressed anger and frustration more freely, and were better able to express inner feelings. In addition, patients were more likely to want to make changes so that they could live a more normal life. Those receiving the intervention also became more articulate, had more appropriate affect, and complained less often about somatic symptoms. Again, there was no evidence of psychotic symptoms worsening as a result of discussing spiritual matters. This was not a randomized trial; a standardized outcome measure was not used; and statistical tests were not performed.

Raguram and colleagues at the National Institute of Mental Health and Neurosciences in Bangalore, India, describe the effects of living in a healing temple in South India.[43] The temple was built in the middle of a graveyard over the tomb of a Hindu holy man who lived in the village a century ago. This had become a popular place of healing, according to reports by people living in the area, and benefits seemed to be especially notable in people with serious psychiatric disorders (as for the shrine of St. Dymphna in Gheel, Belgium). In this study, investigators examined 31 consecutive subjects who came for help and stayed at the temple over the course of 3 months. All subjects had chronic mental disorders: 23 were diagnosed with paranoid schizophrenia, 6 with delusional disorders, and 2 with bipolar disorder with a current manic episode. The severity of psychopathology on the first and last day of their stay was measured using the Brief Psychiatric Rating Scale (BPRS). The 3-month stay at the Hindu temple resulted in nearly a 20% reduction in BPRS scores. Interviews with family caregivers also indicated that subjects had improved during their stay at the temple. The authors stated that this level of improvement was similar to that seen with psychotropic drugs, and hypothesized that such improvements might help to explain the better outcomes for schizophrenia reported in low-income, traditional societies.[44] Again, this was not a clinical trial and there was no control group.

Involving a leader from the faith community in treatment may help in the management of persons with severe mental illness. Sam Tsemberis, executive director of Pathways to Housing in New York City, and Ana Stefancic, in the Department of Psychology at New York University, discuss the case of a 68-year-old homeless, mentally ill Puerto Rican man who believed he was possessed by evil spirits causing his mental problems.[45] He was involuntarily committed twice to stabilize his medical illness, but refused to cooperate with treatment and was soon back on the streets. Given his spiritual beliefs, doctors made efforts to arrange for a visit with a spiritist *(espiritista)* to see if this would help. After one visit with the spiritual healer during his second hospitalization, which involved a spiritual history and rituals to rid the man of demons, he began to participate in his medical treatment and after three years has not been back in the hospital. This demonstrates the power that traditional beliefs may have over a person's mental state and the importance of including culturally sound spiritual input in treatment. Given that there are over 3 million Puerto Ricans in the United States and that 30% to 60% have consulted spiritist mediums at some point in their lives, inquiry about spiritual concerns is an essential component of mental health treatment.[46]

In summary, sensible religious interventions in persons with mental disorders do not appear to worsen psychiatric illness or psychotic symptoms. In some patients, these interventions seem to produce benefit, especially if patients are religious to begin with. Thus, there is sufficient evidence to move cautiously ahead in designing psychiatric interventions for the treatment of specific disorders that consider and possibly utilize the religious beliefs of patients to promote healing. This applies to both persons with emotional problems and those with severe, persistent mental illness.

Limits and Dangers of Religious Treatments

Mental health and religious professionals need to be aware of the limitations and dangers of using religion in mental health treatments.[47] Problems can result if mental health professionals step beyond their boundaries of competency by addressing issues that lie in the expertise of religious professionals, or alternatively, if religious professionals overstep their level of expertise in mental health matters. The responsibility of the therapist lies primarily in helping patients understand how their religious beliefs either help or hinder their way of coping with problems. Asking questions to help patients clarify their thinking about religious struggles is almost always better than giving advice about religion. When there are similarities in religious background, the therapist may be tempted to resolve ideological problems for the patient by providing correct religious views.[48] However, this is not recommended. Experience suggests that attempts to correct patients' religious views can result in religious debates or overextension of the therapist into a position that he or she cannot defend due to lack of religious expertise.

Furthermore, therapists must we aware that their own religious beliefs can hinder their ability to objectively evaluate patients' problems. On the one hand, the therapist with conservative religious views may consciously or unconsciously impose those views on a patient intent on getting an abortion, having sex outside of marriage, cheating on a spouse, or having a homosexual affair. Such behaviors by patients may elicit feelings of distain or disgust in therapists, interfering with their ability to address problems objectively and rationally. On the other hand, nonreligious therapists may dismiss the fundamentalist or conservative religious views of patients as regressive or prudish, and thereby seek to alter patients' religious beliefs that may ultimately undermine an important source for coping. These "counter-transference" reactions are very common and must always be guarded against by both religious and nonreligious therapists alike.

Until they have taken a sufficiently detailed spiritual history, therapists should not assume that a patient is religious or that a religious patient has a good relationship with his or her religious community. This is particularly true if a religious or spiritual intervention is being contemplated. It is always important to obtain uncoerced consent from the patient before delving into religious matters or using religious therapies. Religion is an intensely private matter for many patients, who are often skeptical that they can trust mental health professionals with this important area of their lives. Therefore, therapists without religious training should always approach this area with caution and sensitivity.

When Religion Conflicts with Treatment

How does one handle situations where religious beliefs conflict with psychotherapeutic or medical treatments? A cardinal law in such cases is "always keep lines of communication open." The therapist should try to enter into the worldview of the patient in order to understand the logic behind the patient's views. There is almost always a clear, reasonable explanation why a religious person prefers religious practices to the treatments offered by the therapist. The therapist's job is to find out why. Unfortunately, the first and natural response for most of us is to become offended. To the therapist it seems like the patient has chosen a totally irrational treatment instead of a scientifically proven therapy. This creates anger in the therapist and sometimes leads to rejection of the patient, resulting in arguments and a breakdown in communication. The patient, too, may be reluctant to disclose the reason for his or her decision to the therapist until a trust relationship has developed.

Again, no matter what the patient decides, the most important therapeutic task is to keep lines of communication open between therapist and patient. The therapist may need to accept a religious patient's decision to forego psychiatric treatment and follow the patient carefully, if this can be done without putting life in danger. If patients feel their beliefs and decisions are respected, they will be much more likely to trust and confide in the therapist, and if their own way of dealing with the situation fails, they will be much more likely to try out what the therapist is offering. On the other hand, if patients feel they need to defend themselves and their religious beliefs against an unaccepting therapist, it is likely they will delay seeking professional care even when they recognize the need for it.

In situations where religious beliefs conflict with psychiatric care, the therapist should consult with the patient's clergy (after obtaining consent from the patient). This will help the therapist learn more about the patient's religious belief system and will align the therapist with the patient's religious authority. This may involve including the clergy in a session with the patient. This will help to clarify misunderstandings about religious beliefs and help the patient to understand when he or she is inappropriately using beliefs defensively or neurotically.

Role of Religious Communities

As discussed earlier, religious communities can be important sources of support and care for those with severe mental illness. Sometimes very simple kinds of activities can make a dramatic difference in the lives of such persons. Consider, for example, the study by Katkin and colleagues who examined the effects of a community volunteer program on course of illness among schizophrenic patients.[49] Volunteers for the program in Cincinnati, Ohio, spent a couple hours each week to ensure that patients with schizophrenia took their medication, were coping adequately with life problems, and were successful in find housing and jobs. One year following the institution of this program, re-hospitalization for the 36 patients with schizophrenia in the study was 11% for the group treated by volunteers, compared with 34% for the control group receiving traditional treatments alone. After the first year, volunteers decreased the frequency of their visits to once a month. After two years, re-hospitalization of patients who received volunteer visits was 33% compared to 56% for patients in the control group.

These results have clear implications for the effect that religious volunteers spending only a few hours per week might have on the quality of life of persons with a serious mental illness. Although volunteers in this study were not specifically obtained from churches and there was no mention of religion being the reason for their volunteering, it is likely that religious motivations played at least some part. As I discussed in chapter 3, researchers have found that the strongest predictors of volunteering are religiosity, religious identity, religious socialization, extent of religious social networks, and, especially, level of involvement in church activities.[50] Volunteers are also more likely to have strong moral values about helping those who suffer.[51]

Encouraging persons with mental illness to become involved helping others with mental illness, as John of God did, is also likely to produce benefits. John's efforts to help others may have contributed to his own healing, as did Anton Boisen's. As noted earlier, there is good evidence that helping others contributes positively to mental health.[52] One research study, however, suggests that persons with severe mental illness do not value and do not expect to fulfill roles in the future that might include helping others. Boyer and colleagues in the School of Rehabilitation at the University of Montreal interviewed 29 persons with severe mental illness about their participation in occupational roles, importance of occupational roles, and patterns of occupational roles throughout their life span.[53] Although the number and variety of roles fulfilled in the past seemed very similar to those mentioned by persons in the general population, the roles that were most valued and desired for the future were that of friend, family member, home maintainer, and worker. Valued least were roles as participant in organizations, religious groups, or volunteering. This is a single study, however, and did not assess the potential that spiritually inspired volunteering might play in the lives of these persons.

Summary

In this chapter I described ten ways that religious faith can contribute to mental health. I discussed how a religious perspective on mental illness can give it meaning and purpose and have a positive impact both on the individual and on the faith community. I reviewed clinical trials that have examined the effectiveness of religious psychotherapies from Christian, Muslim, and Buddhist perspectives, and discussed clinical interventions that use religious or spiritual approaches to treat mental illness. The limits and dangers of religious interventions were discussed, especially countertransference reactions by religious and nonreligious therapists. Approaches for dealing with situations where religious beliefs conflict with psychological or medical treatments were described. Finally, the role of the faith community in providing support to those with mental illness was examined. For the remainder of this book, we now focus on what the faith community has done and what it can do to help those with emotional problems and severe mental illness.

PART III

FAITH-BASED MENTAL

HEALTH CARE

CHAPTER 7

CARING FOR THE EMOTIONALLY AND MENTALLY ILL

In this second half of the book, I move away from research on the relationship between religion and mental health, and begin to focus on the role that clergy and religious organizations play in caring for those with emotional problems or severe mental illness. Before discussing the current situation, however, I will provide some historical and theological background information that will provide important insights into the patterns of care provided by faith communities to be discussed later. Then I will examine what words such as *faith-based* and *mental health services* mean, and break down these terms into categories.

Faith-Based Social Services

Prior to 1850 in the United States, the family and the church provided all social services.[1] As reviewed in chapter 2, the concept of caring for the needy had biblical and early Christian roots: the care of widows and orphans in the Hebrew Testament, the care of the needy in the Book of Matthew and the Book of Acts, the care of ill pilgrims by monastic orders during the Crusades, the care of the poor and lepers by the Franciscans, the care of the mentally ill by religious orders such as the Hospitallers of St. John of God, the care of the poor and sick by female religious orders, and so forth. Beginning in the early 1700s, Catholic Charities was the first example in the American colonies of a faith-based organization caring for the poor, the sick, and other discarded members of society.[2]

Protestant religious organizations in Europe, such as the Young Men's Christian Association (YMCA) and the Salvation Army, sprang up in the second half of the nineteenth century in response to the growing poor population. YMCA founder George Williams came to London in 1841 as a sales assistant in a draper's shop. He and a group of fellow drapers organized the first YMCA in 1844 to address the unhealthy social conditions in big cities at the end of the Industrial Revolution.[3] They offered an alternative to the poor and to young workers: Bible study and prayer instead of life on the streets. By 1851 there were 24 YMCAs in Great Britain with a combined membership of 2,700. The first YMCA was started in the United States in 1851 in Boston. After the end of the Civil War, there were more than 700 YMCAs in full operation in the United States.

About the same time in 1852, William Booth began walking the streets of London preaching the Christian gospel to the poor, homeless, hungry, and destitute.[4] Thieves, prostitutes, gamblers, and drunkards became his first converts, and his ministry organized into what later became known as the Salvation Army. To congregations who were desperately poor, he preached hope and salvation and recruited volunteers to help them. In 1867, Booth had only 10 full-time workers, but within seven years, the number had grown to 1,000 volunteers and 42 ministers. In 1879, the first meeting of the Salvation Army in America was held in Philadelphia and rapidly grew from there. The organization had grown to such a degree that President Grover Cleveland received a delegation of Salvation Army officers, giving the organization a warm personal endorsement in 1886. Besides evangelism, the trademark of this organization was, and continues to be, its provision of services to the poor and needy (and mentally ill), especially those located in urban communities.

Another religiously motivated social action program, the Settlement House Movement, originated in England in the early 1880s and spread to the United States in 1890s.[5] This began as a religious response to the extreme poverty brought on by the industrial revolution. Volunteers lived and worked in settlement houses (which were often converted buildings in poor, urban neighborhoods) with the goal of improving the lives of poverty-stricken families by providing needed social services. These might include clubs, educational classes, and social gatherings, as well as playgrounds, education in the arts, sports and summer camps, clean-milk stations, well-baby clinics, and other programs. These settlement houses were to become precedent setting for the development of a future U.S. philosophy on providing social services.[6]

Growth of Government Services

During the 1850s and 1860s, the U.S. government first started to support programs such as the Freedman's Bureau for newly emancipated slaves (a federal program) and mental asylums, poor houses, and orphanages (state programs). In the 1870s the government responded to a major economic depression by giving direct relief to ease the depression's severity. Church and charity workers, however, discouraged direct relief, fearing that it would lead to the moral demise of the poor by encouraging dependency. Instead, they suggested addressing "personal deficiencies" so that people could help themselves. Direct government involvement, however, would soon escalate despite these early warnings.

Between 1900 and 1920, the federal government set up the Children's Bureau and the Maternal and Infant Health Services. Between 1920 and 1930, the states took over many of the services previously performed by private and religious charities. During the Great Depression years of 1930–1940, Democratic President Franklin Roosevelt offered Americans the New Deal, which created many new government-funded social programs, including the Civilian Conservation Corps (to provide jobs for young men), Works Progress Administration (to provide jobs for millions of people in civic construction projects), and especially, the Social Security Act (to provide working people with some economic guarantees and ensure benefits for the elderly and disabled).

Thus, from 1900 to 1940, social services previously provided by religious organizations or religious volunteers were slowly taken over by federal and state governments. In the 1960s, Democratic presidents Kennedy and Johnson began Job Corps, Vista, Community Action Programs, Head Start, legal services for the poor, Foster Grandparents, Department of Housing and Urban Development for low-income housing, Medicaid, Medicare, and the food stamps program. By the mid-1960s, the role that religious organizations had played in caring for the poor, the needy, the elderly, and the mentally and physically ill had become almost entirely replaced by government programs.

Social Services vs. Evangelism

The decline in social service delivery by religious organizations and religious volunteers was also a response to theological forces. After the latter part of the nineteenth century, a split occurred among religious groups within Protestant Christianity on whether or not to provide social services to the needy.

Walter Rauschenbusch, a liberal Baptist minister and later professor of church history at Rochester Theological Seminary, wrote an influential book entitled *Christianity and the Social Crisis*.[7] In this widely read volume, he described the responsibility and duty of the Christian church to provide for the physical, mental, and social needs of a growing class of poor, disenfranchised people often living in urban areas, who had been made powerless by America's switch from an agricultural to an industrial economy. Rather than emphasizing the traditional goals of evangelism, namely, the spreading of Christianity both at home and abroad through preaching and missionary endeavors with a view toward winning converts, Rauschenbusch claimed that an equal or even greater responsibility of the church should be to meet basic human needs. Rauschenbusch probably saw his "social gospel" as a type of evangelism, seeking to combine Christian faith with committed social action. He believed that Christians were charged with bringing the kingdom of God onto the earth, and one of the chief means of achieving that was through social action (based on the kingdom of God theology of Albrecht Ritschl). Out of this social gospel arose a Protestant theology that focused on the provision of social services to meet the practical needs of people, and to some extent deemphasized conservative Christian teachings on evangelism.

In reaction to the movement that Rauschenbusch championed, the more conservative branches of Protestant Christianity during the early twentieth century began to refocus their mission on maintaining correct doctrine, with a particular emphasis on evangelism. Thus, although evangelical Protestants sought to feed the hungry and clothe the poor, this was done specifically in order to convert them—not simply to provide for their basic needs. Conservative Protestant groups such as the Southern Baptist Convention today focus primarily on evangelism and mission work.[8] Although they also provide social services to the needy, this is done largely with the purpose of gaining converts or leading to spiritual transformation.[9] The same is true for the Assemblies of God,[10] the Church of God, and other conservative Christian bodies, as well as nontraditional movements such as the Church of Jesus Christ of Latter-Day Saints.

In contrast, moderate and liberal Protestants, inspired by Rauschenbusch's social gospel, were beginning to feed the hungry and clothe the poor for its own sake, whether they converted or not. As a result, "mainline" Protestant churches began large social service programs (e.g., Lutheran Services in America and, to a lesser extent, the Methodist General Board of Church and Society and the Episcopal Charities), supported by government funding in recent years.[11]

The Catholic Church, on the other hand, took a somewhat middle-ground approach in this regard. While maintaining relatively conservative Christian views (concerning the sanctity of life, and the divinity, birth, death, and resurrection of Jesus) and low-key evangelism, Catholic Charities USA (founded in 1727) has become one of the largest religious social service agencies in the United States.[12] Affiliated with it is the Catholic Health Association (founded in 1915), which is composed of more than 2,000 Catholic health care sponsors, systems, facilities, and related organizations.[13] By not pushing its evangelical mission, evangelizing by actions not words, and focusing on its social services mission, Catholic Charities has for years received large amounts of federal funds to accomplish its social service goals.

As evident from the historical review above, the divergent priorities of the different theological camps may also be reflected in the political structure of the country, with one party tending to emphasize the responsibility of the central government in providing social services and the other political party wanting to reduce central government in favor of more local control. As noted above, large social programs were instituted during Democratic presidencies following the Depression years (and also earlier in response to abuses of workers by large industries). Christians who advocate more liberal theologies have traditionally found more affinity with the Democratic Party's social agenda. Republicans, on the other hand, have emphasized the role of the individual and conservative Protestant values that tend to de-emphasize government-funded social service delivery (such as welfare, etc.).

Interestingly, the current Republican administration's emphasis on faith-based and community initiatives is viewed by some as a way to avoid

government responsibility for providing social services by putting this responsibility back on the churches. This effort has been opposed by both
ends of the religious spectrum, including even some conservative Christian
elements (i.e., Pat Robertson) threatened by the possibility that their primary mission of evangelism might be affected by government regulations.
On the other hand, Catholic Charities and Lutheran Social Services and
the Salvation Army have long been receiving federal funds under both
Democratic and Republican administrations. In 2000, these three religious
groups alone received over $4 billion in government money to provide a
range of services from assisting pregnant teens to helping the dying
through hospice services.[14] In fact, federal funding of faith-based organizations goes back to just after the Revolutionary War in the 1780s, when the
government paid the Philadelphia Bettering House, a Quaker hospital, to
provide care for wounded soldiers.[15]

The general lack of enthusiasm for social programs by fundamentalist
and some evangelical Protestant groups is a bit surprising given that it is
from the lower social classes that a significant proportion of their membership often has come. Alcoholics, drug addicts, the mentally ill, and other social outcasts are often prime targets for evangelism by these groups.
This may be particularly true for those with emotional problems and severe mental illness. A Duke University study of 853 "baby boomers" and
1,826 "non-boomers" participating in Wave II of the NIMH Epidemiologic Catchment Area Survey compared mental disorders in persons from
conservative and mainline Protestant affiliations with those in persons
from Pentecostal affiliations.[16] This study showed that Pentecostal baby
boomers had higher current and lifetime rates of mental disorder across
the board, and a similar although less striking trend was also seen among
middle-aged and older adults (see Tables 7.1 and 7.2).

Further analysis, however, revealed that the differences between religious groups on rates of psychiatric disorder were found primarily among
those who attended religious services less frequently. In fact, low-attending Pentecostals had the highest rates of lifetime psychiatric disorder of
any religious group (52%). Even more important, and especially relevant
to the discussion here, is that despite high rates of lifetime psychiatric disorder, not a single (0%) low-attending Pentecostal baby boomer had seen
a mental health professional within the previous six months. This raises
the concern, then, that such Protestant groups may go to great lengths to

TABLE 7.1 Baby Boomers (born between 1945 and 1966)

Mental/Emotional Disorder	Pentecostal	Mainline	Conservative
Depression (current)	14.5%	4.9%	2.7%
Depression (lifetime)	16.1%	9.3%	3.5%
Anxiety (current)	19.0%	5.4%	12.2%
Anxiety (lifetime)	28.9%	14.0%	17.2%
Alcoholism (current)	3.6%	2.8%	4.9%
Alcoholism (lifetime)	17.1%	9.9%	10.2%
Any Disorder (current)	27.3%	11.5%	16.2%
Any Disorder (lifetime)	42.8%	28.1%	24.9%

TABLE 7.2 Middle-Aged and Older Adults (born between 1889 to 1944)

Mental/Emotional Disorder	Pentecostal	Mainline	Conservative
Depression (current)	2.4%	3.0%	3.5%
Depression (lifetime)	4.2%	4.6%	4.8%
Anxiety (current)	7.2%	5.6%	7.4%
Anxiety (lifetime)	16.6%	11.3%	14.3%
Alcoholism (current)	7.4%	1.4%	1.4%
Alcoholism (lifetime)	17.9%	7.7%	7.4%
Any Disorder (current)	15.0%	8.6%	10.7%
Any Disorder (lifetime)	32.4%	19.2%	21.9%

"save" such people, but then tend not to follow up to ensure that they are included in the faith community and that their mental health needs are met.

Some conservative Protestant groups, such as the Mennonites and the Salvation Army, have maintained more of a balance between providing social services and evangelism. Likewise, the African American church in America has traditionally maintained both a conservative doctrine that emphasizes personal regeneration and evangelism while supporting progressive social service efforts in the community as well.

Bear in mind, also, that now in the twenty-first century the lines of division between the evangelical Christian and the mainline Protestant religious traditions have become less distinct. There are many fundamentalist groups and strongly conservative Christian congregations today that pro-vide social services by sponsoring inner-city programs for the poor, soup kitchens, shelters for the homeless, while at the same time many mainline Protestant groups are now placing a renewed emphasis on evangelism as their memberships have dwindled. Nevertheless, while many of the differ-ences described above have softened over the years, they still have consid-erable influence on the kinds of faith-based efforts toward mental health service delivery that I will describe below.

Finally, while many persons with severe and persistent mental illness and their families have experienced rejection from traditional religious communities (as noted in chapter 1 and elsewhere), studies do indicate that the attitudes of religious congregations toward the mentally ill are less negative and rejecting than attitudes of the general population.[17] No doubt, though, much work remains to be done in educating faith commu-nities about these illnesses and also allaying concerns about dangerousness and unpredictability that prevent many people of faith from reaching out to those with mental illness.

Definitions

Before going on, I would like to define what I mean by terms such as *mental health services* and *faith-based organizations*.

MENTAL HEALTH SERVICES

Under *mental health services* (see Table 7.3) I include counseling and support for anyone experiencing emotional distress. That distress could be from depression, anxiety, or stressful circumstances such as bereavement, divorce, job problems, or economic loss. Counseling and support may be for time-limited emotional problems, or may be directed at severe, persis-tent, long-term mental illness. Mental health services also include both outpatient and residential treatment programs that provide psychothera-py, pharmacological therapy, or other biological treatments for mental ill-ness, as well as case management and social services needed by those with serious mental illnesses. Social services include housing, food, job search,

TABLE 7.3 Types of Mental Health Services

Conditions	Services Needed
Emotional distress (stress, depression, anxiety, family discord)	Counseling (individual, marital, family) Friendship and support Medication management Outpatient psychiatric care Psychiatric hospitalization
Severe and persistent mental illness (schizophrenia, bipolar disorder, severe recurrent depression, severe personality disorder, severe mental retardation)	Counseling (individual, marital, family) Friendship and support Medication management Outpatient psychiatric care Psychiatric hospitalization *In addition:* Case management services Social services (shelter, food, job search and employment maintenance, legal services, family services, preventative and acute healthcare services, advocacy)

health care, and family services. Finally, mental health services also involve education of service providers, education of the general public, organization and networking of groups that provide mental health services, and advocacy for those with mental illness (at local government, national government, and health organization levels).

FAITH-BASED ORGANIZATIONS

A *faith-based organization* (FBO) is either a religious organization or a group with administrative or financial ties to a religious organization or organizations. I include groups that support and coordinate faith-based delivery of mental health services by providing contacts and educational resources to religious congregations. I also include here organizations that are not religious organizations and are not administratively tied to a religious organization, but that have as their primary mission the delivery of health services from a faith perspective. That faith perspective, however, must be rooted within an established and recognized religious tradition (Christianity, Judaism, Islam, Hinduism, Buddhism, etc.). FBOs should be distinguished from secular organizations that provide health services sensitive to the religion of clients or that utilize the religious beliefs of patients as part of the treatment they offer, although their primary mission is not faith based.

FBO CATEGORIES

FBOs that deliver mental health services may or may not include religion as part of the treatment they offer, and this helps to distinguish the various categories of FBOs that I will describe below. There are also two levels of services that FBOs provide: (1) direct care services, or (2) educational, professional, organizational, and networking services at a local or national level. Based on these considerations, I have categorized FBOs into five major groups, drawing heavily on the work of Roger Fallot. Note, however, that any particular organization may have characteristics of more than one group and that overlap is probably more the rule than the exception:

(A) Local churches, synagogues, mosques, and temples that provide counseling and other mental health and social services to members and sometimes to the broader community.

(B) Mainline and conservative Protestant groups that provide support and educational resources to religious congregations to enhance faith-based delivery of mental health services.

(C) Mainline religious groups that have set up relatively autonomous national agencies to provide social and mental health services that are largely secular in nature, but are provided because of religious mission or values.

(D) Trained religious counselors that utilize a combination of both secular and religious treatment strategies depending on the religious orientation of the patient.

(E) Conservative and/or evangelical groups within Protestantism, as well as similar kinds of groups in other religions (Islam, Judaism, etc.), who focus on the religious beliefs of patients and utilize them as a primary way of treating mental illness.

TABLE 7.4 Classification of faith-based organizations (FBOs) that deliver mental health services

Class	FBO Category	Service Provided

I. Local religious congregations	FBO category A:
	Protestant churches
	Catholic churches
	Other Christian churches
	Jewish synagogues
	Buddhist or Hindu
	   temples
	Muslim mosques
		Clergy counseling
		   Individual
		   Marital
		   Family
		Congregational volunteers
		   Companionship
		   Support
		Social services
		   Shelter
		   Food
		   Advocacy
		Spiritual & pastoral care

II. Networking and advocacy groups that support and educate religious congregations to help those with severe mental illness	FBO category B:
	Pathways to Promise
	Virginia Interfaith
	   Committee on Mental
	   Illness
	   Ministries (VICOMIM)
	   Local NAMI (National
	   Alliance for the
	   Mentally Ill) groups,
	   such as Faithnet in
	   California, that are
	   faith based
		Networking for religious
		   congregations, mentally
		   ill persons, and their
		   families
		
		Educational and referral
		   resources for religious
		   congregations
		
		Advocacy

III. National organizations tied financially/ administratively to religious group, that provide mission-driven social services	FBO category C:
	Catholic Charities
	Lutheran Social Services
	Mennonite Mutual Aid
	Salvation Army
	Association of Jewish
	   Family & Children's
	   Agencies
		Social services
		   Food & Shelter
		   Job search & support
		   Legal services
		   Family services
		   Health care services
		   Advocacy
		Counseling (usually
		   secular, but not always)
		Med management (occ.)

(table continues)

(TABLE 7.4 continued)

Class	FBO Category	Service Provided
IV. Groups that deliver faith-based mental health services, but are not connected to a local or national religious group	FBO category D: Religious counselors who mix secular and religious therapies Chaplains Pastoral counselors Samaritan counselors FBO category E: Religious counselors who focus on religious therapies Christian counseling Jewish counseling Muslim counseling	Counseling

Table 7.4 places these five FBO groups that deliver faith-based mental health services into four major categories and describes the kinds of services that they provide.

Summary

In this chapter, I have provided historical and theological perspectives on how social services once delivered by faith communities became taken over by government agencies, a change that took place in the United States during the past 150 years. I then define terms such as *mental health services* and *faith-based organizations* as they will be used in the rest of this book. This chapter is rounded out by a description of five different categories of faith-based organizations that deliver mental health services. In the following chapters, I will focus on each category of FBO, providing details on their organization and mission and examples that illustrate their functions.

CHAPTER 8

LOCAL RELIGIOUS
CONGREGATIONS (FBO CATEGORY A)

Perhaps the largest FBO category, this consists of local churches, syna-gogues, mosques, and temples that provide counseling and support prima-rily to their members, and includes mental health services delivered by pastors, priests, ministers, rabbis, imams, and other local clergy and staff, as well as companionship and support provided by volunteers from within the religious congregation.

Clergy Counseling

Clergy deliver an enormous amount of mental health services to needy persons and families. These mental health services are seldom recognized or acknowledged by mental health professionals, who are often surprised by how much mental health care clergy actually provide. In reality, clergy are often the first line of defense for emotional problems in the popula-tion. To get a sense of the magnitude of clergy-delivered mental health services, consider the following.

In 1998, according to the Department of Labor, there were approxi-mately 353,000 clergy serving congregations in the United States. This fig-ure includes 4,000 rabbis, 49,000 Catholic priests, and 300,000 Protes-tant pastors.[1] A recent review of 10 separate studies found that clergy report spending between 10% and 20% of their 40- to 60-hour work week counseling those with emotional or marital problems.[2] A quick cal-culation comes up with the following statistic.[3] Clergy spend 138 million hours delivering mental health services each year, which amounts to the entire membership of the American Psychological Association (83,000)[4] delivering services at a rate of 33.2 hours per week. Not included in the former figure is counseling done by chaplains or pastoral counselors, by nearly 100,000 full-time Catholic sisters,[5] by thousands of brothers in religious orders, or by clergy from Buddhist, Hindu, Muslim, and other religious traditions in the United States.

Evidence for the enormous volume of clergy-based mental health services has been around for decades, although seldom is highlighted in professional mental health circles. Twenty years ago, Veroff and colleagues examined the pattern of help seeking for *personal problems* in the United States between 1957 and 1976.[6] In 1957, 43% of Americans sought help from a clergyman, 30% from a physician, 18% from a psychiatrist or psychologist, 14% from some other mental health source, and 3% from a social service agency. In 1976, 39% saw a clergyman, 21% a physician, 29% a psychiatrist or psychologist, and 24% some other mental health provider.

Information on help seeking for mental *disorders* (as opposed to personal problems) has been available since the 1980 Epidemiologic Catchment Area (ECA) surveys. This was the first population-based survey of mental disorders in the population based on *Diagnostic and Statistical Manual* (DSM) definitions, and was supported by the National Institute of Mental Health. The ECA surveys determined the prevalence of psychiatric disorders and assessed use of mental health services in a sample of over 18,000 Americans in 1980–1981. According to this survey, conducted primarily in major urban centers such as Los Angeles, Baltimore, and St. Louis, 2.8% of respondents sought help for mental disorders from clergy, 12.1% from mental health professionals, and 2.8% from both.[7] What was particularly notable about this study was that the types of mental health disorders that people sought clergy for were remarkably similar to the conditions that led them to see mental health specialists. This underscored how common it was for persons to seek help from clergy even for serious psychiatric disorders—not just for worries or minor personal problems.

Joan Lafuze and colleagues from Indiana University conducted a relatively recent survey of what pastors knew about mental disorders.[8] Three conference offices of the United Methodist Church distributed surveys to pastors in Indiana and Virginia, asking them about the causes of mental disorders and their perceptions of people with mental disorders. Sixty percent (n=1,031) of those contacted completed the survey. The results indicated that most Methodist pastors had well-informed views about the causes of mental disorders, which were felt to be more likely due to chemical imbalance, excessive use of drugs or alcohol, or inherited genes, rather than inconsistent parenting, social pressure, or lack of deep religious commitment. Furthermore, 86% agreed or strongly agreed that medication helps people control symptoms, deal with day-to-day stresses, manage their relationships, and feel better about themselves.

Note, however, that 47% of pastors disagreed with the statement "Mental patients are no more dangerous than an average citizen" (only 24% agreed). This likely reflects the prevalent negative stereotyping of individuals with mental disorder. On the other hand, research does support pastors' concern about the potential for violence among those with mental disorders. That risk of violence, however, is increased only for certain disorders.[9] According to systematic reviews on the topic, there is only weak evidence that psychiatric patients pose a danger to others, particularly when patients are not psychotic and are taking their medications.[10] Rather than simply conclude that all mentally ill patients are dangerous, forensic psychiatrist Renee Binder says we should ask, "Which mentally ill, under what circumstances, are dangerous?"[11] Bergman and colleagues at St. Johns University in New York suggest that while it is true that people with severe mental illness are statistically more likely to be violent than members of the community at large, that elevated risk is true only for a small minority of mentally ill individuals, typically those suffering from acute psychotic symptoms, a substance abuse problem on top of their mental illness, multiple psychiatric diagnoses, or a co-existing severe personality disorder.[12] Educating clergy about such issues is necessary to decrease negative perceptions held toward persons with severe mental illness, negative perceptions that are even held by many clergy with four years of college and three years of divinity school (since courses on severe mental illness are not usually included in the curriculum).

There is also evidence that religious persons are more likely to blame those with chronic mental illness for their condition (schizophrenia).[13] This adds to the stigma that these disorders carry and to the exclusion of such person from religious congregations. Despite such a tendency among the religious, 80% to 90% of Methodist pastors in the study reported by La-fuze and colleagues disagreed that people with mental illnesses cause their own problems or can control their behavior and symptoms.[14] Bear in mind, however, that Methodist clergy tend to be well educated and hold mainline Protestant views toward such issues. Views of more conservative or funda-mentalist clergy toward mentally ill persons have yet to be determined.

Congregation-based Volunteers

Congregations often have programs where volunteers, trained in listening and simple counseling techniques, provide support to persons struggling with emotional or mental problems. Perhaps the largest and most widely known church-based program is the Stephen Ministry. The program is based on the biblical passage, "They chose Stephen, a man full of faith and of the Holy Spirit . . . and the Word of God increased; and the number of disciples multiplied greatly in Jerusalem . . ." (Acts 6:5–7). To become a Stephen Minister a person must receive 50 hours of formal training, followed by regular sessions of continuing education and supervision (usually twice a month). This training equips volunteers to supplement the work of the pastoral staff by giving confidential one-on-one care to church members during times of need. Stephen Ministers also serve by volunteering to visit members who are hospitalized, by being present in the church during prayer time, and by acting as support group facilitators. In these ways, Stephen Ministers greatly multiply the pastoral care a church offers to the congregation. The Stephen Ministry program is part of a ministry based in St. Louis. It involves more than 6,000 congregations in all 50 states and 10 foreign countries with 65 denominations represented.

Congregations can provide support and care in other ways, too. Social worker Jennifer Templeton works at a residential care facility in Philadelphia that serves adolescents with serious emotional and substance abuse problems. She notes that many of these young people are struggling because of situational problems due to inadequate home environments. They have often been neglected, abused, or otherwise not shown the attention and respect necessary to develop stable emotional lives. What these young people need, Templeton says, are healing communities that can serve as surrogate families to these troubled youth, providing them with the positive attention they never get at home. Church communities are ideally suited to provide this kind of support and care. The church may enlist volunteers to mentor such youth, or sponsor special educational, recreational, and spiritual programs to meet their needs. The target of such programs is often at-risk inner-city youth.

For example, Kings Park International Church in Durham, North Carolina, sponsors a Life Center that identifies neglected, emotionally or physically abused children and adolescents through the local social services agency. Volunteers from the church run the program and bring the children to worship services on Sundays, include them in the church's recreational activities, provide special recognition and awards to those who do well academically, and even involve them in drama or skit presentations for Christmas and Easter. In this way, the church makes them feel wanted, needed, and thereby meets critical psychological, emotional, social, and spiritual needs, which no doubt helps to ward off the development of later mental problems, substance abuse, and criminal activities.

AFRICAN AMERICAN CONGREGATIONS

Estimates of unmet need for mental health services are particularly high in African American communities.[15] Clergy in minority communities are a key source of mental health services, and are often instrumental in holding such communities together under the pressure of discrimination, socioeconomic deprivation, crime, and substance abuse. A survey of 635 African American congregations in the northeastern United States found that 18% of church-based programs involved some form of counseling for members.[16]

Robert Taylor and colleagues from the School of Social Work at the University of Michigan in Ann Arbor examined the process by which mental health needs are identified and addressed within African American faith communities.[17] They note that very little systematic research has been done on the role that African American pastors play in delivering mental health services. Clergy often serve as gatekeepers to the formal mental health care system,[18] and this is particularly true for the African American community.[19] There is also evidence that people who seek African American clergy first for personal problems are less likely to contact other professionals, particularly if the problem involves counseling for emotional issues.[20] African American ministers provide counseling on such diverse problems as alcohol and drug abuse, depression and anxiety, marital and family conflict, unemployment, and legal problems. Richard Mollica and colleagues at Massachusetts General Hospital (Boston) surveyed the counseling practices of 214 clergy. They found that black ministers were more heavily involved in mental health counseling than white clergy were, with 7 of 10 black ministers spending more than 10% of their time in counseling activities. Such counseling often consists of crisis intervention, as well as helping persons diagnosed with severe mental illness.[21]

Training in counseling, however, is often minimal, even among those who have years of postgraduate education, whether African American or Caucasian.[22] The level of training that clergy receive is usually quite different from that actually needed to diagnose and/or manage individuals with short-term anxiety or depression, provide counseling for those with chronic mental illness, or deliver case-worker services for the chronically mentally ill. However, this is the level and type of mental health services that black clergy often must provide. Theological background and educational training also influence the likelihood of referral of church members to mental health professionals for further treatment. Ministers with more liberal theologies and more education are more likely to do so than those with conservative theologies and less education.[23]

Interestingly, African American clergy are considerably more likely than white ministers to make referrals to community mental health centers.[24] Taylor and colleagues discuss the role of African American ministers in developing church-based programs with linkages to formal service agencies.[25] The black church has long been a leader in providing a wide range of community outreach programs, some of which involve addressing the mental health needs of black persons without access to mainstream professional services.[26]

Given the tight economy and the reduction of community mental health services by many states, which disproportionately affects African Americans, the role of the black church becomes even more important in terms of providing church-based services. There continues to be a strong ethos of community service in African American congregations that provides the motivation to meet the emotional and practical needs of those with mental illness, and their participation in community programs is greater than that by white congregations—especially in those programs that address the needs of the poor.[27] The church often functions as a mediator between African Americans and community service organizations, including community mental health centers and departments of social services.[28] A study by Billingsley and Caldwell found that 50% of African American churches indicated that they collaborated with local mental health service agencies to provide community outreach programs. Twenty-eight percent of the support provided by African American churches was emotional in nature and focused on counseling and support groups.[29]

HISPANIC CONGREGATIONS

According to the U.S. Surgeon General's report on mental health, "In the family/community-centered perception of mental illness held by Asians and Hispanics, religious organizations are viewed as an enhancement or substitute when the family is unable to cope or assist with the problem."[30] There is good data suggesting that Hispanics[31] depend heavily upon their religious faith to cope with adversity, whether that adversity has to do with physical health problems[32] or emotional problems.[33] Furthermore, studies demonstrate the importance of addressing religion and spirituality when dealing with the issues of disease and health in this population.[34]

Information on FBOs that deliver mental health services to Hispanic populations, however, is not readily available. While it is likely that Catholic FBOs in the Southwest and other areas of the country provide such services to Hispanics, there are few groups that specifically advertise faith-based services to this group. There is a national helpline called "Su Familia Helpline," but this does not appear to be faith based.[35] There is a Web site at Baylor University that provides information on Hispanic beliefs that influence health care, including information about religious beliefs.[36] This is not, however, a faith-based organization.

Mark DeHaven in the Department of Family Practice and Community Medicine at the University of Texas Southwestern Medical Center in Dallas provides a number of insights on the delivery of mental health care to Hispanics. He notes that even providing general health care to Hispanics in the Dallas area is a significant and challenging problem. When it comes to providing care for mental illness, the dimensions of the problem are staggering.

According to DeHaven, a U.S. Surgeon General's report released in late 2001 indicated that the rate of mental disorders among Hispanic Americans living in the community is similar to that of non-Hispanic white Americans. However, the rapid growth of the Hispanic-American population (currently approaching 35 million and projected to be 97 million by 2050) has created some dramatic needs. For example, although the percentage of Spanish-speaking mental health professionals is not known, only about 1% of licensed psychologists identify themselves as Hispanic. Another study indicates that there are only 29 Hispanic mental health professionals for every 100,000 Hispanics in the United States, compared to 173 non-Hispanic white providers per 100,000 white persons. Given prevailing patterns of mental health service utilization, it is difficult to imagine the level of unmet need among Latinos. The high numbers lacking health insurance in this group (37% for Hispanics compared to 16% for all Americans) further exacerbate this problem.

Hispanics in Dallas face the same issues related to language and lack of insurance that those in the nation as a whole do. DeHaven says that the National Alliance for the Mentally Ill (NAMI) Interfaith Committee of Dallas has two representatives from the two largest Catholic Churches in the city. Each of these churches conducts five masses on Sunday alone, one that accommodates 4,000 Hispanic parishioners and the other that has over 10,000. The priest at the church of 4,000 is on that NAMI committee, as is a deacon from the church of 10,000. Both of these churches and those who staff them are stretched beyond their limits as they attempt to meet the needs of parishioners. As noted before, Hispanic parishioners tend to be uninsured and low income. There are no formal mental health-related services available in either of these two Catholic churches. Rather, both the priest and the deacon rely on their NAMI Interfaith Committee contacts to help address specific problems and needs as they arise. Thus, there is no systematic approach to addressing the mental health problems of these Hispanic parishioners. Once again, the problem is largely due to the rapid increase in the numbers of Hispanics and the shortage of Spanish-speaking providers. For instance, in the Catholic Diocese of Dallas, out of the 850,000 parishioners, 66% are of Hispanic origin, significantly increased from ten years ago.[37]

DeHaven notes that he recently began working with Maria del Carmen Uceda-Gras, who is establishing a nonprofit organization and applying for local and national funding to develop a comprehensive approach to health and wellness for Latinos. Las Obras is a Dallas-based Catholic Latino health care organization founded in 2002 whose mission is:

To create and/or promote the conditions necessary for Latino families to learn, develop and share their Christian values; to provide consulting services to systems in achieving these conditions; and to create compassionate, new and original healthcare concepts that alleviate suffering of mind, body and spirit through the reclaiming of human dignity.[38]

The largest component in Ulceda-Gras's faith-based program will be mental health treatment, since her experience is that this is the area of greatest need among Hispanics in Dallas and elsewhere. Between March and September of 2003, Las Obras conducted a survey among four Catholic parishes to assess unmet needs among Latino families. They reached an estimated 3,260 Latinos in parishes located in south, north, west and far north Dallas with a 31% response rate. The survey listed symptoms indicative of unresolved past traumas, depression, and family conflicts. Results emphasized a need for Las Obras to develop replicable educational and healing models of prevention, early intervention, and aftercare services.

Uceda-Gras is currently a consultant for several of the largest providers of mental health services in Dallas and is charged with developing Hispanic-sensitive approaches to treatment. One of the components she is introducing into treatment is that of Living Scriptures, which incorporates therapeutic psychological techniques with spiritual ritual, imagery, and meditation/reflection on biblical passages. Participants are given spiritual assessments that identify their "root" problems. Groups with similar health issues embark on a five-month emotional and spiritual healing process with family enrichment psychoeducational programs to strengthen families in Christ. As a Catholic, Uceda-Gras says mental health care should be approached as a process that is, first and foremost, a journey of faith where one encounters the love of the Divine Father.

Generally speaking, the context surrounding access to and delivery of mental health services for Hispanics in Dallas appears to be one of desperate need with limited ability to respond. If anything is going to happen in the faith community, says DeHaven, it will occur through the Catholic Church, since he has not heard of other FBOs addressing this need.[39]

Model FBOs at the Local Congregation Level

Providing even basic mental health services to those with emotional problems, especially for minorities, seems to be an enormous challenge for many religious organizations. Providing services to those with severe and persistent mental illness raises the challenge to a new level. Nevertheless, model church-based organizations do exist that have successfully taken on this role. The booklet *New Models for Ministry: Serious Mental Illness and the Faith Community* provides examples of numerous such FBOs.[40] These include:

- Andrew House in Washington, D.C. (started by two Presbyterian churches)
- Ascension Homes in northeast Baltimore (started by seven churches, including Episcopal, Baptist, Presbyterian, Lutheran, Catholic, and United Methodist)
- Presbyterian Campus Ministry at New Mexico State University
- Center City Churches in Hartford, Connecticut (started by a coalition of eleven churches, including Baptist, Lutheran, Presbyterian, Catholic, and Methodist groups)
- Church Women United in Minneapolis, Minnesota
- Ecumenical Ministries of Oregon in Portland
- Gould Farm in western Massachusetts (a coalition of Brethren, Mennonite, Lutheran, Methodist, United Church of Christ, and Catholic congregations)
- Luther Place in Washington, D.C.
- New Mexico Conference of Churches
- Institute of Human Services in Honolulu, Hawaii (started by an Episcopal priest)

- San Jose Urban Ministry (sponsored by nine local churches)
- St. Francis House in Boston, Massachusetts
- 7-2-9 Club sponsored by the New York Avenue Presbyterian Church in downtown Washington, D.C.
- Women of Hope in Philadelphia (sponsored by Catholic Social Services)

According to attorney and mental health specialist Diane Engster, FBOs should not simply provide a mental health program (i.e., case management and medication management), but rather provide a *ministry* to people with chronic mental illness.[41] In addition to case management and medication, they also need religious counseling and support—*pastoring*. This might involve hospital visits, birthday cards, prayer with the pastor or pastoral staff, discussions about faith, Bible study, or involvement in church-related activities. FBOs should not simply repeat services that already exist in the formal mental health care system, or attempt to replace them.

Engster says that a program in her local church, called Agape Reservoir Ministry, operates on such a model.[42] They have a Friday night dinner to which persons with severe mental illness are invited along with volunteers from the church congregation. On this evening, no distinctions are made between volunteers and those with severe mental illness. The Friday night dinner group also subsidizes other church functions that involve persons with severe mental illness, and volunteers may go with them to church or otherwise act as friends or companions. The governing group of this church program consists of a mixture of persons with and without severe mental illness. There is an attempt to identify the gifts of these persons and utilize those gifts to truly integrate them into the program. Members of the Friday night group often do services for the community, which might include making earthquake kits to send to Central America, for example.

Another model of a local faith community that provides services to those with mental illness is the Ballard Ecumenical Homeless Ministry in Seattle, Washington. It is an outreach performed through the cooperation of about twenty churches to provide shelter, food, and socialization for a limited number of homeless, mentally ill people. It was established about eight years ago and continues to function well. For more information about this organization, contact Duane Glasscock.[43]

These are just some examples of the role that the local faith community can play in meeting the needs of persons with severe mental illness, the most neglected of all those needing faith-based mental health services.

Summary

In this chapter I describe FBO category A, the first grouping of FBOs that delivers mental health services. This category consists of local clergy, volunteers within congregations, and local faith communities who are active in delivering mental health services, either alone or together with other local congregations. I noted the huge volume of mental services that clergy provide, and how they serve at the front line in helping people deal with both personal problems and serious psychiatric disorders. Lack of training on how to diagnose and treat mental disorders seems to be a problem for many clergy, who seldom get adequate training to prepare them for this role. Minority communities (African Americans and Hispanics) appear at particular risk for being underserved by traditional mental health services, making religious organizations particularly important in filling this gap. Congregational resources for delivering mental health services also appear to be limited, although several model programs exist that have made real headway in developing effective outreach to those with severe mental illness.

CHAPTER 9

NETWORKING AND ADVOCACY

ORGANIZATIONS (FBO CATEGORY B)

Besides FBOs that actually deliver mental health services, there are national and local networking, education, and advocacy groups that exist to help religious congregations deliver services more effectively, especially to those with severe and persistent mental illness. I will now discuss some of these groups.

National Alliance for the Mentally Ill (NAMI)

NAMI is a secular organization that provides education, networking, and advocacy for patients with chronic mental illness and their families. Although a special lecture that focuses on the topic of religion and mental health is sponsored by NAMI at its annual conference, the organization is not faith based and is not an FBO. While NAMI is not faith based, it has local and state affiliates that vary in the degree to which religious faith is a recognized component of the services they offer and is part of their underlying mission. For example, the Indianapolis NAMI has a Faith Communities Mental Illness Education Committee that offers year-round educational resources (speakers, books, curricula, videos, an annual conference, an annual interfaith service, etc.) to churches in the area.[1] Most local and state NAMI organizations, however, do not have a formal committee that targets faith communities. I describe a few notable exceptions below.

NAMI OF COASTAL GEORGIA

An example of a local NAMI that works with churches is NAMI of Coastal Georgia, which serves the southeastern corner of Georgia (about three counties). Their board of directors agreed in 2002 to offer free mental health consultations to the community through the offices of Christ Episcopal Church (912-882-5308) in St. Mary's, Georgia, and King of Peace Episcopal Church (912-510-8598) in Kingsland, Georgia. These two churches have sponsored NAMI programs to help reduce the stigma and ignorance associated with mental and emotional disorders. Mental health consultations are available to anyone who calls and at no cost, although contributions are appreciated if the client is able. Other services that the NAMI of Coastal Georgia provides include: consultations to clergy; assessment, diagnosis, and recommendations; and referral for counseling and communications with the referred agency. Such help is offered without religious promotion, since churches sponsor these services for the benefit of the community. With regard to improving their outreach, physician Bryan Warren (executive director of NAMI of Coastal Georgia) suggests that the federal or state government could help by providing grant support for advertising to let the public know about their program.

NAMI-CALIFORNIA

Another example is NAMI-California, which launched its outreach to churches, synagogues, and mosques several years ago. This outreach is called FaithNet NAMI, and was started under the direction of Gunnar Christiansen, a retired ophthalmologist and past president of NAMI-California.[2] FaithNet NAMI reaches out to many different religious organizations, mainly in southern California. According to its Web site, it was established in 1994 by NAMI Orange County and in 1997 was co-sponsored by NAMI-California with the goals of: "(1) facilitating the development within the Faith Community of a non-threatening, supportive environment for those with serious mental illness and their families, (2) pointing out the value of one's spirituality in the recovery process from mental illness and the need for spiritual strength for those who are caretakers, (3) educating clergy and congregations concerning the biologic basis and characteristics of mental illness, and (4) encouraging advocacy of the Faith Community to bring about hope and help for all who are affected by mental illness."[3] FaithNet NAMI represents an online model for other state and local groups to follow.

Interfaith Compeer

Associated with FaithNet in California is Interfaith Compeer, a local organization that recruits, trains and supports volunteers from the faith community and matches them, one-to-one, with adults and children with mental illness in the Santa Cruz County area.[4] *Compeer* means a companion who is also a peer. The Interfaith Compeer team consists of the volunteer, the person with mental illness, a mental health professional, and an Interfaith Compeer staff person. Volunteers commit to an hour or two a week (or two to four hours every other week). Interfaith Compeer is connected with an international organization called The International Affiliation of Compeer Programs (IACP).[5]

IACP was started in 1973 in Rochester, New York. In 1982, the National Institute of Mental Health chose Compeer as a model program and funded the development of similar programs throughout the nation. There are now about 120 programs in the United States, Canada, and Australia. Compeer seeks to decrease isolation and loneliness, reduce the number and the length of hospitalizations, instill self-confidence, independence, and trust, and improve treatment compliance. According to its Web site, there are now 3,600 Compeer volunteers pared with 5,750 children and adults diagnosed with mental illnesses. Volunteers gave over 229,000 hours of support during 1997 at an average cost of $1,240 per volunteer. This organization (Compeer), however, does not have a faith focus or faith motivations, and therefore is not a FBO.

According to its Web site, Interfaith Compeer staff believe that friendship is priceless and therefore they charge no fees. The program is funded by foundation grants, local donors, and fundraising events. Interfaith Compeer includes on its Web site a list of mentally ill persons who need matching and a short description of each person. Most of those who volunteer have no prior knowledge or experience with mental illness. Some, however, have experienced the symptoms of mental illness themselves and have recovered to the point that they want to help someone else. Friends and family of those with mental illness may also become volunteers. Volunteers spend time with their Interfaith Compeer friend doing whatever they might do with any other friend, including have coffee and conversation, go for a walk on the beach or at the park, go out for lunch or a snack, talk on the telephone, go to a movie, window shop at the mall, or attend an Interfaith Compeer group activity.

The role that faith plays in this program is primarily as a motivation to provide comfort and support to those in need. Recall that systematic studies have shown that providing support to those with mental illness, such as that provided by Interfaith Compeer, measurably impacts the need for mental health services and acute hospitalization.[6] In fact, the Compeer Web site indicates that those matched with a Compeer volunteer experience a 70% reduction in psychiatric hospitalization, 75% reduction in use of emergency services, 78% increase in compliance with usual treatment plans, and 69% increase in compliance with medications.[7] This makes sense. People with mental illness who have a friend to talk with and encourage them are better able to cope with life problems and less likely to experience prolonged stress that precipitates illness relapses.

Interfaith Compeer is also associated with the Faith in Action program sponsored by the Robert Wood Johnson Foundation. Faith in Action is a national program started in the mid-1990s to provide support for local programs that train and coordinate volunteer caregivers to help families caring for a loved one with chronic health problems or mental illness. Faith in Action provides start-up funding ($35,000 for 2½ years) and sometimes ongoing support to programs that have started up through their funding.[8] A coalition of different religious organizations (representative of the faith groups within a community) may get together and apply for such a grant. Programs that include mental health services usually involve volunteers to provide in-home support, transportation, friendly visiting, and phone support to those with mental illness.

Pathways to Promise (PTP)

PTP is considered "the" national resource center for religious groups needing education, advocacy, or other services that address severe and persistent mental illness. Headquartered in St. Louis, Missouri, they have links to major denominational and other religious offices, and provide information about where mental health service concerns are addressed in each major denomination. Fifteen faith groups and three mental health organizations created Pathways to Promise in 1987 and continue to work with it.[9] According to its chairman, Robert Dell, Pathways sees itself as a technical assistance resource center that offers liturgical and education materials, program models, and networking information to help congregations minister to people with mental illness and their families. Dell indicates that his organization is unique both in the scope of faith groups represented and the resources they have developed. The Web site (www .pathways2promise.org) is an incredible resource for information about severe mental illness and has links to other resources, including programs in all major religious groups that address mental health issues.

At the time Pathways to Promise was starting, the New York Avenue Presbyterian Church in Washington, D.C., published the booklet referred to in chapter 8 titled *New Models for Ministry: Serious Mental Illness and the Faith Community.*[10] This report details the results of a nationwide survey of the 60 largest religious bodies in the United States, the National Council of the Churches of Christ and its 31 constituent bodies, and non-Christian groups such as Muslim, Baha'i, Buddhist churches of America, and Jewish organizations. The survey asked what kinds of services these religious bodies provided to those with severe and persistent mental illness. Of the 60 religious bodies, 22 replied: Presbyterian USA, Lutheran (two divisions), American Baptist, Episcopal, Mennonite, Brethren, Salvation Army, Christian Reformed, Assemblies of God, Reformed, Reorganized Church of the Latter-Day Saints, Christian Science, Seventh-Day Adventist, United Methodist, Christian and Missionary Alliance, Church of God, Congregational Christian, Church of the Nazarene, National Catholic Office for Persons with Disabilities, International Council of Community Churches, and Baha'i. At that time, six denominations had no policy statements or programming specifically related to serious mental illness. Only two of the 22 (Evangelical Lutheran Church in America and the Mennonite church) had years of extensive programs for meeting the needs of the severely mentally ill.

According to one of its authors, Diane Engster, this book really started the ball rolling. Prior to that time, Engster reports that the Mennonite Church was the group that did the most for those with severe mental illness. Around the time of World War II, Mennonite groups began to explore the conditions in mental hospitals. Because of the deplorable conditions, they decided to build their own mental hospitals. This history has been documented in a book by Alex Sareyan entitled *The Turning Point: How Persons of Conscience Brought about Major Change in the Care of America's Mentally Ill*, published by American Psychiatric Press.[11] Mennonite aid for persons with severe and persistent mental illness dates back to somewhere between 1910 and 1927, when a psychiatric hospital was established in Bethania, Russia. In 1947, the Mennonite Central Committee voted to establish three homes for those with severe mental illness in the eastern, western and mid-western United States: Brook Lane Farm in Hagerstown, Maryland, King View Homes in Reedley, California, and Prairie View Hospital in Newton, Kansas. In 1963, Mennonites built Oaklawn Psychiatric Center in Elkhart, Indiana. By 1989, the number of Mennonite mental health centers in the United States had increased to eight. Mennonites continue to lead other religious organizations in their commitment to the needs of this group.

Virginia Interfaith Committee on Mental Illness Ministries (VICOMIM)

In contrast to the national scope of PTP, VICOMIM provides an example of a local FBO network that seeks to increase the awareness among churches of the needs of those with mental illness.[12] Directed by dynamo Margaret Ann Holt, this United Methodist organization has been in operation since 1995. Every two years they offer a six- to ten-hour event, workshop, or conference that focuses on such questions as "Why should the church be concerned about mental illness?" "What can the church do to respond to the needs of persons within their congregation who have a mental illness, and to the needs of their families?" and "Creating a Caring Community with Persons with Mental Illnesses." In 2000, they put on an event that described the organizational structure and funding framework that faith communities need in order to carry out such ministries. In May 2002, they sponsored an event called "Dialogue with Seminaries" in which a number of seminaries sent a panel member to discuss the kind of education they are providing to seminarians to help them minister to mentally ill persons in and outside of their congregations.

VICOMIM also operates a speaker's bureau of experts willing to talk to faith communities or congregations who requests a speaker. Their Web page has many congregation-specific resources on severe, persistent mental illness.[13] Resource pages list books, pamphlets, newsletters, audiotapes, videotapes, courses, relevant Web sites, and sermons. VICOMIM works primarily at the state level, although it has made an impact at the national level as well. Articles by VICOMIM organizers have been published in the *NAMI Advocate* magazine and in the Pathways to Promise newsletter. VICOMIM has a large list-serve that sends e-mails concerning its activities to people around the United States, and publishes booklets for clergy such as *A Guide to Mental Health Care in Virginia* and *American Psychiatric Association Clergy Guide*. VICOMIM is presently in dialogue with the United Methodist Church General Board of Global Ministries to get information about mental health and mental illness into their *Congregational Health Ministries* notebook. Finally, they are lobbying to have denominational bookstores (such as the Methodist store Cokesbury) offer materials to educate clergy and laity on the topic of mental illness.

What kind of resources would help them expand their efforts? The majority of funding for VICOMIM comes from the Virginia Conference United Methodist Church, although individuals, Sunday school classes, churches, and the Virginia Diocese of the Episcopal Church also provide support. VICOMIM director Margaret Holt indicates that this ministry could use a full-time paid position, since its staff is currently made up entirely of volunteers.

Other Faith-Based Networking Groups

The Presbyterian Church also has a network that focuses on meeting the needs of those with chronic mental illness called the Presbyterian Serious Mental Illness Network, directed by Brenda Gales.[14] Several other Protestant denominations have mental illness networks that provide educational resources and consultation to member churches. While the role of the Catholic Church in meeting the needs of those with chronic mental illness has not been emphasized in this section, such efforts have been going on at many different levels for nearly 1,500 years and will be described more in the next chapter.

Summary

Networking and advocacy groups make up this FBO category B. These groups are different from local clergy and congregations that deliver services (FBO category A) and different from large faith-based social services agencies that include secular mental health care as part of what they do (FBO category C). Their unique role exists in helping to educate local faith communities and serve as resource centers that faith communities can turn to for information and guidance. Some groups (like Interfaith Compeer) provide practical ways for members of faith communities to help those with serious mental illness.

CHAPTER 10

MISSION-DRIVEN FAITH-BASED

SERVICES (FBO CATEGORY C)

Several mainline religious groups have set up relatively autonomous agencies to provide social services. They are similar to and often linked with religiously affiliated medical centers and hospitals, which would also be included in this FBO category. Such groups provide services to all those in need regardless of their religious beliefs or commitment. Services do not depend primarily on the religious belief of the patient and, in contrast to FBO category E, they do not typically utilize religious beliefs or practices as part of the treatments they offer. While respecting and sometimes utilizing the religious resources of patients to facilitate emotional healing, this is not their primary goal. Their actions are more driven by their faith-based mission to care for the poor and needy, rather than a desire to mobilize persons' spiritual resources for healing. Examples of such groups at the national level include Catholic Charities, Lutheran Social Services, Mennonite Mutual Aid, and Association of Jewish Family and Children's Agencies. Included here are nondenominational and interfaith organizations such as the Salvation Army. All of these groups have both local chapters and a national organization that help to fund, administrate, and monitor the activities of local groups.

Catholic Charities USA

Catholic Charities' national office in Alexandria, Virginia, seeks to provide leadership, technical assistance, training, and other resources to assist local agencies to more effectively serve their communities. According to their Web site, Catholic Charities addresses human needs and social injustices, and advocates for social policies that reduce poverty, improve the lives of children and families, and strengthen communities. At the local level, Catholic Charities staff and volunteers seek to help people become self-sufficient. The kinds of mental health services they offer include counseling, emergency financial assistance, emergency shelter, housing assistance, job training, prison ministry, refugee and immigration assistance, soup kitchens and food pantries, and treatment of substance abuse.

Catholic Charities USA serves nearly 10 million people each year through 1,400 local Catholic Charities organizations, ranging from providing a bag of groceries at a food pantry to individual and family counseling, to providing child care to needy families so that parents can work.[1] In 1999, Catholic Charities had 50,488 paid staff and 201,034 volunteers and board members. Its income was $2.34 billion and expenditures $2.26 billion. Sources of income included state and local government (53%), program fees (18%), church/community support (12%), federal government (9%), United Way (3%), and other sources (4%). Nearly 90% of expenditures went to support programs. In 2000, Catholic Charities and its network of 175 diocesan agencies reported providing 547,732 clients with counseling/mental health services.[2] Local branches of Catholic Charities are present in all 50 states, four U.S. territories, and throughout Canada.[3] For example, Catholic Social Services of Muskegon (CSSM) serves six counties in western Michigan.[4] They provide two areas of mental health service: behavioral health and child welfare services. In operation since 1947, their mission is to serve all people in need. The Behavioral Health Services (BHS) division serves both individuals and families (approximately 900/year), and includes substance abuse services to both adults and children. BHS is funded by government dollars, private pay, insurance, and charity dollars (both United Way and the Catholic Church). CSSM is accredited by the Council on Accreditation and does not use religious beliefs or practices as part of mental health therapy. The major barrier they face in delivering mental health services is access to Medicaid reimbursement, which is driven by the local community mental health agency and has nothing to do with their being a Catholic agency.

Lutheran Social Services

Faith-based mental health services have been provided by Lutherans for the past 150 years, dating back to the sponsoring of orphanages during the Civil War. They have had U.S. government contracts to serve the poor since 1920. The umbrella organization, Lutheran Services in America (LSA), was formed about five years ago. The network under LSA is now the largest nonprofit in the country based upon their combined operating revenues ($6.9 billion/year).[5] Of course, if Catholic Charities USA and the Catholic Health Association combined forces, they would be much larger than LSA. However, with regard to faith-based social service agencies, LSA ranks first in size.

LSA is an alliance of the Evangelical Lutheran Church in America, the Lutheran Church-Missouri Synod, and their 280 human service organizations that operate in over 3,000 communities across the United States. Their mission is to "support members' ministries of service and justice by creating a unified system to build and maintain relationships and resources." According to their Web site,[6] LSA serves over three million people annually regardless of race, gender, or religious beliefs, and works through more than 138,000 employees and over 130,000 volunteers. LSA does not have control over all of the 280 organizations within its umbrella, but rather networks with them, seeks to influence public policy, and helps with leadership development and determination of best practices.

Lutheran Social Ministry Organizations offer a wide spectrum of services to children and families, to older people, and to people with disabilities. Some of the services they offer include:

- adult day care
- advocacy
- alcohol and substance abuse services
- addiction counseling
- AIDS ministries
- care team ministries
- chaplaincy
- children's residential services
- consultation and development programs for pastors
- congregations and community groups
- counseling/behavioral health
- employment services
- food
- shelter
- emergency aid

- foster care
- adoption
- hospice
- housing

- ombudsman services
- prison ministries
- refugee resettlement

They also provide services to older persons (including senior companion, assisted living, and nursing care), residential (or long-term hospital) care, and other services for people with disabilities. According to LSA's 1999 annual survey, approximately 60% of services were for hospital care, 25% for social services, 3% for residential care (long-term care), and 13% for emergency assistance. In 1999, more than 130,000 people received mental health counseling services through LSA.

Many different organizations are included in the umbrella organization LSA, some with special niches such as providing nursing care for the elderly, residential treatment for kids, help for refugees, and other services. Some organizations serve only specific counties or regions. According to Jill Schumann,[7] president of LSA, a number of groups work specifically with persons who have severe and persistent mental illness. They provide housing and residential treatment as well as inpatient care when needed. Persons from all religious faiths are served. LSA organizations are located in every state in the union except Hawaii, although the range of services varies by state. Mental health care is funded by fee for service (private pay), third party payers, foundation grants, government contracts (social service block grants, county mental health monies, state monies), and contributions from local churches. Sources of support are broken down as follows: 52% from client fees, 39% from government, 4% from investments, 2% from community support (including United Way and Lutheran church support), and 3% from other sources.[8] Patients are served regardless of ability to pay, and when they do pay, the amount is determined by a sliding scale. Service providers in the Lutheran system are all well credentialed, typically with a Ph.D. or M.S.W.

Is religious faith used as part of the treatment for mental health problems? This varies across groups within LSA. Although faith tends to be the motivation for the organizations' existence, religion is not part of what is delivered to clients. Even in chemical dependency programs, they may refer to Alcoholics Anonymous but will not insist on the person's definition of their "higher power." Mental health counseling is often congregationally based, where the congregation hosts the agency's counseling office in a church. This is similar to how Catholic Charities operates. Some organizations within LSA define their service providers as pastoral counselors and extend to people the opportunity to deal with religious issues. This, however, would not be done under government contract, but rather through private pay or congregation-subsidized services (several congregations might get together to hire a pastoral counselor). Currently, LSA is struggling with what it means to be a faith-based organization, what differentiates it from other service providers, and how to show respect for non-Christian therapists and clients. Patients are probably more likely to be asked the question, "And what about your faith?" taking into account an understanding of their spiritual resources in treatment, although those resources would not typically be used as part of the therapy.

LUTHERAN CHILD AND FAMILY SERVICES OF ILLINOIS

An example of a local LSA organization is Lutheran Child and Family Services of Illinois. According to its director of clinical services, Brent Diers,[9] this is a statewide social service agency certified by the Council on Accreditation and affiliated with the Lutheran Church-Missouri Synod. Founded in 1875, their annual budget is now about $20 million. They provide a wide range of social services, including adoption, foster care, food and clothing distribution, mentoring, and in-home services to families. The services that fall into the mental health category include family counseling and residential treatment. The residential program provides intensive services to severely emotionally disturbed children and their families, services that are funded through Medicaid.

Family counseling is available in about twenty-five sites across the state of Illinois. All counselors have master's degrees in social work, counseling psychology, marriage and family therapy, or related fields. The counselors are licensed by the State of Illinois. The majority of these counselors are based in offices in Lutheran churches. About 1,500 clients received services from these counselors in the past year. They provide counseling to a wide range of clients, including those with depression, anxiety, end stage of life, marriage, family, and parent-child issues. In most cases, therapy is relatively short term, although they may also have clients who have been in treatment for months or even years. Counselors often coordinate services with psychiatrists when clients require medication. However, they don't generally treat persons with severe and persistent mental illness.

This program serves all persons who seek help regardless of religious affiliation. Their counselors are comfortable providing therapy within a Christian framework for those who request it. However, clinicians provide therapy that is appropriate for wherever religious background the client may be coming from. Their funding comes from a highly diverse mixed-payer base. Clients may be private pay, have insurance coverage, or be supported by United Way or Lutheran church donations. They also have a variety of contracts with companies and schools. Services are paid on a sliding scale, sometimes as low as $25 per session.

LUTHERAN COMMUNITY SERVICES NORTHWEST

An example of another local program is Lutheran Community Services Northwest (LCSN), which covers Oregon, Washington, and Idaho, and has been in existence for over seventy-five years. According to its director, Bruce Strade,[10] LCSN provides an entire range of services, from counseling those with acute mental health problems to treating persons with severe and persistent mental illness. In some areas, they have the contract in the counties to operate as the Community Health Center. In other areas, they are a Medicaid service provider. In some cases LCSN may be the only mental health service provider in town. In most offices mental health professionals offer medication management. However, 24-hour crisis and case management are only provided in offices where they are the county mental health authority and LCSN provides no residential services for those with severe mental illness. Their active caseload is between 8,000 and 10,000 patients, and services are provided to all persons who seek help. LCSN also has the largest refugee program in the Lutheran system. They are funded through client fees, government contracts, insurance, private donations, congregational and denominational support, United Way, foundations, and other sources.

When asked whether the patient's religious faith is utilized as part of the mental health services they offer, Strade says that LCSN's religious beliefs determine their values and are part of the motivation for providing services. However, religious faith or beliefs would only be used within the therapy process if that were part of a client's worldview. They do not impose their belief system on patients because they believe this would be exploitive, especially at a time when the client is vulnerable, and therefore unethical. They provide services "because they are Lutheran, not to turn people into Lutherans."

GLADE RUN LUTHERAN SERVICES

A third local LSA program is Glade Run Lutheran Services in Zelienople, Pennsylvania. According to executive director Charles Lockwood,[11] this is a JCAHO-accredited mental health organization that primarily serves children (ages 6 to 18), but also provides care to adults and families. Their programs run along two continuums. One continuum is degree of structure, from very supervised to more independent functioning. The most highly structured program is the residential treatment facility that requires a psychiatric diagnosis for admittance. They currently have a capacity of 61 in that program and are moving to a capacity of 117. Less structured programs include community mental health services and therapeutic animal and horticulture programs. They also have a private licensed school that serves residential treatment facility clients. The second continuum is the kinds of mental health services that are provided. Glade Run has residential services where clients live in the facilities and also have in-community services that are provided in an outpatient center or a family's home. In addition, they provide social services such as foster care and independent living assistance that are not funded with mental health dollars. Glade Run has about 400 employees with varying levels of education and credentials.

HELPING THOSE WITH SEVERE MENTAL ILLNESS

Among Protestant denominations, the Lutheran and Mennonite churches have been at the forefront in meeting the needs of persons with mental illness. Prior to 1983, however, there was no focused effort by Lutherans to help those with severe mental disorder. At that time, the Lutheran Church began a new initiative by contacting and bringing together persons with severe mental illness, their families, representatives from congregations with ministries to the mentally ill, and representatives of Lutheran social service agencies. The "Initial Consultation on Chronic

Mental Illness" convened for the first time in October 1983, and began a national effort to increase education and awareness about severe mental illness. It did so with regional meetings, newsletters, pamphlets, and videotapes, as well as by encouraging clergy to obtain training in seminary and continuing education (CE) courses.

In 1987, the Lutheran Charities Foundation (LCF) provided financial support for an interfaith conference in St. Louis that involved the National Council of Churches and the National Alliance for the Mentally Ill. Five post-conference seed grants were offered by LCF to implement projects in order to meet the objectives of the conference. There was a second national conference in 1988, which helped give birth to Pathways to Promise (see chapter 8). This occurred about the same time that Harris and colleagues put together their 1989 report referred to in chapter 11 (*New Models for Ministry: Serious Mental Illness and the Faith Community*).[12] According to Diane Engster, Lutherans (Church of the Missouri Synod) provided total funding support for Pathways to Promise during its first two to three years of existence. However, I was unable to acquire further information available on LCF mental health activities between 1988 and 2004.

Mennonite Mutual Aid (MMA)

MMA is a church-related organization that helps Mennonites and Anabaptists to practice biblical stewardship. MMA offers expertise in pursuing stewardship solutions through insurance and financial services as well as charitable-giving programs and fraternal benefits. Within the fraternal benefits section is the Mental Illness Consultant Ministry (MICM). MICM provides education and resources to all Anabaptists and other faith groups across the United States on mental illness. This is accomplished in a number of ways. First, workshops are held in local congregations (with titles such as "Mental Illness and OUR Church," "Understanding Depression," and "Supporting the Family in Need"). Second, two retreats per year are held for family caregivers of those with mental illness ("Streams in the Desert Weekend Retreat"). Third, there is an Anabaptists Mental Health Provider Network created for persons who want a mental health provider with professional expertise, Anabaptist connections, and Christian-based practice. A list of providers in this network and detailed information about them can be acquired from MICM or their Web site.[13] Fourth, MICM produces several print resources for local congregations to help them better understand mental illness (e.g., "A Christian View of Mental Illness," "Mommy Stayed in Bed This Morning," "Becoming an Accessible Congregation"). Fifth, MICM provides resources on specific diagnoses. Sixth, it provides consultation to pastors, families, and individuals who are trying to understand mental illness. Finally, it has Sharing Fund programs that provide financial assistance to congregations for mental health services to individuals and families in need.

MICM's ministry to the mentally ill is from a Christian perspective with an Anabaptist focus. All resources, workshops, and events are presented from a Christian perspective (so in this respect it is similar to FBO types D and E). Even though the ministry is designed for Anabaptists, it is accessible to all denominations. The Mental Illness Consultant Ministry is funded by MMA. Anabaptist mental health organizations include: Association of Brethren Caregivers,[14] King View Mental Health System,[15] Oaklawn,[16] Meadow Lark Homestead,[17] Prairie View,[18] Brook Lane Health Services,[19] Ben-Ela Child Development Center,[20] Penn Foundation,[21] Philhaven,[22] Family Life Resource Center,[23] and No Longer Alone Ministries.[24] The Mennonite Church has long been a leader in providing mental health services, especially to those with severe mental illness.

Salvation Army (SA)

The Salvation Army is a Protestant, nondenominational, interfaith, international Christian organization, one of whose purposes is to provide services to those in need.[25] A recent book entitled *Red-Hot and Righteous: The Urban Religion of the Salvation Army* details the origins of this organization, which is perhaps best known for its used-clothing stores.[26] It is difficult to decide whether SA should be categorized as an FBO-type C or an FBO-type E, given its strong evangelical emphasis. From the start, however, the SA's goal has been to minister to the physical/mental as well as to the spiritual needs of people, including the running of soup kitchens and other projects designed to provide physical assistance to the poor.

Founded in 1878 by William Booth, a Methodist minister, the SA took the form of a military organization in its war against evil. With that came uniforms and a chain of command. The first branch of the Salvation Army in the United States was established in Pennsylvania in 1880 by a small group of followers from England. In 1934, the SA became an international organization with Booth's daughter, Evangeline Booth, as the acting general. The SA now has 14,000 centers of worship in 100 countries throughout the world, with its international headquarters in London and a local headquarters in New York City.

SA corp officers have the same professional status as ordained ministers and work on a full-time basis committed to their religious duties and serving others in need.[27] Officers must spend two years at a Salvation Army training college and on graduation receive a rank of "lieutenant," which increases to "captain" after five years of service and "major" after fifteen years of service. Both men and women are equally accepted as officers in the SA. Officers may also serve outside the church in social service agencies, Goodwill community centers, or in administrative roles in central offices. They are expected to be "ready for duty at any time of day or night, when people turn to them for help." The tasks of SA officers include preaching, evangelism, hospital visitation, prison work, counseling, conducting religious ceremonies, and administering church programs.

In keeping with its military form, regular members of the SA are called "soldiers." Soldiers must accept a standard of moral behavior that includes avoidance of smoking and alcohol. It is up to them whether they wear uniforms as a witness to their faith, unlike officers who are required to do so. Many have their own jobs out in the community like members of any other religious denomination. If, however, they accept responsibilities in the SA, then they must wear uniforms, comply with the doctrine of the SA, and provide their services free of charge. There is also a category of members called "adherents" who attend services and SA gatherings, but who do not wear uniforms or take on the responsibilities of a soldier.

The SA provides a vast array of social, medical, and community services to those in need.[28] Volunteers and full-time personnel meet both emergency and nonemergency situations as they arise. The SA provides a place to sleep for nearly 30,000 homeless people each year in its 539 hostels, and runs more than 2,000 food distribution centers and feeding programs.[29] The SA operates 300 occupational centers that provide job rehabilitation to people trying to put their lives back together. It has 780 residential care centers that house over 16,000 older persons, 352 hospitals that provide care to over 27 million patients, 30 convalescent homes, and 30 special homes that provide accommodations for 1,600 physically handicapped persons each year. They even have 2 leprosaria that treat over 360 leprosy patients. In addition, the SA helps more than 2.5 million families each year and runs 130 centers for the care of refugees without resources.

With regard to mental health, the SA runs 152 centers for alcoholics and drug addicts, helping more than 15,000 people a year. Members of the SA assist in over 200,000 police court cases, visit 450,000 prisoners per year (and help after their release), and run 106 probation programs that accommodate over 4,000 youth offenders. The SA provides anti-suicide counseling that helps more than 220,000 people and provides mental health counseling to an additional 235,000 people per year. Because of their evangelistic focus, the SA may be more likely than Catholic Charities, LSA, or AJFCA to utilize religious beliefs as part of its services. However, mental health expert Roger Fallot[30] puts the SA in the same category as Catholic Charities and Lutheran Social Services.

Association of Jewish Family and Children's Agencies (AJFCA)

AJFCA is an organization consisting of over 145 Jewish family, children's, and specialized human service agencies throughout the United States and Canada.[31] AJFCA indicates that it is a vital force in Jewish life, providing social and human services to the most vulnerable in the community.[32] The organization, which has been in existence for 30 years, helps Jews wherever there is a need. Governed by a board of 65 lay and professional leaders, the organization represents a wide spectrum of interests and orientations. AJFCA has an operating budget of over $900,000, and in the year 2000, its member agencies spent over $400 million on families, including over $23 million on resettlement services.

AJFCA encourages Jewish communal assistance for Jewish refugees and immigrants from other countries, developmentally disabled adults and children, adults and children with psychological or social problems, Holocaust survivors and their families, the elderly and their caregivers, and individuals with addictions and illnesses such as AIDS. AJFCA advocates for the Jewish family and community, supporting local agencies in their efforts to sustain and enhance the quality of Jewish life. It facilitates local agency involvement in organizations such as the Conference on Jewish Material Claims against Germany and the National Center for Jewish Healing. It provides consultation, executive search services, and information resources on programming and administration, including resettlement. It sponsors conferences, institutes, and small group education and training opportunities, and seeks to influence public policy with legislative monitoring and advocacy. Finally, it publishes the *Tachlis* newsletter, the *Professional Opportunities Bulletin*, and the *Executive Digest*. The AJFCA directory contained on its Web site includes current information about every AJFCA agency, such as the services it offers and a link to a local agency's Web site if it exists.

Summary

In this chapter I discussed several national organizations that exemplify mission-driven FBOs: Catholic Charities, Lutheran Social Services, Mennonite Mutual Aid, Salvation Army, and Association of Jewish Family and Children's Agencies. Mission-driven FBOs usually provide services to those with mental illness out of a desire to care for the poor and needy, rather than to mobilize the persons' spiritual resources for their healing. Nevertheless, some organizations such as Lutheran Social Services and the Salvation Army will take the patient's religious beliefs into consideration when providing psychological care and also provide pastoral care services for those who desire them. The distinctiveness of this particular category of FBO, however, is that religious values provide the motivation for delivering the services, and they do not usually use religion in the treatment process. This is quite different from the next FBO group, which seeks to use and integrate religion into treatment itself.

CHAPTER 11

FAITH-INTEGRATED

COUNSELING (FBO CATEGORIES

D AND E)

While FBOs in chapters 8, 9, and 10 provide counseling either by local clergy (FBO category A) or by trained secular counselors (FBO category C), there is not usually an attempt to combine faith-based and secular therapies. FBO category D consists of clergy who undergo the training necessary to certify them as professional counselors and have the acquired skills to fully integrate religious therapies with secular psychotherapy (chaplains or pastoral counselors). FBO category E consists of trained counselors, usually without professional religious training, who emphasize faith-based therapies in the treatment of their patients (Christian counselors, for example).

Chaplains and pastoral counselors are often a blend of FBO categories C and E, providing a mixture of secular and religious treatments depending on the patient and the condition. They include chaplains, pastoral counselors, and Samaritan counselors, and other religious professionals who are certified by their national organizations to provide mental health and counseling services.

Chaplains

Chaplains have provided counseling and support to hospitalized patients on a widespread basis since the end of World War II. They also provide such services in the military, prisons, psychiatric hospitals, and nursing homes. It is important to realize that chaplains do not displace local clergy, but rather fill specific needs related to intense medical or psychiatric settings that complement the activities of congregation-based clergy.[1] Because of the high prevalence of depression, anxiety, and other mental health concerns of medical patients when hospitalized, these needs often overwhelm the social and psychiatric services available in the hospital to meet them. Consider the fact that nearly 50% of medically ill hospitalized patients have either major or minor depressive disorder,[2] many of whom receive no treatment at all—neither psychotherapy nor antidepressant drugs.[3] The situation is even worse in nursing homes, where emotional problems and severe mental illness are even more common than in the acute hospital setting, and mental health services are not readily available.[4] It is the chaplain in many cases who meets the psychological and spiritual needs of these patients.

Today in the United States there are approximately 10,000 chaplains in full-time practice or training programs. The four largest organizations are the Association of Professional Chaplains (APC) (with 3,700 members, formed in 1998 by the merging of the College of Chaplains and the Association of Mental Health Clergy), the National Association of Catholic Chaplains (NACC) (4,000 members), the Association of Clinical Pastoral Education (ACPE) (1,000 members), and the National Association of Jewish Chaplains (NAJC) (400 members). Other chaplain organizations in the United States include American Protestant Correctional Chaplains Association, Chaplaincy Commission of New York Board of Rabbis, Council on Ministries in Specialized Settings, International Conference of Police Chaplains, National Conference on Ministry to the Armed Forces, and National Institute of Business and Industrial Chaplaincy.

In order to be certified by the Association of Professional Chaplains, a person must complete four years of college, three years of divinity school, and anywhere from one to four years of clinical pastoral education (CPE). This involves a minimum of 1,625 hours of clinical supervision counseling persons with health problems—4 units of CPE. In addition, certification requires a written and an oral board examination. Thus, chaplains are highly trained professionals able to address the psychological, social, existential, and spiritual needs of persons with physical or mental illness. Chaplains provide 10 to 15 million hours of counseling each year.

The benefits of chaplain services have been documented by systematic research. In a survey of 432 patients at six hospitals in Pennsylvania that examined how patients felt about the helpfulness of various hospital personnel, Parkum found that more patients reported visits from chaplains as helpful (67%) than visits from social workers, patient representatives, and volunteers combined (51%).[5] In this study, patients indicated that chaplains were also more likely to meet their need for individual expression (called "expressive needs") than were social workers, patient representatives, or volunteers.

Chaplain visits have been shown to predict a decrease in pain and stress level,[6] less need for medication, and shorter hospital stays.[7] Chaplains also meet the psychological and spiritual needs of hospital staff. One study found that 73% of intensive care physicians and nurses indicated that providing comfort for staff is an important role of the chaplain, and 32% believed chaplains should be available to help staff with personal problems as well.[8] Despite the demonstrated relationship to patient satisfaction, reduced use of health services, and low cost ($2.71 to $6.43 per patient visit,[9] which costs the same as two hospital Tylenol[10]), chaplain programs are being downsized or eliminated in many institutional settings. In a recent survey of 370 randomly sampled pastoral care department directors, 27% reported budgetary cutbacks.[11] The State of Georgia eliminated all full-time chaplaincy positions in state prisons and psychiatric facilities in 1991 because of state budget problems.[12] Chaplains tend to be clinically oriented, and therefore seldom conduct research that documents the benefits they provide to patients. In the cost-conscious hospital environment of today, *that* can be a liability.

CLINICAL PASTORAL EDUCATION

Training programs for chaplains exist in hospitals affiliated with academic or large regional medical centers and/or universities with a divinity school. These are called clinical pastoral education programs and are members of a national organization called the Association of Clinical Pastoral Education (ACPE). ACPE describes itself as "a multicultural, multifaith organization devoted to providing education and improving the quality of ministry and pastoral care offered by spiritual caregivers of all faiths through the clinical educational methods of clinical pastoral education (CPE)."[13] ACPE has 3,300 members, approximately 350 accredited centers, and 600 certified CPE supervisors. It also has 118 theological schools and 21 faith groups who have officially partnered with ACPE to provide CPE training.

CPE exposes clergy (seminary students or ministers who go back for such training) to patients in hospital settings and teaches them how to address the issues that these patients grapple with.[14] Many seminaries (although not all) require 1 unit of CPE training before students can receive their master's of divinity degree (necessary for ordination in some mainline denominations). If seminary students wish to go on and specialize in chaplaincy, they require 3 additional units of CPE training (which typically takes about one year to complete). Those who wish to be CPE supervisors may need to take anywhere from one to three additional years of training. CPE training involves direct contact with sick patients and feedback from peers and supervisors on how to meet these patients' needs. In this way, the student develops skills in interpersonal relationships with patients and inter-professional relationships with health care providers.

CONTRACT PASTORAL CARE

In 1999, an entire issue of the *Journal of Health Care Chaplaincy* was devoted to describing a new trend of freestanding pastoral care and CPE training organizations that provide chaplains on contract to local hospitals.[15] The *Journal* describes nine such organizations:

The Ecumenical Institute (Cherokee, IA)
The Foundation of Interfaith Research and Ministry (Houston, TX)
The HealthCare Chaplaincy (New York, NY)
Interfaith Healthcare Ministries (Providence, RI)
Lutheran Chaplaincy Service (Cleveland, OH)
The McFarland Institute (New Orleans, LA)
Marketplace Ministries (Dallas, TX)
The Northern Rockies Clinical Pastoral Education Center (Billings, MT)
Rocky Mountain Pastoral Care and Training Associates (Littleton, CO)

Many of these organizations started up in response to the changing structure of the health care system in the mid-1990s, with many pastoral care departments based in hospitals being downsized and chaplains losing their jobs. Typically, chaplains are trained and hired by hospitals, and receive their retirement income from this source as well. The financial base for chaplains, however, has become unstable in the current health care environment. Out of this anxiety and desire by chaplains for more security arose the freestanding centers. The founders of these centers were typically a single individual or a group of persons with commitment and vision who saw that the reduction in chaplain services due to hospitals efforts at cost containment had to be countered because many patients had spiritual needs and no one was addressing them. These freestanding centers train chaplains and then contract them out to local hospitals, nursing homes, or rehabilitation centers—institutions that either don't have their own chaplain service or have a service that is inadequate to meet the needs of their patient population.

HEALTHCARE CHAPLAINCY

The largest, nondenominational, freestanding pastoral care and education center in the United States is located in the heart of New York City and in 1999 provided chaplains to 22 local medical facilities.[16] Besides providing contract chaplains, the HealthCare Chaplaincy (HCC) is a multi-faith chaplain-training program with over 300 CPE students. It is also the only Jewish and Muslim CPE training program in the United States, according to CEO Walter Smith. HCC is also involved in an extensive array of research activities (formerly directed by Andrew Weaver, Ph.D.), and serves an advocacy role for chaplains and pastoral counselors in public policy arenas. The growth of HCC has been largely attributed to the marketing expertise of its founders, who were able to tap into the philanthropy world of New York City. Private fundraising is the key to the success of all the freestanding centers, since the contracts with health care institutions pay only part of the cost of the chaplain services provided.

HOLLYWOOD VISITING CHAPLAINCY PROGRAM

An example of a local group that provides chaplain services to meet the mental health needs of persons in nursing homes is the Hollywood Visiting Chaplaincy Program (HVCP).[17] The initial idea for this program came from a community-based multidisciplinary team that focused on elder abuse and neglect. The team included senior center case managers, adult protective services, law enforcement, clergy, nursing home and board/care licensing agency personnel, community leaders, emergency response fire department personnel, and a real estate long-term care expert. After an extensive and depressing review of local nursing homes' public files, the team attempted to find ways in which the community could get involved in improving the quality of its nursing homes and providing a positive presence in some institutions. The result was the creation of a visiting chaplaincy program. The initial funding for a part-time chaplain came from the Queen's Care Foundation, a foundation created when a major, local, nonprofit hospital was sold to a for-profit corporation. The new program started in spring 2000. Within three months, HVCP was accepted in 7 (out of 22) Hollywood nursing homes, thus reaching and stretching the limits of the part-time chaplain. Under this grant, the visits were limited to patients at the poverty level, thus placing a lot of pressure on the chaplain, since other patients wanted her to visit them also (visits that were often done on her own time). They also received a small grant from Wheat Ridge Ministries, which did not allow them to operate more than half time but did allow the extension of services beyond the first year.

When the time came to renew their initial grant from Queen's Care, a conflict between board members ended its funding. Disappointed that other mental health proposals did not qualify for support, some board members of Queen's Care argued that HVCP was a mental health program and should not be funded either. Due to this controversy, the funding was not renewed. However, a $30,000 grant from the Guenther Foundation came just in time to save the program in the summer of 2001, giving them funds to operate another year, but still at a part-time level. Other grants have been denied because of the faith-based component. They continue to struggle to find funding to expand and meet the needs in their community. The dual faith-based and mental health components are seen by many as controversial and make funding a challenge.

Examples provided by HVCP Vice President Anne Marie Lardeau concerning the effectiveness of this program include the following. One patient, who had stopped speaking for several months, said her first words to greet the chaplain after a few visits. Other patients started to feed themselves again after refusing food or requiring to be fed. Many patients reported less pain or more progress during physical therapy. Often, the chaplain was the first person that patients had had a conversation with in a long time. Some patients indicate that this was the first time they had been able to talk about their fear, anger, or depression. Doctors, nurses, and orderlies are too busy and rushed to engage in this type of conversation. The rare "friendly visitors" tend to focus on happy talk and patients do not want to scare them away with a dark and depressing conversation. A chaplain is a safe person with whom even patients without strong religious beliefs can share their despair and isolation. Patients with a deep faith find additional strength from the chaplain's visits.

Pastoral Counselors

According to the national membership organization and certifying body for pastoral counselors, the American Association of Pastoral Counselors (AAPC), "Pastoral counseling is a unique form of psychotherapy which uses spiritual resources as well as psychological understanding for healing and growth. Pastoral counselors are certified mental health professionals who have had in-depth religious and/or theological training. . . . Pastoral counseling moves beyond the support or encouragement a religious community can offer, by providing psychologically sound therapy that weaves in the religious and spiritual dimension."[18] Founded in 1963, AAPC sets the standards for pastoral counseling and provides credentialing. It has a membership of about 3,000. An AAPC-certified pastoral counselor typically has four years of college, three years of divinity school or seminary, and a master's or doctoral degree in counseling or psychology. The latter must consist of at least 1,375 hours of supervised clinical experience involving individual, group, marital, and family therapy, and 250 hours of direct approved supervision working in both crisis and long-term situations. According to the AAPC Web site, pastoral counselors deliver approximately 3 million hours of treatment annually in institutional and private settings. This Web site also provides the ability to search the AAPC membership for a local pastoral counselor anywhere in the United States.[19]

AAPC-certified pastoral counselors provide a wide range of services, from marriage and family therapy to addressing a full range of mental health concerns. Where pastoral counselors focus their therapy depends on the extent and scope of their training. AAPC's code of ethics stresses practicing only in areas of competence, and otherwise referring to appropriate professionals. Major depression or bipolar disorder would normally be managed together with a physician who is evaluating and likely prescribing medication. Pastoral counseling centers typically have one or more psychiatric consultants, as do pastoral counselors in solo practice. Some pastoral counselors see persons with severe and persistent mental illness, but most clients have more acute mental health needs. Pastoral counselors do not provide residential services but frequently work with those who do, and many have privileges to follow their clients if they require hospitalization. Pastoral counselors are funded by a variety of means, principally by private pay or through provider status with managed care organizations. In pastoral counseling centers, community congregations often contribute funds to offset the loss of fees that results from seeing low-income clients at a reduced fee. The general working principal is to see all persons regardless of ability to pay, so sliding scales or discounted fees are generally used. Most centers need approximately 20% of their budget contributed from other sources in order to follow the principle of seeing all who come.

Is religious faith utilized as part of the mental health services the pastoral counselors offer? According to AAPC's Executive Director Roy Woodruff,[20] clients' religious beliefs and practices are an integral part of the therapeutic process. Disciplined, therapeutic integration is the core of the integrity of certified pastoral counselors. It is what distinguishes pastoral counselors from those who have no training in therapeutic integration and who therefore may use religious beliefs and practices in less than helpful ways. Equally important is the spiritual depth, commitment, and integrity of the pastoral counselor, and his or her spiritual formation that training stresses. In order to be certified, AAPC also requires endorsement by one's faith community.

According to Woodruff, AAPC has been recognized by a number of federal health agencies, such as the Center for Mental Health Services (part of the Division of Health and Human Services), the National Institutes of Mental Health, Federal Employees Health Benefits, the Bureau of Primary Health Care, the Armed Services through provider recognition under TRICARE (formerly CHAMPUS), and others. AAPC is currently working to achieve provider recognition under Medicare and is being reviewed by MedPAC under a mandate from Congress. They are also in the process of developing a Pastoral Counselor Provider Network of AAPC-certified pastoral counselors (see their Web site). AAPC is an active member of the Mental Health Liaison Group in Washington and supports mental health legislation such as the Dominici-Wellstone Mental Health Parity Act. Thus, AAPC also serves an advocacy group for pastoral care at the public policy level.

PITTSBURGH PASTORAL INSTITUTE

An example of a local pastoral care group is the Pittsburgh Pastoral Institute (PPI), directed by Doug Ronsheim.[21] In addition to being accredited as a service and training center by AAPC, it is licensed by the state to operate as an outpatient psychiatric clinic. PPI provides about 12,000 hours of outpatient services each year through its 17 clinical sites in four counties. These offices are located in congregations and four primary care sites. Although PPI serves a broad socioeconomic spectrum, 90% of the budget is hard-funded both commercially and by Medicaid. According to Ronsheim, PPI has been instrumental in building comprehensive models for health care delivery in underserved communities. PPI's Coordinated Care Network provides integrated service delivery by using a sophisticated business plan to sustain the network. They have gone to Medicaid HMOs and negotiated cost savings agreements that pay the network a percentage of the cost savings that they generate for the HMO. Ronsheim indicates that the network has reduced utilization of hospital bed days by 22% and emergency room visits by 24% for their outpatient population. The network is able to increase access to a variety of psychosocial, medical, and behavioral health care programs, provide prevention services, keep the population healthy, and reduce costs. Rather than contain medical costs by decreasing supply of services, Ronsheim says that that they are keeping people healthy, thus reducing demand. The network has received support from national and local foundations and federal grants.

CHRISTIAN COUNSELING CENTER
OF PAINESVILLE, OHIO

An example of a smaller pastoral counseling center operated by Marcy Sacchini, LPCC (licensed pastoral care counselor) is the Christian Counseling Center of Painesville, Ohio, which has been in operation since 1984. Sacchini provides outpatient counseling for people with a variety of psychosocial complaints such as anxiety, depression, anger, and marital problems. She serves approximately 100 people per year. Her clients are Christians and anyone else who wishes to receive services, including non-Christians, in the Lake County, Ohio, area. Funding comes from private pay, insurance plans, and some church-supplemented sponsorships. In her therapy she utilizes the client's religious beliefs, with the Bible being the foundation (in this respect she uses religion in therapy and borders on being an FBO type E). Barriers to the delivery of mental health services, according to Sacchini, include not been recognized by either Medicare or Medicaid, which prevents many persons insured under these programs from receiving services.

Samaritan Counselors

The Samaritan Institute was established in 1979 after years of observing that ministers, therapists, and physicians could be especially effective in providing whole-person health services if they worked together. Called Samaritan counselors, these professionals are trained in both theology and psychology and are certified or licensed similarly to pastoral counselors. The Samaritan Institute is a nonprofit organization devoted to developing counseling centers, providing a network to help reduce the cost of services by centralizing management, and maintaining high-quality standards using an accrediting process. Today, there are nearly 500 Samaritan centers in 340 cities in the United States and abroad. The centers offer counseling at about two-thirds the cost of other providers. According to their Web site, Samaritan counselors "understand and respect the religious perspectives of each counselee and, if appropriate, incorporate these views into the therapeutic process."

Samaritan counselors tend to be linked with local physicians and provide assessment and consultation as needed. The kinds of services that these centers offer include outpatient counseling, wellness programs, consultation, and mental health training for clergy. The Samaritan Web site indicates that they are supported by 5,000 congregations from 40 denominations. They attribute their growth over the past 30 years to the expanding needs of congregations related to coping with increasing stress levels.

National Interfaith Coalition for Spiritual Healthcare and Counseling (NICSHC)

NICSHC is a national organization that represents chaplains and pastoral counselors. Its focus is on research, education, and advocacy.[23] They have conducted several research studies, funded by both private and government sources, to examine the effects of spiritual interventions on mental health outcomes. Since chaplains and pastoral counselors are primarily clinical in their orientation, as noted before, they seldom conduct research to assess the effectiveness of services they provide. This organization helps to rectify that weakness. It not only conducts research but also holds conferences and symposia in order to educate clergy, mental health professionals, and physicians on the role and value of chaplains and pastoral counselors.

Faith-Based Counseling

Counselors in this next category of FBO (category E) tend to be more conservative and/or evangelical in their doctrinal emphasis, and are often affiliated with Protestant Christian groups (although may also be associated with Muslim, Jewish, Hindu, or other religious groups; see chapter 12). They typically serve the mental health needs of persons who are already religious, although they may often reach out to those who are only marginally tied to religion, to the homeless, and to the poor. In contrast to FBO-type C, they use a specific religious belief system as part of the mental health service they deliver. Depending on the particular faith group, this may include prayer, meditation, and readings from the Bible, Torah, or Qur'an. Counselors will use the patient's religious beliefs to help change unhealthy cognitions, behaviors, and emotions, and may or may not integrate this with secular counseling techniques. Examples include the following faith-based counseling ministries that provide mental health services and/or other support for people with mental disorders. These can be divided into nonprofit and for-profit groups.

CHRIST COMMUNITY MEDICAL CLINIC (CCMC)

Formed by four Christian doctors in 1995, CCMC is a nonprofit organization devoted to providing medical and mental health care to inner-city neighborhoods in Memphis, Tennessee (which is the most medically underserved area in the mid-South). During the first four years of operation, the clinic increased its client load to over 10,000 patients. Religious beliefs are utilized as part of mental health treatment, as the clinic's mission statement includes the purpose of "knowing Jesus and making him known, in the context of top-quality health care."[24] Serving in three locations around Memphis, it now has at least eight primary care doctors, two nurse practitioners, a few physicians who specialize in obstetrics-gynecology, and a Ph.D. psychologist. Their Web site indicates that all providers are Christians committed to their mission statement. CCMC also supports a home visitation program.

Their psychologist, Alex Galloway, was hired in 1997 to help address the mental health problems they were seeing in Memphis. According to Galloway, the TENCare state health insurance program in Tennessee, a pilot program started under Clinton, has been terrible in terms of reimbursement for mental health services. Few if any psychologists in the state are seeing patients on TENCare, which pays about $40/session. Apparently, the low reimbursement rate is not so much of a problem as the time necessary to complete the paperwork necessary to receive payment, which takes nearly an hour for every hour spent counseling. Galloway sees patients referred to him from the medical clinic or receives referrals from pastors in the community for cases they are not able to handle. Patients who can pay privately or have insurance are referred to mental health professionals in the community. If they do not have insurance or if they have TENCare, then Galloway sees them—basically free of charge.

In an attempt to empower the churches to provide counseling, part of Galloway's job is to train people within churches (pastors and church leadership) to provide needed mental health care. Pastors were doing a lot of counseling anyway, but aside from the Bible and brief experience in seminary, they had little mental health training. Furthermore, many pastors in the area didn't even go to seminary and so had no formal mental health training at all. Galloway is now teaching a course in a local college that pastors can take to get credit toward a bachelor's degree—introduction to pastoral counseling, and marriage and family counseling, which includes just the basics of counseling.

With a little education and training, Galloway has found that pastors can provide a lot of quality mental health services. In the last three years, he has trained approximately 70 ministers or church leaders and conducted about 30 seminars in churches (almost all being African American congregations). These services were privately funded from nonprofits, donors, and foundations, without any support from state or federal sources. Recently, however, the organization was designated a Federally Qualified Healthcare (FQHC) "look-alike" and is now able to receive funds from the federal government for health services. They were assured that they would not have to compromise their mission statement to qualify.

PINE REST CHRISTIAN MENTAL HEALTH SERVICES (PINE REST)

Started in 1910, Pine Rest has been providing Christian-based mental health services for nearly a century. According to its mission statement, "Pine Rest Christian Mental Health Services is called to express the healing ministry of Jesus Christ by providing behavioral health services with professional excellence, Christian integrity, and compassion."[25] Pine Rest provides a full range of mental health services, from outpatient to home visits to day treatment to inpatient care, and includes 18 outpatient sites around western Michigan and in Iowa. Affiliated with Spectrum Health System, its main campus and inpatient unit is located in Grand Rapids on approximately 220 acres. Pine Rest has the region's largest staff of psychiatrists, who work with nurses, psychologists, social workers, educators, and clergy. Pine Rest describes itself as a nonprofit organization dedicated to serving the community, to providing professional services to people of all faiths and walks of life, to respecting all individuals, and to embodying Christian ethics and values (in this respect it overlaps with FBO type C).

Pine Rest has child, adolescent, adult, and older adult inpatient and partial hospitalization programs. It also has residential programs for the developmentally disabled (81 beds) and an adolescent program for boys and girls (48 beds). Specialty services include an attention deficit disorder (ADD) program, eating disorders program, consultation services for older adults, co-occurring mental health and substance abuse programs, employee assistance and church assistance programs, medical hospital consultation programs, nursing home consultation, psychiatric medical units, psychiatric residential services, psychological consultation centers, and school counseling centers. In 1998, Pine Rest joined with St. Mary's Mercy Medical Center to form a day treatment and inpatient hospitalization program available to all patients regardless of ability to pay or insurance status (Pine Rest Mercy Care). This inpatient program has 162 licensed beds with 150 usually active.

TEEN CHALLENGE (TC)

According to Dave Scotch, TC's accreditation manager, TC doesn't provide any mental health services. However, it is apparent that they do seek to meet the emotional and mental needs of the people they serve. TC has two programs that are licensed by the state and maintain licensed drug and alcohol counselors (in Pennsylvania and Puerto Rico). The rest of the 156 drug and alcohol centers in the United States are required by TC Standards to make referrals. Standard 52 indicates that they will identify mental conditions or behaviors that exceed the ministry's intervention capabilities so that appropriate and timely referral may be made. Standard 53 says that there must be mental health professionals designated for this purpose and referrals must be documented.

The 156 TC centers in the United States fall under a variety of headings depending on the particular state. Scotch indicates that they advise their centers to stay away from clinical or therapeutic terms unless they have qualified staff. TC fulfills its purpose through religious discipleship training. "Where, within this training, qualified ministries choose to employ general therapeutic vocabulary such as but not limited to therapy, patient, client, psychosocial, treatment, plan, etc., ministries do so at their own discretion while adhering to the principles of Biblical consistency.

Ministries should be aware that in many states the use of these terms by anyone other than licensed counselors or psychotherapists is not legally permissible. Further, where a ministry chooses to adapt specific tools or instruments (e.g., personality and temperament inventories, treatment plans, etc.), it shall be done in a Biblically consistent manner with personnel trained or certified where appropriate." This statement comes directly out of TC's standards' manual.[26]

A nonprofit organization, TC currently maintains about 4,500 beds in the United States and Puerto Rico, with 86 centers for males ages 18 or over, 37 centers for females ages 18 or over, 13 centers for females ages 12–17, and 11 centers for males ages 12–17. Over 8,000 people entered TC residential programs in 2001, and 2,901 completed them. The criteria for entry into a TC facility are the presence of a life-controlling problem (predominantly drugs and/or alcohol), willingness to complete the program (normally 12–18 months), and willingness to submit to the guidelines of the program (the religious nature of the program is explicit). Scotch indicates that a conversion or Christian experience is not required either for entry or graduation from the program. If a student does not want to believe what is taught, that is fine, but it is necessary that a person not sabotage another student's experience with arguments concerning what is taught. Religious studies and services are mandatory and an essential part of the program.

What areas of the country do they serve and how long have they done so? TC centers draw from all parts of the United States and its territories. There are TC centers in every state except Delaware, including Alaska and Hawaii. In addition, TC maintains over 180 centers in 67 countries around the world.[27] TC started out in Brooklyn, New York, in 1958 and grew as graduates went out and started new centers. It is only within the past 15 years or so that standards have been developed to define and regulate TC centers.

How are the services of TC supported? TC is under the Assemblies of God religious denomination but is not funded by it. Funding primarily comes through individuals and churches that support the program. Other significant sources of funding are work projects in the centers (they differ depending on the opportunities available), as well as fees. Adolescent centers, because they double as Christian boarding schools, are more regulated. They typically cost $1,500 a month. Adult centers may charge an intake fee of $200–500, but this can be waived if the person is unable to pay.

Is religion used as part of the treatment? TC shares a statement of faith with the Assemblies of God. Religious faith is the motivation for the program and an integral part of the treatment itself. There are parts of the program that are nonreligious in nature such as vocational training, GED, and ABE programs. Scotch indicates that the program could be segmented between religious and nonreligious if government funding was made available for certain activities or education. TC classes also include training on money management, job skills, and personal relationships that are not inherently religious in nature.

What are some barriers that TC faces? According to Scotch, the greatest barrier to delivering mental health services is a philosophical difference between TC and the regulating community (i.e., the government). TC is not a clinical program and does not subscribe to the disease model as the standard for treatment. If the government would allow and be willing to fund people with addictions who want to choose this type of program over the clinical approach (via a voucher system, for example), this would help. Scotch admits that there is need of a study of TC effectiveness. Catherine Hess, from the National Institute on Drug Abuse, headed the last study of TC over 25 years ago.[28] The abstract of the project indicates that they collected follow-up data during a seven-year study of TC program participants (TC is described as "a national program for youthful drug abusers based on Pentecostal Protestantism that emphasizes the need to become a 'born again' Christian"). They collected information on the characteristics of program participants, program effectiveness, dropout rates, and success in the community after completion of the program. Unfortunately, I was unable to locate the actual results of this study. Scotch says that funding is needed for another assessment of program outcomes. Additional funding for these programs is needed, along with greater consistency in local availability of food stamps and financial aid for TC students.

MINIRTH-MEIER AND RAPHA
MENTAL HEALTH CENTERS

Growing out of the Christian psychiatry movement in the mid-1970s and 1980s, a network of Christian psychiatry units in hospitals and independent treatment centers started in the late 1980s and early 1990s. These for-profit centers target evangelical Christian patients. Among the best known are the Minirth-Meier New Life treatment centers and Rapha mental health centers. Christian mental health professionals staff these centers, and provide "Christ-centered professional counseling [that] can help Christians struggling with emotional and substance abuse problems, restoring God's peace and joy to their lives."[29] Christian counselors often refer patients to these centers when inpatient treatment is needed. Frank Minirth and Paul Meier, who started the first of these organizations, wrote a series of best-selling Christian self-help books that widely popularized the centers.[30] There is an article posted on the Internet that details the checkered history of the Minirth-Meier clinics.[31] The article is quite critical of the now greatly reduced ministry. To what extent their accusations or criticism is warranted remains unclear.

Rapha treatment centers also have their critics,[32] although they are not as passionate as those of the Minirth-Meier clinics. According to its Web site, Rapha was founded in 1986, in response to the need for an inpatient psychiatric environment in which persons could receive high-quality mental health care from a Christian perspective by Christian practitioners.[33] Five inpatient treatment centers now exist in Chicago, Little Rock, Louisville, Shreveport, and Tulsa.

NYSTROM & ASSOCIATES' CHRISTIAN
COUNSELING CENTER (CCC)

A number of individual, private treatment centers also exist that are not connected with any particular regional or national chain such as Rapha or Minirth-Meier. According to president Brian Nystrom, CCC is a Christian-based, outpatient mental health clinic licensed under the State of Minnesota.[34] They have an in-home family therapy program as well. Licensed staff members (psychologists, clinical social workers, marriage and family therapists, and psychiatrists) are Christian, and seek to integrate Christian values into their approach. He says they do not use a cookie-cutter approach with everybody, and the treatment approach varies from patient to patient based on the situation and what the patient is looking for. However, there is definitely a "faith" component in the service rendered.[35] Payment for services is through commercial insurance, managed care organizations, and they offer a sliding scale fee for those without coverage.

With regard to barriers, Nystrom notes that when he began in the mental health field twenty-two years ago, a clinician was chastised for even using the word God. Religious faith was definitely split off from mental health care. Now, he observes, it has almost become fashionable to integrate faith into therapy. One obstacle that Nystom faces is when trying to hire new staff. For example, the *Minneapolis Star Tribune* won't let him use the word "Christian" in his ads, even though he is paying for the ad. While the *Star Tribune* says it is their policy, this impedes recruitment.

Professional Organizations

In addition to category E faith-based groups that actually deliver mental health services, there are professional organizations at the national level that provide education, advocacy, networking, and research for these groups.

AMERICAN ASSOCIATION OF
CHRISTIAN COUNSELORS (AACC)

According to its Web site, AACC is a professional organization devoted to helping professional, pastoral, and lay persons provide effective, Christ-centered counseling and direction to those in need.[36] AACC is committed to assisting Christian counselors whether they are licensed professionals or simply caring church members with little or no professional training. It does so by equipping them with biblical, theological, and psychological therapeutic principles designed to heal emotional wounds and bring about wholeness, competence, stability, and spiritual maturity. Its statement of faith focuses on belief and commitment to Jesus Christ. With nearly 50,000 members, this is clearly the largest and best known of the

Christian counseling national associations. Their quarterly magazine, *Christian Counseling Today*, has a wide circulation.

CHRISTIAN ASSOCIATION FOR PSYCHOLOGICAL STUDIES (CAPS)

CAPS describes itself as a professional association of Christians who serve as psychologists, marriage and family therapists, professional counselors, pastoral counselors, psychiatrists, professors and researchers, social workers, psychiatric nurses, guidance counselors, students, and professionals in training.[37] They (1) encourage understanding of the relationship between Christianity and the behavioral sciences at the clinical/counseling and theoretical/research levels, (2) promote networking among Christians in psychological and related professions, (3) foster the spiritual, emotional, and professional well-being of members themselves, and (4) sponsor educational and research opportunities. CAPS was founded in 1956 by a small group of Christian mental health professionals and has grown to over 2,000 members in the United States, Canada, and twenty-five other countries. According to the CAPS Web site, members represent a variety of denominations, professional groups, and theoretical orientations, and are united in their commitment to Jesus Christ and to professional excellence. Unlike AACC, this organization is primarily for licensed mental health professionals (regular members), although it does have an "associate member" category for those who may not be licensed.

ASSOCIATION OF CHRISTIAN THERAPISTS (ACT)

ACT is a Christian professional organization with strong Catholic healing roots that began in August 1975 at a Catholic charismatic healing retreat.[38] It is made up not only of mental health professionals but of other health care professionals and nonprofessionals as well. The common bond is a commitment to Christ and being open to the gifts of the Holy Spirit, especially the gift of healing. While the majority of the members identify with the Catholic Church, ACT encourages membership from all Christian denominations. Members include physicians, nurses, medical technicians, dentists, psychologists, psychiatrists, counselors, therapists, social workers, chiropractors, chaplains, clergy, religious, and lay persons.

CHRISTIAN MEDICAL AND
DENTAL ASSOCIATIONS (CMDA)

The Christian Medical Association (CMA) and the Christian Dental Association (CDA) are combined under this umbrella organization. CMDA has a number of goals that include taking positions and addressing policies on health care issues; conducting overseas medical evangelism projects through its mission arm, Global Health Outreach; coordinating a network of Christian doctors for fellowship and professional growth; sponsoring student ministries in medical and dental schools; distributing educational and inspirational resources; hosting marriage and family conferences; providing Third World missionary doctors with continuing education resources; and conducting academic exchange programs overseas. Founded in 1931, CMDA now has a membership of over 14,000. According to its Web site, "By being the 'hands of Jesus' to needy people, CMDA seeks to fulfill His Great Commandment (Matthew 22:39; 25:36) and His Great Commission (Matthew 28:19)."[39] This organization's magazine, *Today's Christian Doctor*, is colorful and informative.

CHRISTIAN COMMUNITY HEALTH
FELLOWSHIP (CCHF)

Christ Community Medical Clinic (described earlier) is actually one of about eighty similar groups that make up a national network of Christian health providers called Christian Community Health Fellowship. The mission of this loosely affiliated network is to provide health care (including mental health services) to underserved populations in the United States. It emphasizes spiritual, social, and psychological effects on physical health, and stresses the need to address all of these factors in whole person care. Jerry Stromberg is director of the parent organization based in Chicago, Illinois.[40] The organization is Christian oriented and biblically based and has both a general membership of health professionals and also a student membership composed mostly of medical students.

A recent survey completed by 80 of 260 members attending a national CCHF conference found that 34% were physicians, 25% nurses or nurse practitioners, 6% miscellaneous health care practitioners, 18% administrators, and 15% other interested persons.[41] Two-thirds (66%) worked for organizations with an explicitly Christian identity. Two-thirds had provided health care to underserved populations for between one and five years, and 24% had been involved in such work for the past ten years or more. Over 80% practiced in urban areas in organizations that provided services to approximately 750 patients per month. Nearly 70% of respondents indicated that their organizations had a mental health practitioner on staff or an ongoing consultation relationship with one; 39% of mental health practitioners were social workers, 31% were master's level counselors, and slightly less than 20% were psychiatrists or psychologists.

CCHF has received a grant from the Bureau of Primary Health Care as part of the Bureau's "Best Practices Program." The aims of the grant are to (1) identify and document existing effective programmatic practices among CCHF-related ministries; (2) plan, implement, and prospectively evaluate new and current programmatic efforts among CCHF-related ministries; and (3) plan and initiate a central coordinating and data collection infrastructure for a faith-based practice research and evaluation network. Documentation on over twenty "best practices" programs is now available.[42] A few of these programs have included mental health-related targets, such as substance abuse treatment and outreach to homebound older adults.

Summary

In this chapter I described the last two types of FBOs that deliver mental health services (categories D and E). FBO category D consists of chaplains, pastoral counselors, and Samaritan counselors who are trained clergy who have also completed further training in counseling or psychology that certifies them to practice as chaplains or as licensed pastoral counselors. These groups seek to fully integrate patients' religious beliefs with secular counseling in order to address their mental health needs. FBO category E is made up of nonprofit and for-profit counseling centers that provide faith-based counseling that focuses on using the religious beliefs of patients (based on biblical principles for Christians) to achieve mental healing. For both of these groups there are professional membership organizations that prepare and sometimes certify members to provide services. For chaplains, there are four major national organizations (APC,

ACPE, NACC, NAJC); for pastoral counselors, there is a single national organization (AAPC); for Samaritan counselors, there is the Samaritan Institute; and for Christian counselors there is AACC. In the next chapter, I describe non-Christian FBOs that provide counseling services to members of their own faith. While such groups may not always use the religious faith of patients in treatment (as a strictly FBO type E would), a particular religious faith is usually foundational and may be necessary in order to receive treatment.

CHAPTER 12

NON-CHRISTIAN FAITH-BASED
SERVICES

The previous chapters referred primarily to members of Christian groups and their efforts to provide faith-based mental health services. In a country where nearly 85% of the population consider themselves Christian, this makes sense. Nevertheless, Native American Indian, Muslim, Jewish, Buddhist, and Hindu religious groups offer similar services to the mentally ill. Although less is known about these groups, they provide many services in less formal ways.

Native American Indians

There are nearly 50,000 persons in the United States who claim a Native American Indian religious faith.[1] The modest scientific literature on this topic suggests that American Indians require a unique mental health approach based on cultural norms specific to their religious belief systems.[2] In her doctoral dissertation based on a study conducted in upstate New York, Katharine Earle found that there was a significant difference in the rate of mental health services received by American Indians (1%) compared to white, non-Hispanics (11%). In a second study, Earle found that while 38 American Indian subjects were more likely to have alcohol problems, they were substantially less likely to receive mental health treatment compared to 38 white, non-Hispanic subjects matched by age, gender, and program. When asked to rate factors important to good mental health, American Indians were more likely to rate high the ability to have visions,

see things others could not, and guide life according to spirits. These findings underscore the importance of integrating the American Indian patient's belief system with the therapeutic process when delivering mental
health services, a conclusion supported by others.[3]

Information is not easily obtained about faith-based organizations
within the Native American Indian community that deliver mental health
services. However, *Well Nations Magazine* is a Native American Indian
magazine that addresses mental health and substance abuse issues and is a
treasure trove of information.[4] This magazine contains articles about Native Americans struggling with mental health problems and describes programs designed to address such problems. There is also a video (83 minutes, VHS) called *Counseling the Native American Indian Client* (1995)
that is available from the California State University Learning Technology
Center, which discusses cultural issues likely to affect counseling sessions
with Native Americans and strategies for addressing them.[5]

Several counseling centers exist specifically for Native Americans. The
Los Angeles County Department of Mental Health sponsors an American
Indian Counseling Center.[6] There is also an All Tribes Counseling Center
in Mariposa, California, that offers counseling services and community
activities and incorporates respect for American Indian values.[7] Personal
and family counseling services are provided for marital problems, personal problems, child and parenting problems, anxiety and depression, crisis,
anger, and grief. Home visits are made if needed. Crafts, creative writing,
pow-wow dancing and drumming classes, and an honored elders program
are also offered. Fees for services are determined on a sliding scale. The
extent to which services at these counseling centers integrate Native American religious teachings into therapy is not known. These services are designed to meet the needs of Native Americans in Mariposa County.

Muslims

There are approximately 4.1 million Muslims in the United States,
making it the largest non-Christian religion in the country.[8] Dr. Abdul Basit, president of the American Islamic Association of Mental Health Professionals, is affiliated with the Department of Psychiatry at the University
of Chicago.[9] He has written extensively on faith-based delivery of mental

health services to and by Muslims in the United States, and for years has chaired the Center for Mental Health Services' National Advisory Council.[10] Basit also chaired the First Annual Islamic Society of North America's Community Development Conference titled "Islamic Perspective on Counseling," held in Plainfield, Indiana, in June 2000.

Basit says that there are many Muslim mental health or social service centers in Chicago, New York, Los Angeles, Detroit, and Ann Arbor, but these organizations do not necessarily provide faith-based services. The reason is that most clinicians who are working in the field have been trained in the West. Consequently, they have maintained a strictly secular viewpoint. He says that Christian mental health professionals realized a long time ago that thinkers who were either atheists or agnostics dominated modern psychiatry, and therefore Christian therapists did their best to introduce their beliefs and values into counseling. This phase has not started yet in the American Muslim community, Basit notes. There is only one national Muslim mental health organization, and that was established only a few years ago (American Islamic Association of Mental Health Professionals). Other Muslim organizations may soon be influential in this area. For example, the Islamic Society of North America (ISNA), which is the largest Muslim organization in America, is planning to establish an ISNA Center for Health and Human Services. That center plans to provide an array of mental health services that will definitely be faith based, says Basit.

What types of services do Muslim-based counseling services provide? The majority of people seen at Muslim mental health or social service centers show symptoms of anxiety, depression, or adjustment disorders. Marriage counseling is also very common, says Basit. Figures for the number of clients served at these centers are not readily available, so the following are only estimates. In Chicago, Muslims receiving services are mostly from India, Pakistan, and the Middle East. The three Muslim mental health centers in Chicago serve more than 500 clients each year. Muslim communities fund these centers, and some of them receive state and/or federal support. Again, Islamic beliefs and practices are not utilized as part of the therapy. The same secular approach is used that dominates the general field of mental health care in the United States. These FBOs, then, belong to category C organizations like Catholic Charities and Lutheran Social Services.

With regard to barriers to delivering faith-based services, Basit emphasizes the training of clinicians who are well entrenched in the secular approach. They do not believe that faith has any role in the well-being of individuals, says Basit. Though modern research during the past two decades has brought some basic change in attitudes, it has not yet completely filtered through the Muslim mental health community. He stresses the need to collect data from faith-based Muslim organizations that provide mental health services. He believes that an important role of the government is to help fund these faith-based programs and also to conduct rigorous research to determine how their approach is different from others and whether they really work or not.

Psychotherapist Uzmar Mazhar and a number of colleagues operate a Web site at www.crescentlife.com that seeks to disseminate information from sociological and psychological perspectives of interest to Muslims, to raise social awareness, to encourage self growth, to encourage Muslims to reach out to Muslims in need of help and support, and to provide an open forum for discussion and dialogue. One part of the Web site gives the names of psychiatrists and contact information, and allows readers to submit questions about mental health issues. The Web site has information about activities of the Islamic Society of North America (ISNA), and has links with many other organizations and Muslim groups that provide mental health services. Examples include the following.

ALL DULLES AREA MUSLIM
SOCIETY (ADAMS)

ADAMS is part of the FEMA project "Resilience," operating in Fairfax County, Virginia, to provide outreach and crisis counseling to those affected by the events of, and following, 9/11.[11] Muslim therapist Salma Abugideiri provides mental health services using an Islamic perspective in the ADAMS Center and works closely with its director/imam, Mohamed Maged.[12] A description of her practice provides a glimpse into how an Islam-based FBO operates.

Abugideiri is employed by a private, nonprofit multicultural agency that works with ADAMS, and serves a Middle-Eastern population, mostly Muslim. She provides individual and family counseling for a broad range of mental health needs. As a practicing Muslim, Abugideiri says she integrates her belief system into her counseling practice. Her religious values guide her philosophical approach and ethical application of counseling principles. However, as an employee and as a provider to clients who may not practice Islam to the same extent as she does, she does not use Islam explicitly with all clients. Abugideiri says that it is beneficial to turn to the Qur'an for some clients, while not for others. In this role, then, she acts like a pastoral counselor (FBO category D).

Abugideiri uses a similar approach in her private practice, which is relatively new and still small. So far, most of her referrals are from the mosque (ADAMS Center), so that people who come to her have asked for a Muslim therapist and are expecting to benefit from the Islamic worldview as part of the counseling process. The ADAMS Center is both a mosque and a community center that provides a wide range of services. Abugideiri is not employed by the center, but does some volunteer work and accepts referrals from there. The ADAMS Center is a place for prayer, social events, social services, and educational activities. Many types of classes (religious, parenting, etc.) are held there. The director, Mohamed Maged, provides spiritual counseling, premarital counseling, and marriage counseling. When he identifies an underlying mental health issue (depression, anxiety, etc), he refers that person to Abugideiri. If patients need medicine or have unusually complex cases, she refers them to Muslim psychiatrists for evaluation or monitoring. Maged and Abugideiri do cotherapy for couples experiencing domestic violence or other complex issues when it is necessary to have therapists of each gender present. In some cases, Maged works with the male batterer and Abugideiri works with the female victim. Abugideiri notes that they are creative and flexible and willing to use whatever approach may be most beneficial to the family within the parameters of Islam and counseling ethics.

ADAMS has been in operation for about 10 years and has a membership of over 400 families. Any person is welcome to receive services from ADAMS, and they have in the past provided financial assistance through their social service committee to non-Muslims who have requested it. Of course, most people frequenting the mosque are Muslim and come from all over the world. The primary area that they serve is Northern Virginia, especially Fairfax and Loudoun counties. Their services are funded by private donations. When mosque director Maged does counseling, he does so as a member of the clergy (FBO type A). When appropriate, Qur'anic

verses and sayings of the Prophet Muhammad *(hadith)* will be used for education, encouragement, and motivation of the client. This is also the approach that Abugideiri takes in this setting (as would occur in FBO category E, where a trained counselor uses religious faith as part of the
therapy).

According to Abugideiri, several barriers have slowed down or prevented the ADAMS center from delivering mental health services. These
include lack of awareness in the community about the need for mental
health services, stigma attached to mental health problems, lack of understanding about the concept of counseling (there is no equivalent in the
Middle East, for the most part), and no distinction in the community's
mind between psychiatric services for "crazy" people vs. counseling for depression, anxiety, intergenerational conflict, and other personal problems.
Resources are needed to help overcome these barriers. Abugideiri indicates
that they need financial support to pay staff and hold educational events
that could build awareness of mental health issues. They also need more
Muslims trained in the mental health field, and could benefit from written
materials (psychoeducation) such as brochures and pamphlets, especially
those translated into Arabic, Urdu, and Farsi.

Community Healing Centers (CHC) are nonprofit Islam-based psychotherapy centers in San Francisco and Novato, California. Most therapists are Sufis and, while they do not use the center to promote Sufism and
Islam per se, all are profoundly influenced in their work by their spiritual
practices, says director Uzmar Mazhar. There is an opportunity for clients
to incorporate issues of Islamic spirituality into their psychotherapy. Similarly, therapists are sensitive and responsive to cross-cultural issues related
to Muslims seeking mental health services.[13]

According to Jamal Granick, a counselor at CHC, they provide individual, couple, child, and family outpatient psychotherapy for a wide
range of mood and relational issues. In operation for about five years,
CHC does not serve the severely mentally ill, nor do their therapists provide case management, inpatient, residential, day treatment, medication,
or other adjunctive services. They do have programs under development
to expand their client base to include underserved populations. CHCs are
open to clients of any race, religion, and nationality, according to Granick,
although most therapists are Sufis and therefore likely to be particularly
skilled in meeting the mental health needs of Muslim patients. Services

provided to approximately 50 clients per center annually are supported by private pay and insurance, although CHC is applying for grants and government funding to further develop their programs. Religious faith is not part of the services per se, according to Granick, although therapists are responsive to clients' faith issues. A barrier to growth has been finding a niche that makes their services available to people with faith-related issues without deselecting potential clients who are not Muslim or Sufi. This sounds like an organization that could fall either into the FBO C or D categories.

OTHER MUSLIM COUNSELING CENTERS

Another example of an Islamic FBO delivering mental health services is the Islamic Health and Human Services, which offers a full range of psychological services including psychotherapy, substance abuse treatment, and even support services to returning prisoners (including ongoing counseling). While their services are available to anyone who asks, Muslims typically use them because all the services are based on Islam, following the Qur'an and Sunnah (FBO category E).[14] A number of counseling centers like this exist in areas of the United States with large Muslim populations.

Jews

There are 3.2 million Jews in the United States,[15] making it the second largest non-Christian religious group after Muslims. At the congregation level, thousands of rabbis in local communities provide counseling, support, and religious guidance to Jews with emotional problems. In addition, there is the social services agency, Association of Jewish Family and Children's Agencies (AJFCA), which I described in chapter 10 when discussing FBO category C. Jewish chaplains and pastoral counselors provide mental health services and are included with Christian and other religions in the discussion of FBO category D. There are also Jewish counseling services in FBO category E. Finally, many individual mental health practitioners are themselves Jewish (chapter 2) and offer services from a Jewish perspective.

Compared to the large number of FBOs in category E that offer Christian counseling, there are much fewer that advertise specifically Jewish counseling. An advanced Internet search using the search engine Google found 70 hits for the term "Jewish counseling" compared to 70,100 hits for "Christian counseling." For example, Rabbi Aaron Gottesman directs a Jewish Counseling and Fellowship Center in San Diego.[16] This center provides counseling for individuals, couples, and families; visitations to hospitals, nursing homes, and hospice patients; conversion counseling; and workshops and support groups for interfaith couples and families. They also offer consultations with mental health professionals for Jewish life and family issues.

Another example is an interesting organization called Jewish Counseling Service (JCS) that operates online and involves no in-person contact.[17] JCS describes itself as a non-sectarian organization with a long history of providing counseling services to the South Florida community. It combines highly qualified clinical skills with the Jewish values of charity and compassion in order to help individuals and families experiencing difficult life events. While their fee schedule is a bit steep,[18] online counseling reduces the stigma of having to go see a mental health professional and preserves privacy; of course, the down side is lack of face-to-face contact with another human being.

As noted above, there are many individual mental health practitioners who are Jewish and may offer services from a Jewish perspective, although they have not to my knowledge formed coordinated business chains such as Christian counselors have done, nor do many Jewish counselors or counseling centers advertise their services as being faith based. In this sense, they really resemble FBOs categories C and D.

Buddhists and Hindus

The Chinese place a heavy emphasis on morality, social responsibility, respect for authority, and also on restraint in social relations and expression of emotions. It should not be surprising, then, that mental illness in Chinese societies might be heavily censured, difficult to diagnose, and largely dealt with by families in secrecy, so as to avoid the stigma.[19] Even decisions concerning marriage might be affected, in that a family history of mental illness could decrease the chances of getting a good match for a daughter or son. This remains a concern even among many devout Buddhist families and, to some extent, Hindu families as well.

BUDDHIST MENTAL HEALTH CARE

Over 600,000 Americans claim membership in a Buddhist or Hindu temple, making this the third largest non-Christian religious group in the United States.[20] Reverend Kong Chhean from Long Beach, California, is an excellent source of information about Buddhist faith-based mental health services.[21] Reverend Chhean is a Buddhist monk, holds a Ph.D. in psychology, and counsels clients in the Long Beach Asian Mental Health Program, many of whom are Cambodian refugees. Much of the information here about Rev. Chhean was obtained from my personal interview with him and from a series of newspaper articles in the *Long Beach Press-Telegram* that described his ministry.[22]

When Rev. Chhean arrived at Long Beach, California, in 1979, no Cambodian Buddhist temples or monks were there. He set up his first temple in an apartment and his second in a private home. These soon became too small, so he began holding rites at a city park. He eventually raised enough money to buy a former union hall and his temple today (called Wat Willow or Khemara Buddhikaram) is the largest Cambodian temple in Long Beach, both in structure size and number of Buddhists attending. The temple provides activities for youth, an adult day care center, daily meditation sessions, and celebrates religious services. He has brought gang members from the street into the temple and trained them to become monks. Even judges in local courts have ordered teens to stay with Rev. Chhean rather than sending them to juvenile hall. He blends a combination of Eastern spirituality with Western psychology when treating patients at the Long Beach Asian Mental Health Program, part of the Los Angeles County Department of Mental Health.

According to the *Press-Telegram*, many Cambodian refugees (85% of whom are Buddhist) suffer from undiagnosed depression, post-traumatic stress disorder, or other mental illnesses related to experiences in Cambodia's killing fields. The first wave of refugees that came over in 1975 were government officers, ambassadors, members of parliament, senators, professors, and medical doctors, who were unable to find work in their former professions. In 1990, 71% of Long Beach Cambodians were unemployed. They lacked the job skills, language, and opportunity to maintain employment. Many of these people seek help to deal with their losses at Rev. Chhean's temple. The Buddhist temple, according to Rev. Chhean, is viewed by Cambodian people as a place where their religion, culture, education, social, mental, and spiritual health are preserved.

Buddhism teaches that all people go through a cycle of reincarnation and that one's chances for a better existence in the next rebirth are determined by the good deeds accomplished in the current life.[23] According to Theravada Buddhism (an early non-Mahayana form), practiced by many Cambodians, only monks can achieve supreme nirvana. Buddhism's basic belief of karma is that a person's actions determine how their life and afterlife will turn out (and Buddhism includes the idea of hell, which Rev. Chhean points out can exist on earth). Theravada Buddhists may explain current hardships or even mental illness in terms of sins committed in previous lives. As in Hinduism, there is also a strong belief in the caste system. These beliefs influence the Buddhist's understanding of suffering and illness and of treatments for them.

In Theravada Buddhism, the belief is that every deed is motivated by an underlying mental state. Perceptual, cognitive, and affective mental factors fit into either mental *health* or mental *disorder* categories. The judgment of mental health or mental disorder is determined on the basis of the collective experience of the Cambodian Buddhist community. The Cambodian Buddhist center/temple was created to celebrate religious rites, to provide educational programs, and to discuss Cambodian community issues. Reverend Chhean says they provide counseling services to the people at his temple using Buddhist psychology, prayers, rational concentration or meditation, and protective chanting. This is done in order to help people rebuild their self-esteem, dignity, and identity. When the Cambodian has a problem, like stress, depression, insomnia, post-traumatic stress disorder, or family problem, they usually approach Buddhist monks at the temple to discuss their problems. This means that the Cambodian people look to their Buddhist temple as their primary source of mental health care and for solutions to problems in everyday life.

Reverend Chhean indicates that in the Long Beach area there are several Buddhist temples that deliver mental health services. They provide services according to the patient's own culture. For Buddhists from a

Western perspective, they use general counseling and support (as an FBO category C or D). For Buddhists from an Eastern perspective, they use protective chanting (as an FBO category A or E). Chinese, Cambodian, Thai, Burmese, Ceylonese, Vietnamese, Hindu, Japanese, and other Asian temples all provide such services in the area. In Rev. Chhean's temple, they serve approximately 25 to 40 people for group therapy on the 8th, 14th, and 15th days of the waxing and waning of the moon on the lunar calendar. They provide individual therapy to about 6 to 8 patients per day (Rev. Chhean has other monks working with him whom he has trained). He notes that the Cambodian Buddhist temple serves the Cambodian population, and the Chinese Buddhist temple serves the Chinese population. Services are free to people because they donate their charity to support the temple by providing food and clothes for monks.

According to Rev. Chhean, there are many barriers that prevent adequate mental health services from being delivered to Buddhists. Most Asian refugees are not familiar with Western psychiatric and mental health practitioners. Many Asian countries have no psychiatrists or psychologists readily available like in the United States, and Asian patients may not be familiar with mental health treatments. For example, Rev. Chhean reports that he recently visited the Faculty of Medicine at the University of Health Sciences, Department of Mental Health, in Cambodia. The psychiatrist did not provide psychotherapy there, but rather treated patients with medicine. However, there was not enough medicine available to treat all patients, even psychotic patients. When he was there, Rev. Chhean said there were only fifteen trained psychiatrists in all of Cambodia. Despite the fact that nearly 80% of the Cambodian population suffers from depression or PTSD, the Cambodian government has no money to provide mental health care to them. When they come to the United States, Buddhist patients fear that the mental health professional will not share their religious faith and may judge them negatively because of their religious or cultural beliefs, socioeconomic status, or sociocultural choices. In addition, a Buddhist patient may fear being negatively judged by his or her community or peers for seeking help from mental health professionals.

Reverend Chhean makes several suggestions to help overcome such barriers. First, he suggests that mental health professionals should be trained to identify and eliminate negative biases against and/or actions toward Buddhist patients. Second, he suggests that mental health delivery systems work closely together with community members and leaders from both Eastern and Western perspectives to overcome negative biases that Buddhist patients have in seeing mental health professionals. Third, he emphasizes trust, respect, and direct communication be a focus in the therapeutic relationship between a mental health professional and a Buddhist patient.

ASIAN PACIFIC COUNSELING AND TREATMENT CENTERS

Besides those identified by Rev. Chhean, other FBOs exist that deliver mental health services to Buddhist and Hindu populations. For example, Asian Pacific Counseling and Treatment Centers (APCTC) provide culturally and linguistically appropriate mental health services. Established in 1977 as a program of the Los Angeles County Department of Mental Health, APCTC was the first mental health service in Los Angeles County that was developed to meet the unique needs of Asian Pacific immigrants and refugees. In 1990, APCTC became a private, county-contracted agency under the auspices of Special Service for Groups (SSG). Their staff consists of over eighty mental health professionals, paraprofessionals, and support personnel. Professional staff members are fully credentialed psychiatrists, psychologists, social workers, marriage family therapists, psychiatric nurses, case managers, and rehabilitation counselors who are bilingual and bicultural. Their staff speaks Cambodian, Chinese (Cantonese, Mandarin, and Taiwanese), Filipino (Cebuano, Ilocano, and Tagalog), French, Hindu, Japanese, Korean, Laotian, French, Italian, Spanish, Thai, and Vietnamese.

Whether APCTC is actually a faith-based organization is not clear. However, according to their Web site,[24] they provide culturally sensitive mental health services that address the psychological and social needs of Asians. Their professional staff has cultural competence that enables them to work effectively with Asian clients who do not have access to, or who feel disconnected from, mainstream American health care settings. I would assume that "cultural sensitivity" and "cultural competence" indicates respect and value for the religious beliefs of patients. Medicare, Medi-CAL, and private insurance provide funding for these services.

APCTC indicates that no one will be denied service because of inability to pay, since the Los Angeles County Department of Mental Health subsidizes fees for those without medical insurance. Co-payments are determined based on a sliding scale. These services are more typical of those that FBO category C might provide, since religious faith would not usually be used as part of the therapy.

INTERNATIONAL BUDDHIST CENTER

Another example of a counseling center that provides treatment from a Buddhist perspective is the International Buddhist Center in Silver Spring, Maryland.[25] The center is similar to Rev. Chhean's temple, in that it provides Buddhist religious services for the local community, as well as educational activities related to Buddhism. The center's head monk and spiritual director, Bhante Uparatana, does Buddhist counseling. Buddhist teachings form the basis for his counseling and spiritual direction, since Rev. Uparatana has no formal mental health training (FBO category A).

HINDU MENTAL HEALTH CARE

According to the 2000 census, there are now over 1.6 million people of Asian Indian origin in the United States. Asian Indians began immigrating to the United States as early as the turn of the twentieth century. Between 1980 and 1990, the population of Asian Indians in the United States increased by 125%. I was unable to identify any FBOs other than Hindu temples (as Rev. Chhean described for Buddhists) that deliver mental health services. Although several groups similar to APCTC provide mental health services from a culturally sensitive perspective to Hindus, it is difficult to categorize these groups as FBOs, since their origins and motivations are not particularly religious. Google searches using the words "Hindu counseling" or "Hindu mental health care" come up with no hits.

Summary

Mental health and counseling services are provided by a number of non-Christian FBOs in the United States, including Native American Indian, Muslim, Jewish, Buddhist, and Hindu organizations. The types of faith-based services that these groups offer vary widely, making them difficult to place in a particular FBO category. One thing is clear, however. It is essential that mental health services delivered to members of these religious groups be culturally sensitive, respectful, and knowledgeable about their unique religious beliefs and practices. At present, FBOs may be among the only groups that can provide such services.

PART IV

BARRIERS AND SOLUTIONS

CHAPTER 13

BARRIERS TO RESEARCH AND IMPLEMENTATION

Many barriers limit our understanding of the role of religion in mental health and the role that FBOs play in the prevention and treatment of mental disorders. With regard to research, what factors prevent scientists from conducting studies on the religion-mental health relationship? Similarly, what barriers prevent research on the effectiveness and cost of faith-based delivery of mental health services? With regard to implementation, what challenges do FBOs face each day as they seek to meet the mental health needs of people? What keeps them from delivering better and more services? I have already addressed these issues to some extent in my discussion of past research and in my descriptions of Christian and non-Christian FBOs. In this section, however, I focus on the most common and resistant of these challenges.

Barriers to Research

Numerous factors today stand in the way of scientific research on the relationship between religion and mental health. Many of these same issues block research on the effectiveness of faith-based delivery of mental health services. Although many others exist, I have chosen to discuss four types of barriers: methodological, focus/priority, funding, and attitudinal.

METHODOLOGICAL

First, and foremost, there is a lack of trained researchers capable of carrying out high-quality epidemiological and experimental studies on the religion-mental health relationship and on FBO effectiveness. To my knowledge, no training programs exist that are specifically designed to prepare and mentor young researchers to develop and carry out high-quality research likely to pass the National Institutes of Health standards today. The only exceptions are a privately funded two-year postdoctorate research fellowship at Duke University's Center for Spirituality, Theology and Health, and a series of five-day summer research workshops sponsored by *Science & Theology News* and Duke Divinity School's Theology and Medicine Program.[1] Training at the postdoctorate level is needed to:

- Provide researchers with a background in religion-health research
- Familiarize them with research that has already been done
- Provide them with methodological skills to design high-quality studies
- Provide them with the statistical skills to analyze study results
- Teach them to write high-quality, competitive grant applications
- Educate them on where to get funding
- Provide them with experience carrying out such studies under the mentorship of seasoned investigators
- Teach them how to write up the results of their research for publication
- Teach them how to present the results to colleagues at professional meetings
- Teach them how to talk with the media so that their findings can reach the public

Second, there exist many instruments to assess and measure religious beliefs and attitudes.[2] There is no one instrument, however, that is considered a standard in the field. Instead, investigators tend to use many different instruments or often make up their own instrument. Having a single standardized measure capable of accurately assessing religiousness across religions (at least monotheistic religions) would be useful. For a brief measure, the five-item Duke University Religion Index may be useful;[3] for a comprehensive measure, the Fetzer Multidimensional Measure of Spirituality and Religiousness is probably the one of choice.[4] These measures, however, assess religion in a relatively superficial manner. For greater accuracy and depth, measurement of religiousness may need to be both religion specific and culture specific.[5] Such instruments have yet to be developed.

Third, there is no specific religious intervention that is used widely for treating persons with mental illness. Religious cognitive-behavioral therapy (RCBT) has the most promise in this regard, since a standardized format has been developed.[6] RCBT, however, is probably only useful for mild to moderate depression and anxiety. Religion-based psychotherapeutic modalities (including group therapies) are also needed for persons with severe and persistent mental disorders. Although some preliminary work has been done, these spiritual interventions have not been rigorously tested and there is no one therapy that is commonly used. Like religious measures, religious interventions may need to be both religion specific and culture specific to achieve their greatest effect.

Fourth, assessing the effectiveness of FBOs in delivering mental health services in a cost-efficient manner will likely depend on the application of research methods developed for use in studying secular programs. These methods, however, may need to be adapted for studying faith-based programs, rather than simply applying secular methodologies unmodified. Care will be needed so that such modifications do not impair the scientific integrity of the assessment process. For example, faith organizations may find it ethically troublesome to identify persons with mental health problems, but not provide them with immediate treatment if those persons are relegated to "control" groups (this has already been a contentious issue in chaplain research). FBO groups may feel ethically bound to deliver care. Furthermore, FBOs by themselves may be poorly equipped to carry out this kind of research, given their lack of training and experience. This will require collaboration with skilled researchers at academic institutions.

FOCUS AND PRIORITY

Many researchers who may be interested in this area and possess the necessary skills to design studies, carry them out, and get them published often do not know where to get started. Funding organizations, both government and private, also often struggle with where they should direct their scarce resources. Which research questions are in greatest need of answering? Which religion and mental health areas are likely to have the greatest payoff? Where should they direct their limited time and resources in this new and unfamiliar area? Lack of experience and focus will cause frustration, wasted effort, and lack of progress. Investigators and funding agencies need to know which studies need to be done first so they can direct their resources to these areas.

FUNDING

The largest source of funds for doing research is the National Institutes of Health (NIH). Grants at the NIH are reviewed by groups of ten to fifteen experienced scientists drawn from the university community. These are called "study sections," and there is usually a different study section for each particular research area. The first problem is that NIH study sections often do not have scientists who are familiar with the past research in this area, the measurement of religion, or the design of studies to test religious interventions. Lack of expertise among grant reviewers is a serious barrier to the likelihood that a religion-mental health proposal will get a high "priority score" and ultimately be funded. Although there is a National Center for Complementary Alternative Medicine (NCCAM) at NIH, this division focuses on studies that evaluate alternative medical treatments (effects of herbs, acupuncture, etc.) or unusual spiritual approaches and do not typically address issues related to traditional religion or mental health. The National Institute of Mental Health does not have a special section for reviewing research proposals that address religion and mental health, and often sends such proposals to NCCAM.

Second, there is little interest in this area at the Office of Behavioral and Social Sciences Research (OBSSR), NIMH, NIA, or any of the other institutes including NCCAM, since they seldom, if ever, release RFPs focused on religion and mental health. Consequently, few research proposals are developed and high-quality research is often not done. Most of the research completed thus far has been either privately funded (much through the John Templeton Foundation) or done without formal funding (religious variables added onto research funded to study other research objectives).

ATTITUDINAL

Negative attitudinal barriers exist among scientists, academic departments, university and hospital institutional review boards (IRBs), NIH study sections, editors, and reviewers concerning the design, funding, implementation, and publication of religion-mental health research.

First, the negative attitudes of many scientists toward research examining religion and health stems from long-held notions of incompatibility between religion and science, and also from a personal lack of religious involvement by scientists. A recent study published in *Nature* revealed that among the 600 members listed in the 1996 edition of American Men and Women of Science, only 39% indicated a belief in God.[7] Furthermore, among the most prestigious scientists in the National Academy of Sciences, only 4% said they believed in God.[8] Compare this figure to 96% of the American population who say they believe in God.[9] This disparity in belief (and probably in value placed on the importance of religious belief) between the populace and the scientific community is concerning. Furthermore, as we saw earlier in this book, psychologists and psychiatrists are the least likely to believe in God or be involved in religious activities among all health professionals.[10] As a result, proposals seeking to study relationships between religion and mental health stand little chance in the intensely competitive funding environment controlled by traditional scientists. Although some study section chiefs indicate that all proposals are judged purely on the basis of scientific merit,[11] subtle biases and personal prejudice against religion invariably affect such decisions.

Second, university institutional review boards (IRBs) and academic departments tend to discourage scientists from doing research in this area. For decades, academic departments have been so negative toward studying religion and health that this area of research became widely known as the "anti-tenure factor."[12] Because of the low academic prestige and lack of rewards for studying this area, it is not surprising that few mental health professionals focus their careers here. Even if a proposal reaches the IRB, it may experience a difficult time getting approved by scientists who sometimes set an unusually high standard for such religion-health proposals, finding small faults in the study that hold up the research or requesting modifications in study design that make the study impossible to carry out.

Third, journal editors have been reluctant to publish such research, and may doom such submissions by sending the articles to highly critical reviewers who are unlikely to recommend publication. For example, a review of articles on religion and mental health published between 1978 and 1982 in the four best journals in psychiatry found that only 2.5% of all published articles assessed a religious variable.[13] The review was repeated ten years later for the period 1991 through 1995. During that time, the percentage of articles assessing a religious variable actually dropped in half to 1.2%. In other words, only 1.2% of articles mentioned that they had assessed a religious characteristic.[14]

Barriers to Implementation

Although there is much research that needs to be done to understand how religion impacts mental health and to determine the best way for FBOs to help the mentally ill, those who struggle with emotional problems and mental disorders continue day after day crying out for help. Should FBOs stand idly by until all the necessary research has been done—which could take decades to complete? Given the volume of research that has already been done, and the many positive findings, it would seem reasonable to move ahead cautiously with implementation, while at the same time continuing to conduct studies. Barriers, however, stand in the way of even these preliminary first steps. What factors prevent or limit faith-based efforts to respond to pleas for help from those grappling with emotional problems or more serious mental disorders?

RESISTANCE FROM MENTAL HEALTH PROFESSIONALS

According to Gregory Fricchione,[15] a Harvard-trained psychiatrist who works at the Carter Center in Rosalynn Carter's program on mental health, a major barrier resides in the mental health community—resistance from clinicians and those in academia. At a time when mental health professionals feel there is so much to offer those with mental illness, backed up by randomized clinical trials demonstrating the effectiveness of medications and other biological therapies, they see the mental health care dollar shrinking and cost-cutting cutting to the bone. Mental health professionals suspect that recent government interest in faith-based groups as vehicles for mental health services is really a cover-up for cutting the budget even further and making the bottom line look better.

Many recall the "bait and switch" situation that arose when a decision was made to release the mentally ill from state mental hospitals and care for them in the community (called "de-institutionalization"). The promised funding for community mental health centers, however, never materialized. Presumably mental health services delivered by faith-based groups will be cheaper. Whether they are as effective as mainstream psychiatric and psychological services is not the primary interest of policy makers—so say some mental health professionals. If the government is concerned about unmet mental health needs of citizens, it ought to be putting more money into proven mental health care treatments and increasing access to those services. This is their basic attitude.

INADEQUATE TRAINING

Fricchione observes that lack of training puts many FBOs at risk for providing substandard mental health services. Clergy and pastoral staff need basic training in recognition of psychiatric disorders, mental health promotion, mental illness prevention, and triaging cases to the appropriate level of care. They need to become familiar with suicide prevention and learn to ask about suicide. Clergy and faith-based counselors should be aware that neurological illnesses, such as complex partial seizures or nonelectrical seizures, may present as psychiatric disorders. They need to know about the terrible disease burden brought on by child or spouse abuse, and how to prevent it and help victims. FBOs need to recognize their limits in treating cases of mental illness where biology and psychopathology predominate, and yet also recognize the power that faith-based approaches have on the human level for dealing with most life crises (complementing the care that mental health professionals provide).

The services that FBOs offer need to be integrated into traditional models of psychiatric and mental health care delivery. They need to develop relationships with local mental health centers or create such centers themselves. One way to do this would be expand the "parish nurse model" that is now becoming popular in primary care medicine collaborative models.[16]

According to Jill Schumann at Lutheran Social Services,[17] whose central office is in Maryland, the state's mental health care system is a big mess. Many providers are going bankrupt because of difficulty collecting insurance payments and the lack of parity between mental health and medical services. There are long waiting lists to see providers, especially if the person does not have insurance. Medicaid in Maryland is not covering the cost of treatment, paying less than 85 cents on the dollar of what it costs providers to deliver care. Since mental health services are often "carved out" in third party medical plans, even people with health insurance often can't get needed services. Mental health coverage is optional in many of these plans—i.e., employers don't have to offer it (this is what "carved out" means). Furthermore, persons who are self-insured may have physical health coverage, but often have no mental health benefits at all. With regard to the problem of mental illness among the homeless, even Medicaid requires an address. Thus, the question is how can an FBO serve people without resources? Many FBOs cannot grow to serve the increasing needs because they have no profit margin to bring on new staff, staff that may take many months to build up a client base to be self-supporting.

Another barrier is availability of direct care (DC) workers, who are becoming increasingly difficult to find. These workers provide basic care for children or older adults, and this position typically requires a bachelor's degree. The reason for the DC worker shortage is because the pay is low and the work hours are poor. They may have to work two or three shifts back-to-back or entire weekends. Few people with appropriate credentials are willing to work under these conditions. However, this is a common situation under managed care and public contracts. Directors of Lutheran Social Services in other states confirm what Schumann is saying.

For example, Charles Lockwood of Glade Run Lutheran Services in Pennsylvania notes that many of the state facilities that used to treat persons with severe mental illness have now closed. Glade Run is now caring for some of these children—children who are psychotic, low functioning, and often requiring psychotropic medication. In 2002, they increased their DC workers' salaries from an average of $8.30/hour to a starting wage of $10/hour. This action was motivated by their faith-based belief in a livable wage and by their desire to stabilize the high staff turnover. DC workers are typically young college graduates just starting out in life. In the Glade Run program, they are being asked to take care of some of the most disturbed children in society. According to Lockwood, the mental health field does not carry with it the respect it deserves. Because of low pay and lack of respect, this forces Glade Run to hire inexperienced staff who often leave quickly for "greener pastures" or because the job is more than they can handle. This is sad in a field that needs stability for the sake of the children. Glade Run's funding comes through Medicaid directly from the state or through a variety of managed care organizations that manage regions of the state for Medicaid. Any significant renovations or building projects that Glade Run plans require fund-raising campaigns through churches and foundations.

Brent Diers, director of clinical services of Lutheran Child and Family Services of Illinois (LCFSI),[18] notes that even with many different sources of funding, counseling services must be extensively subsidized by the agency because the services are not paying for themselves. United Way and a few other groups provide funding, but it is not sufficient. As a result, LCFSI has had to reduce the number of counselors they employ. Many LCFSI counselors work in relatively isolated communities where the variety of choices for mental health services is limited, particularly services with a sliding scale. The loss of LCFSI services often means that people in need of mental health care will lose access. They also provide counseling in many impoverished communities where insurance is not a payment option. Diers is deeply convinced that the counseling they provide serves a crucial community function, but one that simply can't be continued without more resources.

Bruce Strade of Lutheran Community Services Northwest notes that there is a significant proportion of the population that cannot afford counseling because they either do not qualify for Medicaid or do not have adequate insurance coverage that includes mental health services. The managed care (HMO) system has also had its impact, and does not take into consideration the chronically mentally ill population that may need ongoing services. That system allows only four to six visits per year, which for some individuals is totally inadequate. There is also lack of money for education on mental illness prevention, which in the long run could increase the demand for mental health services.

According to Roy Woodruff, executive director of AAPC, funding is almost always the primary barrier that prevents pastoral counselors from delivering mental health services in underserved areas of the country. In the face of constant financial challenges and strains, pastoral counselors still strive to deliver theologically informed, spiritually sensitive, ethically sound, and clinically competent counseling to persons in need. However, there is a limit to what even pastoral counselors can do for free, since they, too, need to feed their families.

OVER-REGULATION

Jill Schumann from LSS stresses that excessive regulations for the protection of patients are another barrier. This adds costs of complying with regulations to the already money-strapped providers. People have to be paid to complete and review the documents that these regulations require. For some organizations operating on lean budgets, the only possible response has been to declare bankruptcy because they are unable to keep up with the regulations. Regulations that require new technology fixes can also be expensive. For example, the executive director of Lutheran Social Services in Washington, D.C., notes that in order for them to continue to see patients with severe, persistent mental illness on the city's contract, they need to put in a new software system. That software, which involves a new billing system, costs over $100,000. Their group simply can't afford this, and the result will be their having to stop serving this patient population.

Like Schumann, Charles Lockwood of Glade Run in Pennsylvania also considers the issue of over-regulation a major problem. Glade Run must undergo multiple audits, with some regulators saying one thing and others saying another. This includes audits by JCAHO, the Department of Public Welfare, the Department of Children and Youth, the Department of Mental Health, county reviews (Pennsylvania is a county-driven system for children), Medicaid, and others. The layers of reviews have become amazing. Furthermore, interdepartmental coordination in caring for children needing services across county systems appears weak and driven by categorical funding streams.

Roy Woodruff, executive director of AAPC, also emphasizes state regulations as a major barrier, particularly when no relevant licensure is available for pastoral counselors. This contributes to managed care groups consistently refusing to include pastoral counselors as providers.

STIGMA OF MENTAL ILLNESS

Psychiatrist Gregg Fricchione believes that one of the most important barriers within FBOs, perhaps stronger in some faith-based groups than others, is the old bugaboo of stigma. Church members are encouraged in a variety of ways to keep mental health problems hidden and there is a gradient toward denial. Mental illness is still a taboo topic in many places, and even if some clergy are enlightened, there remains a general sense that negative consequences will result if they accentuate the need in the church community for more mental health services. Another barrier is that despite all the research, many faith-based groups still don't recognize that providing social support and other mental health resources can really help prevent, hasten recovery from, or stabilize mental illness.

Like Fricchione, Jill Schumann emphasizes the barrier of stigma from the patient's standpoint, especially among the elderly. People are reluctant to admit to such problems because they are concerned about how others will perceive their need for treatment. This is also true for younger persons, to some extent. They are worried about how receiving mental health services will affect future job opportunities, since many applications require that a person mention whether or not he or she has ever needed mental health treatment. There is also concern about how friends at church will see them.

Thus, barriers to FBOs providing mental health services abound. There is resistance within the mental health community, lack of training in the faith community, problems of stigma and fear, government over-regulation, and most important, lack of adequate funding that prevents religious organizations from becoming more active in this area.

Summary

There are many obstacles that stand in the way of a more complete understanding of the religion-mental health relationship and of greater involvement by the faith-based community in meeting the mental health needs of their own members and those in the general population. While there is great potential here, there are also tall barriers. In the research arena, these include methodological barriers, lack of focus and priority, inadequate funding, and negative attitudes on both sides (mental health professionals and clergy). Researchers need training to conduct high-quality research in this area; they need to become aware of the highest priority areas needing study; funds are needed to support this research; and attitudes of scientists that review the research and control its publication need to change. In the implementation area, barriers include resistance by mental health professionals and clergy, inadequate training of religious caregivers, inadequate government funding for services, problems with over-regulation, and stigma within the faith community against mental illness and mental health professionals. In the next chapter, I will examine ways of overcoming these barriers.

CHAPTER 14

IDENTIFYING POSSIBLE
SOLUTIONS

In this final chapter, I explore possible solutions to the barriers discussed previously, both in terms of conducting the research and in terms of supporting the delivery of mental health services by faith-based groups. How can research in this area be improved and expanded? How can faith-based efforts to deliver mental health services be fostered and expanded? Is it necessary or desirable to wait until all the research has been completed before making preliminary recommendations in terms of implementation? I don't think so. Thus, the focus of this chapter is on overcoming barriers to research and on overcoming barriers to implementation.

Overcoming Barriers to Research

In this section I discuss ways of overcoming barriers to conducting research (methodological and priority issues), funding research, and relating to attitudinal biases among scientists who are against studying the religion-mental health relationship and the effectiveness of mental health services provided by FBOs.

METHODOLOGICAL ISSUES

Training grants, such as the National Research Service Award (NRSA), the Minority Access to Research Career (MARC) Award, and the Career Opportunities in Research (COR) Award, are needed for investigators who wish to learn how to conduct research in the area of religion and mental health. These awards are made under the authority of Section 487 of the Public Health Service Act, but not many have gone to religion-mental health researchers. Training grants would allow universities to bring in postdocs for one- or two-year periods to be trained and supervised (i.e., mentored) by experienced senior investigators. These postdocs (i.e., those who have already received a Ph.D., M.D., or other doctoral degree) could either work on their mentors' projects or develop projects of their own. NRSA training programs already exist for specialized areas such as "aging," and there is no reason why one for "religion and mental health" could not be developed.

Besides the research training awards above, other options include having shorter research training courses that interested researchers could attend to receive intensive instruction on religion and mental health. This avoids the problem of having to relocate for a year or two to a particular area of the country where universities and experts provide the training. Scientists can usually take a week to get this training without interrupting their family lives, clinical work, or teaching responsibilities. For example, over the past couple of years, Duke University's Aging Center and Department of Psychiatry have held several successful summer workshops on research in the area of aging and psychiatry. Modeled after these Aging Center workshops are the religion-health seminars held by *Science & Theology News* discussed in the last chapter.[1]

With regard to religious measurement and the development of religious interventions, the NIMH could offer an RFP (request for proposals) to stimulate research in this area. Prior to the release of such an RFP, it would be wise to hold a series of NIH consensus conferences to establish what is known and what needs to be learned in the area of religion and mental health. Although NIH consensus conferences have been held on religion and health (and published in the January 2003 issue of the *American Psychologist*) and on religion and aging (1995), there has never been one that focused on mental health or faith-based delivery of mental health services.

PRIORITY ISSUES

What are the highest priority studies that need to be done, both with regard to the religion-mental health relationship and FBO effectiveness?

Because of its importance in directing and guiding the field, I will address this "priority" issue at length here.

Scientists have only scratched the surface in their understanding of the links between religion and mental health, and there are many areas in which systematic research is needed. High priority areas include learning more about the religion-mental health relationship and determining the costs and effectiveness of faith-based interventions and service delivery systems.

Religion-mental health relationship

There are four areas relevant to mental health that are especially in need of further study: mechanism of religion's effects, effectiveness of religious interventions, impact of religion on seeking mental health services, and effects of religion on mental health in persons with severe mental illness (schizophrenia, etc.) and in special population groups (children, minorities, etc).

Mechanisms. First, research is needed to better understand how religious beliefs and practices lead to better or worse mental health. Although we have some idea of the mechanisms involved, studies that identify the exact pathways are lacking. This is important in order to isolate the "effective ingredients" of religious faith that foster mental health and well-being, as well as "toxic elements" of faith that may worsen it. Note, however, that a religious belief system that appears to convey benefits or risks in one culture may act entirely different in another culture. This point is particularly important when comparing Western and Eastern faith traditions, where worldviews, living environments, and social histories are so different. Specific questions on mechanism that need answering include:

- What aspects of religion are particularly important in increasing or decreasing susceptibility to mental illness? Are there religious belief systems or practices that are particularly "healthy" or unhealthy?
- What "dose" of religious belief or activity is necessary to increase or decrease susceptibility to mental illness or facilitate coping? Is moderate activity better than very high levels or very low levels, or do benefits accrue in a linear fashion with dose?
- What is the size of effect that religious factors have on mental health

compared to those of other psychosocial or biological factors known to influence mental health (i.e., social support, economic status, education level, family history of psychiatric illness, antidepressant or antipsychotic treatment, etc.)?

• What are the effects of religious involvement at different ages (childhood vs. adulthood, vs. later life, i.e., the timing of exposure), at different levels of stress (high vs. low), and for different types of stress (health-related vs. financial-related vs. family-related)?

• Does severity of psychopathology influence the benefits received from religion? In what way (i.e., strength or weaken benefits) and in what circumstances?

• Does type of religious belief or activity interact with severity of psychopathology, and in what way? Might certain beliefs or activities benefit psychopathology at lower levels, but not at higher levels of severity, or vice versa? Does this effect vary by the particular belief system or practice?

• Do these effects vary in different cultural environments, and in what ways? For example, do strong Hindu religious beliefs have the same benefits for those living in the United States compared to those living in India? What about Jews living in the United States compared to those living in Israel?

• Can particular areas of the brain or neurotransmitter systems be identified that help to explain the effects that religious beliefs and practices have on mental health? Does this vary depending on religious practice or belief, or on type of mental illness?

• How might religious beliefs and practices influence and interact with different medications (anti-anxiety vs. antidepressant vs. antipsychotic vs. mood stabilizers)?

• How might they interact with electroconvulsive therapy and other biological treatments?

• Do these effects vary depending on the particular emotional problem or mental disorder?

Religious Interventions. It is important to conduct randomized clinical trials that study the effectiveness of religious interventions and determine the best way of integrating findings into clinical practice. Specific questions that need answering include:

- Does religious cognitive-behavioral therapy achieve better or worse results than secular cognitive-behavioral therapy? What is the minimum number of sessions necessary to achieve significant results?
- Does this effect depend on the type of religion (i.e., Christianity vs. Islam vs. Buddhism, etc.) or level of religiosity of patients being treated?
- Do nonreligious patients benefit from religious psychotherapy, or are they made worse?
- How does a therapist implement a religious intervention that is sensitive and appropriate, that does not adversely affect the therapeutic relationship, and that does not offend the patient or the patient's family? What approach, or approaches, is most effective?
- What characteristics of patients predict better or worse results from religious psychotherapy? Do men achieve the same benefits as women? African Americans as Caucasian Americans? Educated vs. uneducated?
- What is the most effective form of religious psychotherapy—one that depends on altering unhealthy beliefs, one that focuses on behavioral change, one that focuses on simple support and encouragement, or one that examines psychodynamic aspects of religious belief and practice? Does this vary by religious group or cultural background?
- How much and what kind of training is necessary to deliver effective religious psychotherapy? Is this a skill that can be quickly picked up by secular counselors or does it require in-depth training over months or years? Are certain methods of training more effective than others?
- Does a therapist have to be religious in order to deliver effective religious psychotherapy? Does the training of religious vs. nonreligious therapists differ? If so, in what ways?
- How does the religiosity of the therapist influence the effectiveness of treatments that he or she administers (whether those treatments are secular or religious)?
- How do social, psychological, and religious interventions interact with one another in the treatment of patients with mental or emotional illness?

- What role might clergy or trained religious volunteers play in delivering effective religious and nonreligious treatments?
- How do the results of counseling performed by untrained (or poorly trained) community clergy, compare to simple support provided by lay members of the congregation, trained pastoral counselors, and trained secular counselors?
- Does the effectiveness of counseling depend on the type of mental or emotional disorder for which counseling is being sought? In other words, for persons with milder emotional or mental disorders, does clergy counseling or lay support work just as well as that provided by licensed counselors or psychologists? What about more severe disorders?

Use of Mental Health Services. It is important to understand how religious beliefs and practices influence the seeking of mental health care and the compliance with mental health treatments. Questions that need attention include:

- Do devout religious beliefs and practices increase or decrease the need for professional mental health services?
- Do religious beliefs and practices increase or decrease the likelihood of seeking such mental health services?
- Are there particular religious belief systems that are more or less likely to block the seeking of professional mental health care when necessary?
- Does devout religiousness increase or decrease the likelihood of compliance with psychiatric treatments—either psychotherapy or biological treatments such as antidepressant medication or ECT?

Research in Special Populations. There is relatively little information on the religion-mental health relationship for certain mental conditions and subgroups in the population. Given this lack of information, studies of religion's impact are especially important in these groups.

Persons with Severe and Persistent Mental Illness
- What are the effects of religious beliefs and practices on the etiology and the course of severe mental illnesses such as schizophrenia, severe personality disorder, and recurrent depression or bipolar disorder?

- How are the religious beliefs and practices of persons with severe and persistent mental illness or psychosis different from those of persons without these disorders or with milder forms of them?
- What are the biological and psychodynamic causes of religious delusions and how do they influence the course of illness?
- How do religious conversion experiences (sudden vs. gradual, in one religious group vs. another) influence mental health, and are there any biological explanations for this?
- How can religious communities best support those with severe mental illness? What are the limitations of such support?

Children and Adolescents
- How do religious beliefs, practices, and training of children influence their later susceptibility to mental illness or emotional disorder? What about adolescents? Is there a particular age in childhood when religious training is most effective in influencing later mental health?
- How does degree of religiousness and type of religious belief and practice of parents influence a child's susceptibility to mental illness as he or she grows older?
- What is the role of religious psychotherapy in children with emotional problems or severe and persistent mental disorder? Are there particular approaches that are more helpful? Does type of religion make a difference?

Older Adults
- What role does religion play in helping to prevent or treat mental disorders in older adults?
- What about special populations of older adults, such as those who suffer from chronic medical illness or disability, those who live alone and have few resources, and those in nursing homes or other institutional settings?
- What is the role of religion in the prevention of Alzheimer's disease or other dementias, and does religious activity slow the progression of Alzheimer's disease?
- Do religious activities help to reduce agitation in patients with dementia?

- What role does religion play in end-of-life care? How can religion help to facilitate a "good death" for both patient and family? Does the therapist or helper need to be of the same religion as the patient?

Minority Populations
- Are the relationships between religion and mental health stronger or weaker in minority populations in the United States (i.e., African Americans vs. Hispanics vs. Asians vs. Middle Easterners)?
- Are there specific minority populations for which religion is especially important in either the prevention or treatment of mental illness?
- What religious interventions are likely to be most effective in a particular minority population? Which religious interventions are likely to be least effective?

Other Special Populations
- What role does religion play in preventing or treating mental health problems in homosexuals and others with alternative lifestyles that may conflict with traditional religious doctrines?
- What role does religion play in preventing or treating mental health problems in persons with HIV/AIDS?
- What role does religion play in the quality of life and care of those with Alzheimer's disease and other dementias? What about their caregivers?
- What effects do religious belief and practice have on burnout rates in mental health professionals (nurses, social workers, therapists, and physicians)?

FBO Cost and Effectiveness. Just as research is needed on the religion-mental health relationship, studies are also needed to identify model FBOs that maximize impact and minimize cost. Currently, there are very few studies that have examined FBOs in this regard.

Psychologist Mark DeHaven, in the Department of Family and Community Medicine at the University of Texas Southwestern Medical Center in Dallas, recently reviewed health-related activities of faith-based organizations. His purpose was to identify the organizations and assess their effectiveness.[2] DeHaven found close to 386 articles in the medical, public health, allied health, and nursing literature between 1990 and 2000, of which 105 actually discussed any type of health program, 53 examined a specific program, and 28 examined program effects. Of the latter group, only 2 of 28 examined programs that addressed mental illness in church settings.[3]

Only one other scientist besides DeHaven (to my knowledge) has attempted to review research on the effectiveness of FBOs, and that scientist's focus was not specifically on mental health.[4] Sociologist Byron Johnson at the University of Pennsylvania did a search of the literature using keywords such as *faith, faith-based, spirituality*, and *religion*, and came up with 65 studies. Among these were four case reports that were methodologically poor, noted no specific outcomes, and only made conclusions (no results or findings reported). There were four good, methodologically sound studies that used appropriate statistics (all reported positive findings—two studies on prison fellowship, one on teen challenge, and one on adult care). Johnson concluded that very little research had been done on the effectiveness of FBOs, and explained this lack of research as follows.

First, FBOs don't trust academic researchers to evaluate them because they feel their intentions are strictly to expose them. Also, they often feel researchers are overly skeptical and secular. Second, FBOs feel they are doing something good for people and do not want to "lose time" doing research, because they think research will only point out what they are not doing. Third, financially many FBOs cannot afford to pay for outsiders to study their organizations. Fourth, most researchers have not had any interest in assessing the effectiveness of FBOs.

Johnson recommends that future research focus on longitudinal studies of FBOs. As an example, he describes a new FBO in Philadelphia called "Abachi" that is affiliated with Big Brothers/Sisters that matches children of prisoners with mentors from different faith communities. Many in this group proclaim overwhelming positive effects, although there is no evaluation component to measure how such relationships actually help the children. Second, Johnson says that an overhaul is needed on how data are collected. For example, more religious questions relevant to FBOs should be included in the many large national surveys now being conducted and supported by the NIH and CDC. Third, he suggested that more qualitative research on FBOs is needed despite the fact that it is labor-intensive and expensive. Given these recommendations, what are some important questions that research might answer?

- How many FBOs exist in each of the five categories (chapter 7) that deliver mental health services in the United States? Who are they? Where are they? What kind of services do they provide? How much does it cost?
- What kind of mental health services are FBOs best equipped to deliver? How might such services complement those provided by the existing secular mental health system?
- Can FBOs deliver mental health services (1) to the same or more people, (2) at an equal or greater quality, and (3) at the same or lower cost, compared to secular programs?
- Do FBOs provide mental health services that result in more complete and lasting remission or stabilization of symptoms than secular treatments alone? Which emotional or mental conditions might this apply to (and not apply to)?
- What is the long-term effectiveness of FBOs compared with secular programs in meeting the mental health needs of persons in the community? Long-term studies are needed because benefits may not only be immediate but also may accrue over time and involve not only those receiving services but also those delivering the services (and the families of those receiving and delivering services).
- Are there populations in the United States where mental health services offered by FBOs can meet unique and now unfulfilled needs? Minority communities? Rural communities? Urban communities? The elderly? The uninsured?
- Since FBOs operate largely on the basis of volunteers, what determines decisions to volunteer? What are the costs and rewards of volunteering?
- In what specific ways can each FBO category (A–E) best meet the needs of persons with severe and persistent mental illness?
- Do model FBOs exist that are fully integrated with the secular mental health care system? Partially integrated? If none exist, what might this look like?

Efforts by Mark DeHaven and colleagues in Texas demonstrate how systematic research can guide the development and assessment of programs that involve both faith communities and the formal health care system in identifying and treating mental illness in underserved populations. In his position at the University of Texas Southwestern Medical Center and as chairman of the Interfaith Committee of NAMI in Dallas, Dehaven works with numerous faith-based organizations throughout the area that provide health services to the underserved. He reports that they have ten free medical clinics in the city providing services for the uninsured, the homeless, and other needy groups. These clinics provide access to primary care services and, therefore, theoretically access to screening for mental illness and related disorders. However, primary care physicians generally do a poor job screening and treating mental disorders even among patients with insurance. The situation appears to be no different among at-risk patients who come to the free care clinics. DeHaven and his colleagues recently reviewed the records of one of these clinics over a period of six months. Of the 1,230 patient visits, none were for mental health-related problems. In such settings where time is limited and patient flow is high, care is focused on the primary medical complaint and mental health issues are commonly neglected.

As a result, primary care physicians do a relatively poor job of assessing and treating patients with mental health needs. Likewise, pastors and other church leaders are not very well equipped to counsel congregants when it comes to mental illness, particularly if they lack the necessary training. Thus, DeHaven's approach (as Alex Galloway has done in Memphis) is to work with churches and pastors to promote awareness and education about mental illness and treatment. This is a better way of identifying mental health needs than trying to do so in primary care physicians' offices, and they can reach more people because more visit churches than medical offices in a given month.

DeHaven's approach is twofold. First, he and his team hold two education forums each year for the public that are well attended (one at Southern Methodist University). Second, they are constructing a network of churches designed to reduce the stigma associated with mental illness and provide access to care. The biggest barrier they find is that people simply don't know whom to turn to for care. When clergy place a notice in the church bulletin that there is a confidential source in the church available to discuss possible mental health problems, they indicate that they are often inundated by calls for help.

Mental health professionals are able today to control the symptoms of mental illness with medications and, through rehabilitation, can restore function for many patients. However, DeHaven says that the final component of treatment is that of helping the families and those affected by mental illness to rediscover their place in the universe. Thus, they work through an interfaith committee to reach out to faith communities to help those with mental illness obtain the professional care they need, and then allow churches to provide the compassionate, caring, nonjudgmental, and supportive environment that provides the real, long-term healing. In this way, the strengths of the mental health care system and of the faith community are being used to complement one another.

DeHaven and colleagues are designing a study to test the effectiveness of this faith-based program in terms of case identification, treatment access, and outcome improvement. Reducing the stigma associated with mental illness, facilitating access to care through appropriate referrals, and providing care and support based on love, is something that faith-based organizations can do, want to do, and exist to do. It is important, however, to document the effectiveness of these efforts through systematic study. Good intentions don't always translate into good results.

Finally, since minority groups often have the most difficult time getting services, faith-based efforts to deliver mental health services to these communities are crucial.[5] There is need for research that identifies the type and quality of services provided, assesses the clergy's knowledge about what professional mental health services exist within their local community, and documents the referral practices of minority clergy. Taylor and colleagues in the Department of Sociology at the University of Michigan suggest that rather than expending resources on small, unrepresentative samples, the focus should be on studies that survey large, representative community groups that will improve generalization of results. They recommend such studies examine the role of ministers in addressing the mental health needs of members of their congregation, why members of the congregation seek assistance for mental health problems from clergy rather than other sources, the extent to which there is ongoing collaboration between clergy and mental health service agencies, and the factors that influence the development of outreach programs to congregants and other members of the community.[6] Such research is a necessary first step prior to developing, implementing, and assessing faith-based programs in such communities.

OVERCOMING BARRIERS TO FUNDING RESEARCH

As noted in chapter 13, lack of funding for research is a serious problem. A number of specific steps could be taken to address this issue. First, since most members of NIH study sections are poorly qualified to review such research, it is important that they obtain special training in the area of religion and mental health in order to equip them with the necessary expertise. A Web-based training program could be developed to provide these skills. Having well-trained reviewers on study sections would improve the likelihood that religion-mental health proposals will be funded.

Second, an administrative position at the NIH could be created to ensure that special consideration be given to religion and mental health research (or at least ensure that such proposals do not get rejected because of undue bias or inadequate review). This person could work with NIH study section chairs to ensure that appropriate emphasis is given to these proposals, and that qualified reviewers are assigned to assess them.

Finally, a separate bureau or office could be created within one of the Institutes (NIMH, for example). This new office/division might review all religion and mental health proposals and have a separate budget for funding such proposals. Alternatively, a separate, stand-alone office could be created similar to NCCAM or OBSSR. NCCAM was established because it became evident that alternative therapies were widespread in the United States and needed evaluation. OBSSR was established because people realized that social and behavioral factors had a significant impact on health. Similarly, an office could be established that focuses on assessing the relationship between religion and mental health and the effectiveness of faith-based mental health services.

OVERCOMING ATTITUDINAL BARRIERS

Because attitudinal barriers exist both among scientists conducting the research and clinicians implementing the research, a widespread program for educating both researchers and clinicians is needed. Such an attitudinal shift is initially needed among scientists, researchers, and teachers, and if efforts are successful in these groups, then it will likely trickle down to clinicians as well.

For years, research studies funded by the NIH did not include suffi-

cient numbers of women, minorities, or children that would enable findings from these studies to be applied to these groups. Now NIH applications require that all applicants mention how their studies ensure that
women, minorities, and children are included (when possible and relevant). Something like this could also be required for religion and cultural
factors. Doing so would certainly alert scientists to the importance of con-
sidering such factors in their work. As more and more research is done in
the area of religion and mental health, more scientific papers will be published in peer-review journals and more papers will be presented at scientific meetings. This research should result in residency and doctoral training programs, as well as in continuing medical education (CME) seminars
for practicing clinicians, emphasizing the role that religion plays in mental
health. In this way, attitudes within the field will gradually change.

OVERCOMING BARRIERS TO IMPLEMENTATION

In this section I consider ways of overcoming barriers faced by FBOs
seeking to deliver mental health services. What kinds of resources are
needed to overcome these barriers? How might state and federal governments, or private foundations or businesses, make things easier? What can
FBOs do themselves to contribute to solutions?

Perhaps most important is what should *not* be done. The mental
health services that FBOs provide should not be seen as replacing the need
for professional mental health services. Rather, they should be viewed as
complementing what already exists to provide better, more comprehensive
services, especially with regard to disease prevention. This will ultimately
reduce the cost of mental health care as the need for those services becomes less and less over time. However, this will require an initial investment up front in order to fully prepare and engage FBOs in ministries that
meet the short-term and long-term mental health needs of the population.
That investment should be focused on the following areas.

Educate clergy

Training of clergy in the diagnosis, treatment, and referral of mental
disorders is needed to enhance their ability to identify and competently address mental health needs in their congregations and those outside it as

well. This is especially true for clergy ministering to minority and other underserved populations with limited access to professional mental health services. Education should focus on short-term emotional problems and long-term serious mental illness, as well as address illness prevention and mental health promotion. Clergy education models already exist. Consider the impact that psychologist Alex Galloway from Christ Community Medical Clinic has made on pastors in the Memphis area by holding mental health seminars in local churches. In less than three years, spending only a few hours a month, he has trained nearly 70 clergy to better recognize, treat, and refer people with mental illness. New models are needed for other settings and both new and existing models need outcome assessments to determine how effective they are.

To reduce costs, training programs could be conducted over the Internet and incentives given for completion, including degrees or certificates, and other forms of recognition including financial ones (tax breaks or direct payments). Federal dollars directed toward education of clergy who can then both provide free mental health services and train others in their congregation to do so will be money well spent. Such efforts should be guided by careful research that identifies the type and quality of services now provided by clergy, determines their referral patterns, and assesses their knowledge about mental health issues and professional mental health services (as noted earlier).

Educate congregations

Besides clergy, religious congregations themselves need to be educated about the causes and treatments for emotional problems (depression and anxiety disorders) and persistent mental disorders (schizophrenia, severe recurrent depression, bipolar disorder, personality disorder). This will help to reduce the stigma of seeking mental health services and reduce the fear of including and caring for persons with these conditions.

Educate mental health professionals

Resistance to FBO involvement from mental health professionals needs to be overcome.

As noted in chapter 2, there is a long history of antagonism between the faith community and the mental health profession. Neither group has made extraordinary efforts to show respect for or value the contributions of the other. That needs to change. History demonstrates the role that people of faith and religious organizations have played in the establishment of the kind of mental health care system that we have today. Systematic research is increasingly showing the close connection between religion and good mental health. Not only is research demonstrating to the scientific mental health community the benefits of religious faith, but research is also demonstrating to the faith community the contributions to mental health that modern psychology and medical psychiatry are making. Thus, vigorous efforts to educate both mental health professionals and clergy should lead to a decrease in resistance between these two groups. Rather than compete for scarce government resources, the religious and mental health communities need to find ways to complement one another so that scarce resources are best spent on maximizing the contributions of each group.

Coordinate services

Services provided by FBOs and those by secular mental health organizations are separate and disconnected. As noted above, there may even be competition or antagonism between these groups, since neither recognizes or values what the other has to offer. The losers in this battle are those with mental illness and their families. Incentives are needed to foster greater cooperation and communication between FBOs and secular mental health organizations. This will require both the enlightenment of clergy and intensive education for mental health professionals and primary care physicians. Linkages also need to be encouraged between FBOs and local mental health centers, private and state psychiatric institutions, prisons, hospital inpatient psychiatric wards, hospital emergency rooms, and academic departments of psychiatry, psychology, and social work.

Mobilize volunteers

Volunteers from within the faith community need to be mobilized to run and participate in FBO programs that provide support and companionship to those experiencing short-term or long-term mental health problems. As described previously, model programs in this regard include Interfaith Compeer and Stephen's Ministries. These programs train members of faith communities to provide spiritually motivated human friendship and support to those with short-term conditions such as depression, anxiety, loss, stress, substance abuse, and long-term mental illnesses such as schizophrenia, severe recurrent depression, bipolar disorder, or severe personality disorder, and physical health problems resulting from stroke, arthritis, heart failure, diabetes, and other chronic disabling conditions. This may require initial financial assistance for education, training, and administrative support and guidance in setting up such programs. It may also include marketing campaigns on radio and national television to reduce the stigma associated with mental illness and get volunteers from religious and nonreligious communities to get involved in such programs. If mental health care costs are to be reduced and needs met, it will require large numbers of volunteers from religious communities contributing time and talents toward this end. Other programs should focus on mobilizing volunteer mental health professionals (retired or active) who might donate their services for religious reasons.

Change liability laws

Given the professional liability that many religious organizations face when attempting to deliver mental health services, it is important to remove unnecessary liability barriers that are now preventing FBOs from delivering services—particularly services that rely on volunteers and laypersons from the congregation. Certainly some degree of training and accountability is required even for those who provide simple care, support, and companionship. Nevertheless, realistic worries over the possibility of being sued are discouraging many religious individuals and organizations from offering their services. There should be a "good Samaritan" law passed to prevent suits against volunteers who in good faith provide emotional support and physical assistance to needy persons.

Address over-regulation

The problem of over-regulation needs to be tackled. Representatives from faith communities are needed on regulatory boards so that their input can be considered. State laws may need to be reevaluated. The paperwork needs to be simplified so that FBOs aren't spending all of their time and resources completing forms or seeking reimbursement instead of providing services. This can be extremely frustrating even for FBOs who feel called to minister to those with mental health problems. This does not mean that there should be no monitoring of services or regulations, but only that such monitoring should not become prohibitive to the practical delivery of those services. Forms should be simplified and training should be offered in a central location or over the Internet to facilitate the process. If new software is required for billing systems involving government reimbursement, then this software should be provided free of charge to FBOs expected to acquire such technology.

Jill Schumann at Lutheran Social Services emphasizes the need for performance-based contracting and outcome measurements. However, while awarding contracts for service based on performance is good, it also means the possibility of discontinuity in services if contracts are not continued. Furthermore, it involves determining what is good performance, which may depend greatly on setting and may be influenced by many local factors. This requires that further research be done to determine what is effective treatment and how to measure it in different conditions and different treatment settings. This might lead to less complex and more targeted regulations.

Promote charitable giving

Efforts should be made to promote faith-based charitable giving by individuals (i.e., the public) to FBOs that deliver mental health services. This could be done through public education programs, radio and TV marketing efforts, and other forms of mass media or public service announcements. Charles Lockwood of Glade Run Lutheran Services suggests that the government could provide incentives for faith-based charitable donations to social service agencies that deliver such services. Those incentives, however, would need to be targeted specifically for faith-based programs. Funds could be earmarked for direct care staff (especially those who serve the most disturbed mentally ill populations), a group that deserves more recognition and better pay. Higher pay would also encourage young professionals to enter and stay in a career focused on meeting the needs of this population.

Provide targeted funding

Local and national religious organizations that provide services to those with chronic mental illness need additional financial support to continue or expand their current services. Even small public grants could make a major impact, if carefully directed. One example is the Mental Illness Ministry of the Mennonite and Anabaptist churches. While Mennonite Mutual Aid supports this group, funding sources are needed to help expand this ministry. A small amount of additional support would allow them to hire a full-time staff person or two part-time persons to create mental illness resources such as educational videos for teens, Sunday school curricula for youths and adults about understanding mental illness, and retreats for families who need a place to get away. Since volunteers carry out much of the work that FBOs do, funding a position to coordinate such efforts would be dollars well spent.

Roy Woodruff of AAPC says that federal grants for services to underserved and low-income persons would help pastoral counselors who are sensitive to these needs and who desire to serve these populations. Ironically, populations for whom faith is often a prominent part of their lives, such as the elderly and the near-poor or poor, are the ones who can least afford the out-of-pocket expenses for pastoral counseling. Woodruff is seeking a large grant from the government for AAPC that could then be distributed to programs run by accredited pastoral counseling centers around the country providing faith-based, professional care. While his request was positively received, it has not progressed from that point of inquiry. It makes sense that mental health services provided to underserved populations by certified professionals (master's level counselors and up) working within FBOs should be considered for reimbursement under Medicaid and Medicare. Woodruff has prepared a White Paper on pastoral counseling and Medicare that is available on request.[7]

While government funding to support counseling services in underserved communities would be most helpful, Bruce Strade of Lutheran Community Services Northwest notes that such funding tends to be very trendy, depending on the political winds of the time. A consistent plan needs to be developed for all age groups and then adequate funds arranged to support it. Currently, certain groups of people are often ignored or considered disposable, especially based on age. Early intervention in the young is important, but that should not be done at the expense of systems and support for the elderly. Efforts should also be made to fund prevention and wellness programs, which are designed to have long-range benefits. The present system focuses on simply treating disorders that arise, but does not address the root sources of many mental health problems.

Finally, in order to ensure that the efforts described above are carried out swiftly and effectively, a special federal office or a division within an existing office could be created to oversee the implementation of such a plan. Many national and local organizations already exist that are trying to educate and train religious communities to address the mental health needs of members of the congregation and the community. Such an office could help to network these individuals together and provide support and incentives for such efforts. The office could work with private foundations, businesses, insurance companies, and hospitals to help partner with state, local, and national government in offering small grants to FBOs to help expand their services. The office could also coordinate training for FBOs in research design, grant writing, and other skills necessary to successfully compete for federal funds and raise money through local fundraising efforts.

Summary and Conclusions

This final chapter was about solutions. Efforts to foster research on religion, mental health, and faith-based delivery of mental health services will require addressing methodological issues, prioritizing areas most in need of study, providing funding for such studies, and bringing down attitudinal barriers through education and modeling. Such efforts will require cooperation between the Department of Health and Human Services, the National Institutes of Health, and the scientific community—those groups that control the funding and review of such research. As high-quality research is designed, carried out, and published, this will assist in changing the attitudes of educators and mental health professionals toward FBOs and their potential contributions.

A plan also needs to be developed to provide consistent support for faith-based efforts to deliver mental health services (implementation). This will require careful and targeted allocation of resources (first to those that address the needs of underserved populations), followed by rigorous program evaluation to ensure that goals are being met. Regulations, monitoring, and paperwork, however, cannot be so extensive that this impedes the delivery of services. A division could be set up within the Department of Health and Human Services or the Office of Faith-Based and Community Initiatives to coordinate efforts by government, private, and faith-based groups to deliver needed mental health services to the community.

Solutions should not rest entirely on the shoulders of the government or on the scientific community. FBOs, too, will need to make major shifts in their attitudes toward mental illness and toward mental health professionals, will need to prioritize the education of clergy and faith communities on how to meet the needs of persons with emotional or mental problems, and will need to mobilize members to volunteer their time and talents for such ministry. They will also need to either learn to mobilize funding support from private sources or learn grant-writing skills, so that they can successfully compete for scarce federal, state, and local mental health dollars. In the end, however, success will depend on working together and complementing, not competing, with one another. Only by working together as colleagues, respecting and valuing each other's contributions, can the secular mental health community and the faith community meet the challenges that lie before them.

GLOSSARY

ALTRUISM. In its simplest form, altruism is the selfless caring for others without expectation of reward. Altruism involves giving to others without expecting anything back from them. Altruism is contrasted with egoistic giving, which involves performing acts of service to others with the underlying motivation of getting something in return.

ANTISOCIAL. This involves actions that are willfully performed that hurt other people or that involves an avoidance of other people or activities that involve groups of people.

ANTISOCIAL PERSONALITY DISORDER. A firmly held, sometimes lifelong way of thinking and acting that is hurtful to others. Someone with an antisocial personality disorder feels little guilt when hurting others, but rather feels justified in their actions. Often associated with criminal activities.

ANXIETY. Anxiety is an emotion associated with some type of internal or external threat to physical or emotional well-being. It is accompanied by a sense of fear or worry about the future, whether in response to a distinct event, or to no event in particular. It may include feelings of physical restlessness and tremulousness.

BABY BOOMER. This is the name given to a person born between 1945 and 1967, reflecting the post-World War II baby boom. This group makes up about 70 million in the United States.

BIAS. When personal feelings about a subject influence the opinions or actions taken. This term is applicable to scientists in regard to how they approach the religion-health relationship. Many secular scientists may be biased against religion and religious scientists may be biased for religion. Regardless, judgments are made based on those personal beliefs that are not part of the actual facts being observed. Because most scientists are secular, the bias usually goes against religion in academic environments.

BIPOLAR DISORDER. A chronic mental illness associated with periods of severe depression and manic elation that cycle between one another over time. This has also been called manic-depressive illness. The person may experience depression so severe that he or she may wish to commit suicide, which is then followed by a period of great happiness, joy, energy, creativeness, and lack of need for sleep, which is then followed by severe depression and lack of motivation. During either the depressive or manic phases, psychotic symptoms may be present (delusions or hallucinations).

CHAPLAIN. Chaplains are clergy who provide counseling and support to hospitalized patients in acute care medical hospitals, psychiatric hospitals, the military, prisons, and nursing homes. Chaplains do not displace local clergy, but rather fill specific needs related to intense medical or psychiatric settings that complement the activities of congregation-based clergy.

CLERGY. This term refers to ministers, rabbis, imams, monks, and other religious leaders who may or may not be ordained, but who lead religious congregations.

CLINICAL. Clinical refers to patient-related activities. The clinic is a place where patients are treated. Clinical activities involve the treatment of patients either for medical or psychiatric reasons.

CLINICAL TRIAL. A clinical trial is an experimental study that tests the effectiveness of a treatment. Clinical trials may be either randomized clinical trials or non-randomized in terms of assignment of subjects. Clinical trials may be single-blinded (the patient knows, but investigator doesn't know who is getting the active treatment), double-blinded (neither patient nor investigator knows who is getting the active treatment), or open clinical trials (everyone knows who is getting the treatment).

CONVERSION. As it applies to religious conversion, this term means a complete transformation in beliefs, attitudes, and behaviors with regard to religion. This may occur suddenly and dramatically, or may come about slowly and gradually over time. The end result is that a person who was weakly religious or not religious at all ends up with strong religious beliefs and those beliefs influence and guide his or her actions.

COPING. The thoughts or activities involved in adapting to a stressor of some type, where the stressor is either positive or negative (although usually negative).

COUNSELING. Counseling can be either formal or informal. Informal counseling may involve talking with a friend or trusted person about a problem or situation, where the person is either seeking advice (counsel) or simply is needing to ventilate their feelings. Formal counseling involves seeking assistance usually from a trained professional who is experienced and certified to provide such counseling and charges a fee.

CROSS-SECTIONAL STUDY. This is a type of study design where religiousness or spirituality is measured as the same point in time as indicators of mental health, and the correlations between them are examined. For example, a questionnaire is sent out by mail that has questions about religious attendance, prayer, and other religious activities, along with questions about depression, anxiety, or perceived stress. People fill out the questionnaire and return it to investigators, who then examine the correlations between the religious and the mental health scores. Because these are correlations at one point in time, there is no way to determine if the religious activity is responsible for the mental health of participants or whether the mental health is responsible for the religious activity.

DEPARTMENT OF HEALTH AND HUMAN SERVICES. A division of the U.S. government that controls both research on and delivery of health services funded by the government, and especially public policy decisions regarding those services.

DEPRESSION. A psychological-biological state where a person feels sad, has lost interest in things (including socializing), has little energy or motivation to do anything, has trouble sleeping, concentrating, or eating, and is associated with other symptoms as well, including suicidal thoughts if the depression is severe. Depression exists on a continuum from mild feelings of discouragement or sadness over disappointments common to human life that last a few hours or days, all the way to a life-threatening illness that can last weeks or months or years, and has a 15% lifetime mortality rate from suicide alone.

DOGMATISM. Dogmatism involves the arrogant, stubborn assertion of an opinion or belief.

EATING DISORDER. This is a psychiatric condition that is a disorder of eating. People may starve themselves and lose weight (anorexia) or may binge eat and then purge food from the body by vomiting or use of laxatives (bulimia). Anorexia nervosa is often life threatening and has a poor prognosis once weight falls below a certain level.

EMOTIONAL PROBLEMS. In contrast to mental illness (such as schizophrenia), emotional problems may involve mild to moderate depression, anxiety, fear, or worry, often over situational factors. The condition is not usually severe or persistent, and is usually time limited. There is no loss of contact with reality (as in psychosis), and people remain competent and generally in control of themselves and their lives.

ENLIGHTENMENT PERIOD. This is the period in world history between the end of the French Revolution and the beginning of the modern period (1800–1875). During this time, religious views were rejected and replaced by rationalism.

EVANGELISM. Evangelism is an activity whose goal is the conversion of people to a particular religious belief system. The evangelist seeks to convince the person to believe as he or she believes with regard to religion.

EXORCISM. Exorcism is a religious rite that involves the expelling of demons from someone thought to be possessed. In the late Middle Ages, people with certain types of mental illness were thought to be possessed by demons, and exorcism was used in attempts to rid them of the demons. Even today, certain religious groups use exorcism in attempts to rid people of mental problems (in both developed and non-developed countries), although it is admittedly rare.

FAITH. Faith, as used here, involves religious belief and commitment to those beliefs.

FAITH-BASED ORGANIZATION (FBO). This describes organizations that were established on and operate on religious beliefs, which is their reason for being, or organizations that clearly have a religious mission. A *faith-based organization* is either a religious organization or a group with administrative or financial ties to a religious organization or organizations. Included here are groups that support and coordinate faith-based delivery of mental health services by providing contacts and educational resources to religious congregations. Also included here are organizations that are not religious organizations and are not administratively tied to a religious organization, but that have as their primary mission the delivery of health services from a faith perspective.

FBO CATEGORY A. In this category are local churches, synagogues, mosques, and temples that provide counseling and support primarily to their members, and includes mental health services delivered by pastors, priests, ministers, rabbis, imams, and other local clergy and staff, as well as companionship and support provided by volunteers from within the religious congregation.

FBO CATEGORY B. Included in this category are national and local networking, education, and advocacy groups that exist to help religious congregations deliver services more effectively, especially to those with severe and persistent mental illness.

FBO CATEGORY C. Organizations whose religious values provide the motivation for delivering the services ("mission" driven), and they do not usually use religion in the treatment process.

FBO CATEGORY D. Clergy who undergo the training necessary to certify them as professional counselors and have the acquired skills to integrate fully religious therapies with secular psychotherapy. They use religion in the treatment process. This group consists mainly of chaplains, pastoral counselors, and Samaritan counselors, and their supporting national organizations.

FBO CATEGORY E. Organizations of trained counselors, usually without professional religious training, who emphasize faith-based therapies in the treatment of their patients (Christian counselors, for example, although Jewish and Muslim counselors also fall into this category). They use religion in the treatment process.

GENETICS. Genetics refers to inherited characteristics from family members. The *gene* is a basic building block of chromosomes that transmits both psychological tendencies (temperament) and physical characteristics between generations.

HISPANIC. Persons from Mexico or other Latin American countries (Central America or South America), whose ancestors came from Spain (often with intermarriage with native Indians).

INTERVENTION. A treatment used to help a person recover from an illness or disease. For example, psychotherapy or antidepressant medications are interventions used to treat people with depression.

INTRINSIC RELIGIOSITY. A measure of religious motivation. People for whom religious involvement is the object of their ultimate concern, rather than a means to obtaining something more important to them, are said to be intrinsically religious. Individuals who use religion to obtain something more important to them (social connections, good standing in the community, financial gain) are said to be extrinsically religious.

LONGITUDINAL STUDY (see Prospective Study)

MANIA (see Bipolar Disorder)

MECHANISM. Mechanism as used in this book is the pathway by which something (such as religion) influences another thing (well-being). One mechanism by which religion may influence well-being is by giving life purpose and meaning, or by increasing social support.

MENTAL HEALTH PROFESSIONAL. This refers to a psychologist, psychiatrist, counselor, or social worker who is trained and licensed to provide mental health treatments (psychotherapy, counseling, or medication).

MENTAL HEALTH SERVICES. Counseling and support for anyone experiencing emotional distress from depression, anxiety, or stressful circumstances such as bereavement, divorce, job problems, or economic loss. Mental health services also include both outpatient and residential treatment programs that provide psychotherapy, pharmacological therapy, or other biological treatments for mental illness, as well as case management and social services needed by those with serious mental illnesses.

MENTAL ILLNESS. Mental illness usually refers to people with chronic, persistent problems in social relationships or occupational functioning due to a group of mental disorders. These mental disorders cause the brain not to function right, and may influence emotions, thoughts, and perceptions. There is a wide range of mental illness from either very mild (that is hardly different from normal) to very severe (requiring chronic institutionalization). The most common chronic mental illness is schizophrenia.

METHODOLOGICAL. As used here, this term refers to the way that research is designed and carried out. For example, a methodological issue that stands in the way of further research on religion and mental health is the lack of trained investigators with the skills necessary to design and carry out a successful research study.

MIDDLE AGES. Involves the period in human history between 500 and 1400 CE, especially in western Europe. This was sometimes called the "dark ages" because there was a lull in educational advances and academic learning.

MULTIVARIATE ANALYSES. This is a statistical procedure that "controls" or removes the effects of other possible predictors of an outcome. For example, when studying the effects of religious attendance on health, investigators seek to control for (or take into account) the physical ability to get to church and the social support they receive there. They use multivariate statistics to do so.

NATIONAL INSTITUTES OF HEALTH. Established after World Ward II to support medical research, this is a division of the Department of Health and Human Services that both conducts research (intramural programs) and provides funding to outside medical researchers, usually at established universities, to conduct research studies (extramural programs).

OBSESSIVE-COMPULSIVE DISORDER. A psychological condition associated with obsessions (anxious thoughts that persons cannot rid themselves of) and compulsions (the need to perform certain acts to "undue" or prevent the feared consequences of their thoughts).

OFFICE OF FAITH-BASED AND COMMUNITY INITIATIVES. Established by U.S. President George W. Bush in 2000, this office was started to support and expand the delivery of health services by faith-based and community organizations.

PASTORAL COUNSELOR. Pastoral counselors are different from chaplains, although the differences are subtle. These are certified mental health professionals who have had in-depth religious and/or theological training that enables them to integrate the religious and spiritual dimensions into psychological counseling. They may provide their services on an individual basis, be part of a group of other pastoral counselors, or may occasionally work as part of a secular mental health group.

PERSONALITY. The habitual ways that people think and behave that distinguish them as unique individuals. Personality is influenced by both biological or genetic factors (temperament at birth) and developmental factors (environment in which a person is raised).

PERSONALITY DISORDER. When a person has long-standing problems relating with other people in positive and constructive ways, then a personality disorder may exist. This involves habitual patterns of unhealthy ways of relating to others that cause stress for the individual and other people.

POST-TRAUMATIC DISTRESS DISORDER (PTSD). This is an anxiety disorder that develops after a person has been exposed to a horrible experience involving the death or threatened death of a loved one, or threatened death of the person him- or herself. This condition is often associated with startle responses or avoidance of things that remind them of the traumatic event.

PROSPECTIVE OR COHORT STUDY. A study that surveys a group of people at one point in time and the follows them up for a period of time (from several months up to many years) and re-administers the survey to see whether any changes have occurred. If religiousness is being examined as a predictor, then researchers examine whether degree of religiousness at baseline predicts either positive or negative changes in future health status. In contrast to cross-sectional studies, this type of study includes the element of time. It may be established, then, that religiousness came before the change in health status, providing evidence (but not proving) that the religiousness caused the better health.

PSYCHIATRIST. A psychiatrist is a medical doctor (M.D.) who specializes in the mental health problems that people experience. A psychiatrist may do some counseling, but often focuses on finding the right medication or other biological treatment (ECT, etc.) to treat the person's condition. The psychiatrist can prescribe medication, since he or she is a doctor.

PSYCHIATRY. This is a medical specialty that involves the treatment of persons with emotional problems or mental illness. Psychiatrists are M.D.s and can prescribe medication and take care of patients in the hospital. They may also practice psychotherapy, but this has become less common in recent years.

PSYCHOLOGIST. A psychologist is usually a person with a Ph.D. in psychology who focuses on psychotherapy and psychological testing. A psychologist cannot usually prescribe medication.

PSYCHOLOGY. Psychology is a behavioral science that may either be entirely academic (psychologists who teach and do research) or may be clinical (psychologists who see patients and do psychotherapy or psychological testing). Psychologists usually have a Ph.D. in psychology. They cannot prescribe medications or care for patients in the hospital.

PSYCHOSIS. A mental state where the person has difficulty distinguishing fantasy from reality, and may experience delusions (persistent false beliefs) or hallucinations (auditory, visual, or tactile). It can be caused by chronic mental illnesses such as schizophrenia or mania, or it may result from medical conditions that cause disorientation and delirium.

PSYCHOTHERAPY. Psychotherapy is an advanced form of counseling or talk therapy that uses specific techniques such as cognitive-behavioral psychotherapy, psychodynamic psychotherapy, interpersonal psychotherapy, or psychoanalysis. Psychotherapies are interventions that have usually been tested in clinical trials to determine their effectiveness. Rather than simply support a patient or offer advice, psychotherapy involves changing the way people think and behave that results in less emotional pain and greater satisfaction with life.

QUALITY OF LIFE. Quality of life is defined as a person's overall level of functioning, including psychological well-being, social relationships, and ability to care independently for physical needs. It is most often measured in people with chronic illness or terminal conditions such as cancer, HIV/AIDS, and congestive heart failure that seriously challenge them in each of these areas.

REFORMATION. The Reformation is the period of human history beginning after Martin Luther tacked his 95 theses on the door at Wittenberg Chapel in 1517, and continued through the end of the French Revolution in 1800.

RELIGION. Religion is an organized system of beliefs, practices, rituals, and symbols designed (1) to facilitate closeness to the sacred or transcendent (God, higher power, or ultimate truth/reality), and (2) to foster an understanding of one's relationship and responsibility to others in living together in a community.[1]

RELIGIOUS COPING. Religious coping involves the use of religion to cope with or adapt to stressful life circumstances. This may involve prayer, scripture reading, attending religious services, or speaking with a member of the clergy. The religious activity is designed to reduce stress and bring about a sense of peace and hopefulness.

RENAISSANCE. The Renaissance is the period in human history between the Middle Ages and the Reformation (1400–1517). This refers primarily to western Europe, and involves a renewed interest in the arts and sciences that had been largely dormant during the Middle Ages.

RESEARCH. Research as used here involves scientific, objective study of phenomena such as religion and mental health. It consists of the systematic collection of information based on unbiased observation. Different types of research include epidemiological studies (case-control studies, cross-sectional studies, prospective studies) and experimental studies (clinical trials).

RESIDENTIAL TREATMENT. Care that is provided in an institutional or long-term care setting is often called "residential," since the person lives at the facility (i.e., is a resident).

SCHIZOPHRENIA. A chronic psychiatric disorder associated with delusions (having false beliefs that they cannot be dissuaded from, often paranoid in nature) and/or hallucinations (typically hearing voices or seeing visions). Problems with thinking (difficult to follow line of thought), mood (inappropriately jovial or sad), and decision making (ambivalence) are also common. People with schizophrenia must have the above symptoms for at least 6 months or longer.

SCHIZOTYPAL OR SCHIZOTYPY. This is a personality trait that involves a pattern of social and interpersonal difficulties marked by discomfort with, and reduced capacity for, close relationships with others. It also involves cognitive or perceptual distortions and eccentricities of behavior that are sometimes seen in persons prior to the development of schizophrenia.

SIGNIFICANT. If a correlation is said to be "statistically significant," then it meets the scientific convention for events that would occur outside of random chance. The scientific community says that for a single comparison, if the statistic of association (p value) is less than 0.05, then this is said to be statistically significant. A p value of less than 0.05 means that the event would occur by chance alone in less than 1 in 20 cases.

SOCIAL SERVICES. Social services involve assistance with obtaining shelter (housing) and food, and may involve advocacy and in some cases support and counseling. Many faith-based organizations, such as Catholic Charities or Lutheran Social Services, provide social services of this type on a large scale and many smaller churches do so on a smaller scale.

SOCIAL WORKER. Social workers are often employed by hospitals to assist with discharge planning or by department of social services in local governments. Social workers help ensure that people have the necessary resources to survive in the community. They also often provide counseling, especially if they are associated with a medical or mental health clinic. Social workers typically have a master's degree and are certified.

SOCIOLOGIST. Sociology is the scientific study of human social behavior. A sociologist is often a teacher of sociology or a researcher at a university (or may work for the government). Sociologists study how society works and how it changes over time. Sociologists typically have a Ph.D. that certifies them to teach and do research.

SPIRITUAL WELL-BEING. Spiritual well-being, according to Palouzian and Ellison, involves two components: religious well-being and existential well-being. Religious well-being involves feeling close to God, loved by God, and being satisfied with one's relationship with God. Existential well-being involves a sense of well-being about one's purpose in life and identity, a belief that life is meaningful and positive, and a sense of satisfaction about one's future.

SPIRITUALITY. Spirituality is the personal quest for understanding answers to ultimate questions about life, about meaning, and about relationship to the sacred or transcendant, which may (or may not) lead to or arise from the development of religious rituals and the formation of community.[2]

STIGMA. Stigma involves the negative attitudes that some people have toward others (or themselves) with mental illness. People see mental illness as embarrassing and something to be ashamed of, so they hide their symptoms because of the "stigma" associated with having such problems.

STRUCTURAL EQUATION MODELING. Structural equation modeling is a relatively sophisticated, chiefly linear, chiefly cross-sectional statistical modeling technique that is commonly used in the social and psychological sciences. Its advantage is that it takes into account measurement error in the variables studied.

STUDY SECTION. This term refers to a group of about 10 to 15 people who meet together at the National Institutes of Health (NIH) to review grants that people have submitted to the NIH for funding support. There are many study sections at the NIH, and these are convened around specific health-related topics. These people are usually scientists with extensive experience conducting research, so they can comment on the value and quality of the research proposed.

Substance Abuse. The heavy use of alcohol, illicit drugs, or prescription drugs, particularly when these substances are illegal or taken in large quantities without a doctor's knowledge and adversely affect the mental health, social functioning, and/or physical health of the individual.

Univariate (or Bivariate). This is a type of statistical test or analysis where two characteristics of an individual are correlated, but without controlling for or taking into account other factors (as in multivariate analyses). A univariate correlation may also be called a "zero-order" correlation.

ADDITIONAL RESOURCES

In this section I list additional resources for faith communities wishing to deliver mental health services or meet the spiritual needs of persons with severe, persistent mental illness. Many of these resources will also be valuable for mental health professionals wishing to collaborate with faith communities in their area. Margaret Ann Holt, executive director at VICOMIM, contributed much of the information for this section. That information includes written resources, media resources, information for clergy, efforts by local groups to change public policy, and contact information listed by state for individuals leading organizations already active in this area.

Written and Media Resources

Strength for His People: A Ministry for Families of the Mentally Ill (1994) Amarillo, TX: Westcliff Press, is a book written by Pastor Steven Waterhouse, ThM, DMin, of Westcliff Bible Church in Amarillo, TX. Waterhouse's doctoral dissertation from the Dallas Theological Seminary involved the development of a ministry to Christian families with relatives who have schizophrenia. This is a scholarly book, filled with footnotes and references. Pastor Waterhouse does a masterful job of addressing the spiritual questions that arise when mental illness strikes a Christian family. Six chapters describe how God relates to the devastating illness of schizophrenia. Each chapter is followed by questions for discussion. Chapter 6 tackles the dilemma of how a pastor can differentiate between demon possession and symptoms of schizophrenia. To obtain a copy of this book, mail a $6.00 check made out to "Westcliff Bible Church" to: P.O. Box 1521, Amarillo, TX 79105.[1]

"Faith and Mental Illness," *NAMI Advocate* (Fall 2001): 8–9. This article describes a symposium on "The Healing Power of Faith." Excerpts from Kathy Hyler's talk are printed.

Guideposts (monthly interfaith magazine) (January 2002): 18, begins a new series of articles on "Overcoming Depression." The first article titled "My Darkest Hour," features Mike Wallace, senior correspondent for the CBS show *60 Minutes*.

Touched by an Angel (TV show): "When Sunny Gets Blue," aired December 2001, dealt very appropriately with the issue of when a loved one has schizophrenia. This program is not available for purchase on tape. Margaret Holt encourages calls to CBS to express appreciation for the realistic portrayal of schizophrenia and ask them to show this particular episode frequently and to put it on a video for sale (212-975-3247).

Information for Clergy

An example of a sermon on mental illness and an entire worship service with mental illness as a focus: Pastor Frankie Perdue spoke on a "Restored Life" on October 14, 2001. A copy of his sermon and a copy of the worship service are posted on the VICOMIM Web page cited below. Look also for a sermon from Gunnar Christiansen (retired physician) entitled "Divine Healing." VICOMIM's Web site is http://www.vaumc.org/gm/micom.htm (go to Resources, then Sermons/Messages.).

Other examples of sermons about mental illness can be found at http://www. umc-gbcs.org/csasept2_oct2001.htm; these are written by a Methodist chaplain in Tennessee and a Methodist pastor at General Board Church & Society of the United Methodist Church. They illustrate preaching that includes references to mental illness issues to help the congregation become a caring community for those within their own membership who have a mental illness.

Resources for Changing Public Policy

An example of public policy efforts by FBOs to improve care to the mentally ill is a legislative agenda recently adopted by the Virginia Interfaith Center for Public Policy (VICPP) and by the Virginia Council of Churches (VCC) for the 2002 Virginia state legislative year. It includes health care as one of its five concerns. Included under "Health Care" is an initiative to extend mental health care to all Virginians. Of the 286,000 Virginian adults with a serious mental illness, only 39,000 receive community-based services from the public mental health system. Many of those who have committed misdemeanors and are declared not guilty by reason of insanity are confined to hospitals or treatment facilities indefinitely, frequently as long as a decade. Virginia's prisons have replaced the state's mental hospitals for many of those with mental illness.

VICPP and VCC are arguing for funding for community-based mental health services and quality residential care throughout the state, increasing accessibility of medication for the indigent, limiting the amount of time those who plead not guilty by reason of insanity to a misdemeanor are required to spend hospitalized, and decriminalizing some behaviors caused by mental illness to reduce incarceration of those needing treatment. Contact VICPP by phone at 804-643-2474, or online at www.vicpp.org; contact VCC through the Reverend Jonathan Barton, 804-321-3300, e-mail: barton@VCC-net.org.

Individual Contacts

Listed by state are individuals and their organizations that provide education, resources, or direct services to those with mental illness and their families.

CALIFORNIA

Dr. Gunnar Christiansen: Founded FaithNet within NAMI-California. Christiansen is now developing a FaithNet E-Communication that could serve as a national e-mail linkage for all faith communities on the topic of mental illness. FaithNet hosts large events each year featuring nationally known speakers, and provides free audio and video recordings of these events to anyone who requests. Contact information: gunnar@cox.net.

Reverend Chester Watson: As former vice president of FaithNet NAMI, he has many sermons about and knowledge of special services concerning mental illness. Contact information: 3104 Claudia Drive, Concord, CA 94519-2131; WATSONCORD@aol.com.

Reverend Donald Clark: Pastor of the Capitol City Seventh-Day Adventist Church, P.O. Box 245156, Sacramento, CA 95824. Contact information: dccsda@aol.com.

Reverend Susan Gregg-Schroeder: Leader of Mental Health Ministries, 6707 Monte Verde Drive, San Diego, CA 92119. Contact information: sgschroed@cox.net.

Reverend Chhean Kong: Director of The Cambodian Buddhist Monastery, 2100 West Willow Street, Long Beach, CA 90810. Contact information: kchhean@dmh.co.la.ca.us.

Jay Mahler: Co-chair, Contra Costa Recovery Task Force and leader at Mental Health Consumer Concerns, 3187A Old Tunnel Road, Lafayette, CA 94549. He is very knowledgeable about local resources. Contact information: mahler@hsd.co.contra-costa.ca.us.

GEORGIA

Reverend Gary Gunderson: Formed Interfaith Conference on Suicide Prevention in 1997; author of books examining the role and responsibility of faith-based organizations located in the community. Contact information: ggunder@emory.edu.

ILLINOIS

Dr. Abdul Basit: A Muslim mental health leader associated with the University of Chicago, who heads the Psychiatric Rehabilitation Center at 7230 Arbor Drive in Tinley Park, IL 60477. Contact information: ABasit97@aol.com.

Tom Lambert: Has been in Roman Catholic ministries for several years. Contact information: Our Lady of Mount Carmel Church, 690 W. Belmont, Chicago, Il 60657; 773-525-3533. Mr. Lambert is a deacon in the church.

INDIANA

Carole Wills: Affiliated with the United Methodist Church in Indianapolis, IN, she is involved in providing resources and help to the severely mentally ill. Contact information: 317-299-4570; e-mail: carolejwillis@aol.com.

KENTUCKY

Dr. Harry G. Mills: Actively involved in reaching out to the severely mentally ill. Works to have churches hold Family-to-Family training sessions through NAMI-KY (Baptist). Contact information: 502-245-5284; e-mail: namiky.hgmills@mindspring.com.

Dr. Angie O'Mally: Designed a ministry to those with severe mental illness that is being replicated in churches throughout Kentucky (United Methodist). Contact information: 859-224-1395; e-mail: Ajomall@aol.com.

Paul Weaver: Past director of Consumer Affairs, Kentucky, and also Kentucky Center for Mental Health Studies (Baptist). Contact information: Center for Mental Health Studies, Inc., P.O. Box 12065, Lexington, Ky. 40580-2065; 502-564-4448.

MARYLAND

Bishop Felton May: Methodist bishop of the Baltimore-Washington conference. Has done much to support substance abuse and mental health work.

MINNESOTA

Mary Jean Babcock: The contact person at Faithways in Minneapolis, a resource for faith communities about mental illness. This is a resource to educate, train, and mobilize faith communities to address issues of mental illness and include those with mental illness as part of their congregations. Contact information: mjbab@aol.com.

Kris Flaten: Leader in Minnesota State Advisory Council on Mental Health, 469 Dayton Avenue, #2, St. Paul, MN 55102. Contact information: kflaten@visi.com.

NEW JERSEY

The Honorable DeForest Soaries Jr.: Senior pastor of First Baptist Church of Lincoln Gardens, Somerset, NJ; has developed numerous economic, spiritual, and educational programs for church members and local residents concerning mental illness. Contact information: 609-777-1278.

NEW MEXICO

Gilberto Romero: Leader at De Sol A Sol, P.O. Box 459, Santa Cruz, NM 87567; e-mail: gilbertoromero@la-tierra.com.

NEW YORK

Barbara Outterson: Coordinator for ministries to those with mental illness within faith communities (Presbyterian). Contact information: 231 Mobile Drive, Rochester, NY 14616.

Rabbi Bob Kaplan: Director, Commission on Intergroup Relationship and Community Concerns, Jewish Community Relations Council of New York, 70 W. 36th Street, #700, New York, NY 10018. Contact information: 212-983-4800; e-mail: rabbob1@aol.com. See Web site: http://www.communityuplink.net/.

Jim Forbes: Pastor of Riverside Church in New York City. Well-known Baptist preacher on mental illness and social justice issues. Contact information: 212-870-6700.

OKLAHOMA

Barbara Schneeberg: Has been doing mental illness ministry within the United Methodist Church in Oklahoma for at least 10 years. Contact information:

3105 W. Quincy Street, Broken Arrow, OK 74012; 918-252-2966; e-mail: mourningglory@juno.com.

Tim Reside: Associate pastor of Evangelistic Temple in Tulsa, OK. Emphasizes importance of religion in recovery, obtaining jobs, adequate housing. Contact information: Evangelistic Temple, 5345 South Peoria Avenue, Tulsa OK 74105.

OREGON

Scott Snedecor: Advocate for the mentally ill and involved in previous dialogues with SAMHSA's Center for Mental Health Studies. Contact information: 421 SW 6th Avenue, #500, Portland, OR 97204.

PENNSYLVANIA

Jackie Johnson: With Catholic Charities Spiritual Ministries for People with Disabilities. Contact information: 429 East Grandview Boulevard, Erie, PA 16514.

Hikmah Gardner: A mental health advocate and extremely knowledgeable about local resources. Contact information: 6517 N. 6th St., Philadelphia, PA 19126; e-mail: hamkih@quixnet.net.

Jacki McKinney: Long-term advocate (Muslim) for mentally ill. Contact information: 5124 Newhall St., Philadelphia, PA 19144; 215-844-2540.

TENNESSEE

Rose Ann Briotte: Psychiatric chaplain at Lakeshore Mental Health Institute, 5908 Lyons View Drive, Knoxville, TN 37920. Contact information: 865-584-1561.

TEXAS

Jim Gerhard: Chair of the Lutheran Network for Mental Illness. Contact information: Lutheran ELCA, 2422 Bluffridge, San Antonio, TX 78232; 210-859-0950 or 210-494-0737.

Kevin Dinnin: Director of Baptist Child & Family Services, 909 NE Loop 410, #800, San Antonio, TX 78209. Contact information: kdinnin@bcfs.net.

Kinike Bermudez: Leader in the Mental Health Association of Greater Dallas, 624 North Good Latimer, #200, Dallas, TX 75204. Contact information: KBermudez@mhadallas.org.

Carole Woodard: Executive director of Generation Joshua Community Development Corporation, Williams Temple Church of God in Christ, and co-chair of

Faith-Based Initiative, Texas Southeast First Ecclesiastical Jurisdiction, Church of God (130 churches). Contact information: 281-440-0220.

Larry Mills: Director of Agape Center, a peer-support center in the Amarillo Mental Health Association. Runs one of the few churches in Texas offering ministry for mental health needs (classes, social activities, support groups). Contact information: Buchanan Street Baptist Chapel, 1515 S. Buchanan Street, Amarillo, TX 79101; 806-373-2066; email: gjgaff@arn.net.

VERMONT

William J. Richard: Involved in social justice ministries, visual impairment, and inclusion of people with disabilities. Contact information: 1102 Tri-Town Road, Addison, VT 05491; 802-759-2777, billandrie@mycidoco.com

Linda Corey: Working to involve United Church of Christ activities with NAMI recovery and consumer views. Contact information: vpsine@sovern.net.

VIRGINIA

Pat and Betty Burleson: Lead support groups within the United Methodist Church for persons with mental illness and their families. Contact information: bettyboop22@msn.com.

Kit Carter: Has designed a church-based social club for persons with mental illness (Episcopal). Contact information: P.O. Box 60, Fort Defiance, VA 24437; 540-248-0843.

David Cavanaugh: Coordinates Catholic Charities efforts to provide direct services to persons with severe mental illness. Contact information: 3838 Cathedral Lane, Arlington, VA 22203; 703-841-2531; DCavanaugh@CCDA.NET; alternatively, contact Carole Ann Croll at Catholic Charities, 305 Hanson Avenue, Fredericksburg, VA 22401; 540-371-1124.

Thomasine Cubine: Directs an education awareness program for her Episcopal congregation and the community. Contact information: 757-437-5778; e-mail: tcubine@city.virginia-beach.va.us.

Peter Fetridge: Very knowledgeable about the ministries on behalf of those with mental illness within the Virginia Episcopal Diocese; his group supports a home for persons with mental illness. Contact information: Virginia Episcopal Diocese, 1407 N. Kenilworth Street, Apt. 9, Arlington, VA 22205-2852; 703-534-0350.

Margaret Ann Holt: Leader in Virginia Interfaith Committee on Mental Illness Ministries (VICOMIM), P.O. Box 1719, Room 113, Glen Allen, VA 23060. Contact information: MI_Ministries@excite.com or vicomim2@yahoo.com.

Ginger Schneider: Knowledgeable about The Forum for Integrating Mental Health, Spirituality and Community. Contact information: 703-536-2000, ext. 168.

Pat Fracher: Director of a church-based social club for persons with mental illnesses (Episcopal). Contact information: 1020 Bridge Avenue, Waynesboro, VA 22980; 540-942-2090.

Reverend Keary Kincannon: Pastor at Rising Hope United Methodist Church, which is unique in being a real congregation from the street people that live nearby in Alexandria, VA. Although not a social agency, it does have a food pantry, a clothing closet, helps the mentally ill obtain medications when they lose or run out of them, helps them get psychiatric appointments, etc. Contact information: rising-hope@erols.com.

Reverend Bill Yolton and Diane Engster: Bill is a Presbyterian pastor, and his wife, Diane, is a lawyer. They are strong advocates for the severely mentally ill on a national level and are leaders of Agape Reservoir at Mount Vernon Presbyterian Church. Contact information: 703-360-3657; lwyolton@prodigy.net or dengster @aol.com.

WASHINGTON, D.C.

Dr. James Clemons: Retired professor from Wesley Theological Seminary who started a group called OASSIS (The Organization for Attempters and Survivors of Suicide in Interfaith Services) that holds meetings in the Washington, D.C. area. Contact information: 4541 Burlington Place, NW, Washington, D.C. 20016; 202-363-4224; FAX: 202-3663-4224; jamestclemons@aol.com.

Reverend Jackson Day: United Methodist Church minister knowledgeable about mental health issues and involved in several groups related to severe mental illness. He is a member of OASSI, Methvision, Pathvision, May 8 Alumni, and VI-COMIM. Contact information: 100 Maryland Avenue, NE, Washington, D.C. 20002; 202-488-5608 or 410-964-9620; JDay@UMC-GBCS.ORG.

Rev. Paul Tomlinson: A chaplain at St. Elizabeth's Hospital in Washington, D.C., with lots of insight and contacts. Contact information: St. Elizabeth's Hospital, 2700 MLK Jr. Avenue, SE, Washington, D.C. 20032; 202-373-7035; cpcmentalillness@cs.com.

David Donaldson: Founder of We Care America (WCA), a national network of faith-based leaders committed to better utilizing the faith-based community in providing effective human services. He was also the national director of the well-known organization called Operation Blessing that for years has provided disaster relief and development assistance. Contact information: DaveD@wecareamerica. org.

John Prestby: Leader at Milwaukee County Behavioral Health Division, 9201 Water Town Park Road, Milwaukee, WI 53226. Contact information: jprestby@milwcnty.com.

Sr. Ann Catherine Veierstahler: Mental health leader and advocate. Contact information: Sisters of Charity of St. Joan Antida, 3601 South 41st Street, Milwaukee, WI 53221-1014.

Jan Kwiatkowski: Works with NAMI and other state advocacy organizations to develop more formal resources for clergy, parish members, and families of persons with mental illness. Contact information: Episcopal Diocese of Milwaukee, jikjoy@wi.rr.com.

National Organizations

Crystal Horning: As the national mental illness consultant for Mennonite Mutual Aid, she is the leader within the Mennonite faith for education programs on the topic of mental illness. She has also written a book (*A Christian View of Mental Illness*) and travels across the United States doing presentations for Mennonite communities. Contact information: 3401 Brook Road, Richmond, VA 23227; 804-342-9102; crystalh@mma-online.org.

Dr. John Stumme: Director for Studies, Division of Church and Society, Evangelical Lutheran Church of America. Has done much to help faith communities understand mental illness. Contact information: jstumme@elca.org

Gary N. Johnston: Chaplain with special interest in mental health issues at the Spiritual Ministry Division of the National Institutes of Health. Contact information: gjohnston@cc.nih.gov; 301-340-0908.

Rick Birkel: NAMI executive director, also ordained to the permanent diaconate in the Roman Catholic Archdiocese of Washington. Contact information: 703-524-7600.

TASK FORCE FROM SAMHSA/CENTER FOR MENTAL HEALTH SERVICES

Carole Schauer: Task force director, SAMHSA/CMHS, 5600 Fishers Lane, Rockville, MD 20857. To obtain a copy of the task force's report that summarizes several meetings on the issue of mobilizing faith-based mental health services, entitled "Building Bridges: Mental Health Consumers and Members of Faith-Based and Community Organizations in Dialogue," contact the Center for Mental

Health Services, SAMHSA, U.S. Department of Health and Human Services. Contact information: cschauer@samhsa.gov.

Victoria Marquez: SAMHSA/CMHS, 5600 Fishers Lane, Rockville, MD 20857. Contact information: vmarquez@samhsa.gov.

Paolo del Vecchio: SAMHSA/CMHS, 5600 Fishers Lane, Rockville, MD 20857. Contact information: pdelvecc@samhsa.gov.

Kevin Amani Hicks: SAMHSA/CMHS, 5600 Fishers Lane, Rockville, MD 20857. Contact information: khicks@samhsa.gov.

Chris Marshal: SAMHSA/CMHS, 5600 Fishers Lane, Rockville, MD 20857. Contact information: cmarshal@samhsa.gov.

REFERENCES

INTRODUCTION

1. Guralnik, D. B., ed. *Webster's New World Dictionary of the American Language*. New York: Simon & Schuster, 1974.

CHAPTER 1: PEOPLE AND COMMUNITIES OF FAITH

1. See Web sites http://www.hospitallers.org/noframes/saints/john_of_god.bio.html and http://www.newadvent.org/cathen/08472c.htm.

2. See Web site http://www.sjog.ie/sjog/about/index.html.

3. See Web site http://www.sjog.org.au/heritage/.

4. See Web site http://www.sjog.ie/sjog/about/index.html.

5. Hemenway, J. E. Clinical pastoral education from a historical perspective. See http://www.acpe.edu/acroread/cpehistory.pdf.

6. Jackson, S. W. 2001. The wounded healer. *Bulletin of the History of Medicine* 75:1–36.

7. Boisen, Anton T. 1936. *The Exploration of the Inner World*. New York: Harper & Brothers. See Web site http://www.firstchurchbloomington.org/sermons/010923.htm.

8. Breyer, C. 2000. Pastoral learning at Bellevue Hospital. *The Christian Century* (August 30–September 6): 862–69. See Web site http://www.religion-online.org/cgi-bin/relsearchd.dll/showarticle?item_id=1955.

9. Boisen, *Exploration of the Inner World*, 15 (see http://primal-page.com/mystica.htm).

10. Ibid., page unknown (see http://primal-page.com/mystica.htm).

11. Boisen, *Exploration of the Inner World*, quoted in McKenna, D. L. 1987. *The Whisper of His Grace: A Fresh Look at Suffering Through the Eyes of Job and Jesus*. Nashville: Word Books, 48.

12. Asquith, G. H. 2000. Boisen's method of theological inquiry. *Oates Journal* 3 (see http://www.oates.org/journal/mbr/vol-03-2000/articles/g_asquith-01.html).

13. Association of Professional Chaplains, *About Chaplaincy: History* (see http://www.professionalchaplains.org/resources/curresrch.html.)

14. See the Chicago Theological Seminary Web site: http://www.ctschicago.edu/content/about/thennow/pastoral.php.

15. Srole, L. 1977. Gheel, Belgium: The natural therapeutic community 1475–1975. In *New Trends of Psychiatry in the Community: Proceedings of the Fourth International Symposium of the Kittay Scientific Foundation*, March 28–29, 1976, ed. G. Serbin. New York: Ballinger, Cambridge.

16. Rademaeker, A. 1948. The colony of Gheel. *Mental Health* 8:13–16, and Read, C. S. 1921. Familial care of the insane. *Journal of Mental Science* 67:186–95.

17. See Web site http://www.mncdd.org/parallels/two/3.html.

18. See Web site http://austin.nami.org/newslettermaroo.html#Gheel,%20Belgium.

19. See Web site http://www.geocities.com/TimesSquare/Cave/2944/dymphnabackground.html.

300 References

20. See Web site http://www.newyorkcityvoices.org/apro102.html.

21. See Web site http://www.irishmasscards.com/IMC-Prayer/imc_pr_stdympna.htm.

22. See Web site http://www.geocities.com/TimesSquare/Cave/2944/dymphnabackground. html.

23. See Web site http://www.mncdd.org/parallels/two/3.html.

24. See Web site http://www.irishmasscards.com/IMC-Prayer/imc_pr_stdympna.htm.

25. Sano, F. B. 1932. The care of the insane outside of institutions. *Proceedings of the International Congress on Mental Hygiene* 1:379–91.

26. Tuntiya, N. 2003. The forgotten history: The de-institutionalization movement in the mental health care system in the United States. See Web site http://arc.cs.odu.edu:8080/ dp9/getrecord/oai_dc/oai:USF:etd-05212003-105432.

27. Muller, T. 2002. Spatial concepts of psychiatric family care in France, Belgium and Germany: A comparative study. Presented at symposium titled *Space, Psyche and Psychiatry: Mental Health/Illness and the Construction and Experience of Space, ca. 1600–2000.* Oxford, England: Oxford Brookes University, December 13–15, 2002.

28. Unknown author. 1848. A village of lunatics [an account of Gheel] *American Journal of Insanity* 4 (3): 185–279.29. See Web site http://www.newyorkcityvoices.org /apro102. html.

30. See Web site http://www.irishmasscards.com/IMC-Prayer/imc_pr_stdympna.htm.

31. Baca, Maria Elena. 2003. Churches reach out to people with mental illness. *Minneapolis-St. Paul Star Tribune,* July 12, 2003, mbaca@startribune.com.

32. Copyright 2003 *Star Tribune.* Republished with permission of *Star Tribune,* Minneapolis-St. Paul. No further republication or redistribution is permitted without the written consent of *Star Tribune.*

33. Some details of this case have been changed to ensure anonymity.

CHAPTER 2: HISTORY OF MENTAL HEALTH CARE

1. Pollak, K. 1968. *The Healers: The Doctor, Then and Now.* London: Thomas Nelson and Sons, 10.

2. Porter, R. 1997. *The Greatest Benefit to Mankind: A Medical History of Humanity.* New York: W. W. Norton and Co., 81.

3. Ibid.

4. Ibid., 493.

5. Numbers, R. L., and D. W. Amundsen. 1998. *Caring and Curing: Health and Medicine in the Western Religious Traditions.* Baltimore, MD: Johns Hopkins University Press, 51.

6. Sarton, G. 1931. *Introduction to the History of Science.* Vol. 2. Baltimore: Williams and Wilkins, 245; Granshaw, L. 1993. The hospital. In *Companion Encyclopedia of the History of Medicine,* ed. W. F. Bynum and R. Porter. New York: Routledge, Chapman & Hall, Inc.; and Porter, *Greatest Benefit to Mankind,* 88.

7. Porter, *Greatest Benefit to Mankind,* 87.

8. Numbers and Amundsen, *Caring and Curing,* 49.

9. Porter, *Greatest Benefit to Mankind,* 88.

10. Numbers and Amundsen, *Caring and Curing,* 48.

11. Alexander, F. G., and S. T. Selesnick. 1966. *The History of Psychiatry: An Evaluation of Psychiatric Thought and Practice from Prehistoric Times to the Present.* New York: New American Library, Inc.

12. Fleming, P. 1929. The medical aspects of the medieval monastery in England. *Proceedings of the Royal Society of Medicine* 22:25–36.

13. Kroll, J. 1973. A reappraisal of psychiatry in the Middle Ages. *Archives of General Psychiatry* 29:276–83.

14. See Web site http://www.d.umn.edu/cla/faculty/tbacig/studproj/is3099/pplfrst/ Untitled1.html.

15. For information on Restoration and eighteenth-century studies in English, see http://instruct.uwo.ca/english/234e/site/lndnmpbedlam.html.

16. Gamwell, L., and N. Tomes. 1995. *Madness in America: Cultural and Medical Perceptions of Mental Illness before 1914.* New York: Cornell University Press, 23.

17. See http://instruct.uwo.ca/english/234e/site/lndnmpbedlam.html.

18. Bassoe, P. 1945. Spain as the cradle of psychiatry. *American Journal of Psychiatry* 101:731–38.

19. Kroll, A reappraisal of psychiatry, 282.

20. Foucault, M. 1967. *Madness and Civilization.* New York: New American Library, Mentor Books.

21. Kroll, A reappraisal of psychiatry, 29:276–83.

22. Brouette, E. 1951. "The 16th Century and Satanism," in *Satan.* New York: Ward & Sheed.

23. Zilboorg, G. 1941. *A History of Medical Psychology.* New York: W. W. Norton Co.

24. Gamwell and Tomes, *Madness in America.*

25. Kroll, A reappraisal of psychiatry, 281.

26. Knoll, J., and B. Bachrach. 1984. Sin and mental illness in the Middle Ages. *Psychological Medicine* 14:507–14.

27. Phillips, S. M. 2002. Free to speak: Clarifying the legacy of the witch hunts. *Journal of Psychology and Christianity* 21 (1): 29–41.

28. Thielman, S. B. 1998. Religion in the history of psychiatry. In *Handbook of Religion and Mental Health,* ed. H. G. Koenig. San Diego: Academic Press, 3–18.

29. John of the Cross. 1578. *Ascent of Mount Carmel,* trans. E. A. Peers. Garden City, NY: Image Books (translation published in 1962).

30. Hunter, R., and I. McAlpine, eds. 1963. *Three Hundred Years of Psychiatry 1535–1860.* London: Oxford University Press.

31. Cheyne, G. 1733. *The English Malady: or, a Treatise of Nervous Diseases of all Kinds.* London: G. Strahan and J. Leake.

32. Brecht, M., and J. L. Schaaf, trans. 1993. *Martin Luther: His Road to Reformation, 1483–1521.* Minneapolis, MN: Augsburg-Fortress.

33. Porter, *Greatest Benefit to Mankind,* 497.

34. Ibid., 495–97.

35. Taubes, T. 1998. "Healthy avenues of the mind": Psychological theory building and the influence of religion during the era of moral treatment. *American Journal of Psychiatry* 155:1001–8.

36. Ibid.

37. See Web site http://www.friendshospitalonline.org/History.htm.

38. Gamwell, L., and N. Tomes. 1995. *Madness in America: Cultural and Medical Perceptions of Mental Illness before 1914.* New York: State University of New York at Binghamton and Cornell University Press.

39. Taubes, "Healthy avenues of the mind."

40. The 17th Annual Report of the Officers of the Retreat before the Insane at Hartford. 1841. Hartford, CT.: Case, Tiffany & Burnham, Printers, 24 (quoted in Taubes above).

41. Ninth Annual Report of the Trustees of the State Lunatic Hospital at Worcester. 1842. Boston: Dutton & Wentworth, State Printers, 41 (quoted in Taubes above).

42. Taubes, "Healthy avenues of the mind."

43. Porter, *Greatest Benefit to Mankind,* 503–4.

44. Freud, S. 1907. *Obsessive Acts and Religious Practices.* In *Standard Edition of the Complete Psychological Works of Sigmund Freud,* trans. and ed. J. Strachey. London: Hogarth Press (published in 1962).

45. Freud, S. 1913. *Totem and Taboo: Some points of agreement between the mental lives of savages and neurotics;* 1919. *Psycho-Analysis and Religious Origins;* 1927. *Future of an Illusion;* 1930. *Civilization and its Discontents;* 1939. *Moses and Monotheism.* In *Standard Edition of the Complete Psychological Works of Sigmund Freud,* trans. and ed. J. Strachey. London: Hogarth Press (published in 1962).

46. Freud, *Future of an Illusion*, 43.

47. Ellis, A. 1988. Is religiosity pathological? *Free Inquiry* 18:27–32.

48. Watters, W. 1992. *Deadly Doctrine: Health, Illness, and Christian God-Talk*. Buffalo: Prometheus Books, 12.

49. Ellis, A. 1980. Psychotherapy and atheistic values: A response to A.E. Bergin's "Psychotherapy and religious values." *Journal of Consulting and Clinical Psychology* 48:635–39.

50. Shafranske, E. P., and H. N. Malony. 1990. Clinical psychologists' religious and spiritual orientations and their practice of psychotherapy. *Psychotherapy* 27:72–78; Ragan, C., H. N. Malony, and B. Beit-Hallahmi. 1980. Psychologists and religion: Professional factors and personal beliefs. *Review of Religious Research* 21:208–17.

51. Neeleman, J., and M. B. King. 1993. Psychiatrists' religious attitudes in relation to their clinical practice: A survey of 231 psychiatrists. *Acta Psychiatrica Scandinavia* 88: 420–24; Bergin, A. E., and M. P. Jensen. 1990. Religiosity and psychotherapists: A national survey. *Psychotherapy* 27:3–7; and Neeleman, J., and R. Persaud. 1995. Why do psychiatrists neglect religion? *British Journal of Medical Psychology* 68 (2): 169–78.

52. Princeton Religion Research Center. 1996. Religion in America: Will the vitality of the church be the surprise of the 21st century? Princeton, NJ: The Gallup Poll, 22.

53. Larson, D. B., S. B. Thielman, M. A. Greenwold, J. S. Lyons, S. G. Post, K. A. Sherrill, G. G. Wood, and S. S. Larson. 1993. Religious content in the DSM-III-R glossary of technical terms. *American Journal of Psychiatry* 150:1884–85.

54. Accreditation Council on Graduate Medical Education. March 1994. Special requirements for residency training in psychiatry. Chicago: Accreditation Council on Graduate Medical Education (ACGME).

55. Roskes, E. J., L. Dixon, and A. Lehman. 1998. A survey of the views of trainees in psychiatry regarding religious issues. *Mental Health, Religion and Culture* 1 (1): 45–55.

56. See Web site: http://www.gwish.org.cnchost.com/id41.htm.

57. Grabovac, A. D., and S. Ganesan. 2003. Spirituality and religion in Canadian psychiatric residency training. *Canadian Journal of Psychiatry* 48 (3): 171–75.

58. Bilgrave, D. P., and R. H. Deluty. 1998. Religious beliefs and therapeutic orientations of clinical and counseling psychologists. *Journal for the Scientific Study of Religion* 37:329–49.

59. American Psychological Association. 1995. Guidelines and principles for accreditation of programs in professional psychology. In *American Psychological Association Committee on Accreditation Site Visitor Handbook*. Washington, DC: American Psychological Association, ?Iw-27.

60. Dols, M. W. 1992. *Majnun: The Madman in Medieval Islamic Society*. Oxford: Clarendon Press.

61. National Library of Medicine, Islamic Culture and the Medical Arts. See http://www.nlm.nih.gov/exhibition/islamic_medical/islamic_12.html.

62. Porter, *Greatest Benefit to Mankind*, 105.

63. Ibid., 104.

64. This hospital was different from the Royal Hospital in Granada that John of God was admitted to in 1538. Catholic monarchs Isabel and Fernando of Spain commissioned the Royal Hospital in 1504. While it originally served as a hospital for the poor, for pilgrims, and for soldiers who had been injured during the conquest of Granada, it became used exclusively for housing the mentally ill in 1536 (see Royal Hospital, http://www.granadamap.com/hospitalreal.htm).

65. Porter, *Greatest Benefit to Mankind*, 105.

66. Dols, *Majnun*.

67. Al-Issa, I. 2000. Mental illness in medieval Islamic society. In *Al-Junun: Mental Illness in the Islamic World*, ed. Ihsan Al-Issa. Madison, CT: International Universities Press, Inc.

68. Ammar, S. 1987. Historie de la psychiatrie maghribine. In *Manuel de Psychiatrie du Practicien Maghribin*, ed. S. Douki, D. Moussaoui, and F. Kacha. Paris: Masson, 1–15.

69. Al-Issa, Mental illness in medieval Islamic society, 63.

70. Ibn Qayyim Al-Jawziya. 1978. *Prophetic Medicine*. Publisher unknown. (See pp. 65–66 in *Al-Junun: Mental Illness in the Islamic World*.)

71. Crapanzano, V. 1973. *The Hamadasha: Study in Moroccan Ethnopsychiatry*. Berkeley: University of California Press.

72. Al-Subaie, A., and A. Alhamad. 2000. Psychiatry in Saudi Arabia. In *Al-Junun: Mental Illness in the Islamic World*, ed. Ihsan Al-Issa. Madison, CT: International Universities Press, Inc., 210–11.

73. Vayikra 19:18, *Jewish Publication Society Bible*, http://www.breslov.com/bible/Leviticus19.htm#18.

74. See Web site http://www.mind.org.uk/NR/exeres/732965F2-2980-4D74-A3EA-A11366204C6D.htm?NRMODE=PublishedandwbcpurposeBasicandWBCMODE= PresentationUnpublished.

75. Freud, S. 1989. *An Outline of Psycho-Analysis*. New York: W. W. Norton and Co. ed. James Strachey; and Freud, S. 1900. *The Interpretation of Dreams*, trans. A. A. Brill, New York: Macmillan, 1913.

76. Devarim 28:28, *Jewish Publication Society Bible*, http://www.hareidi.org/bible/Deuteronomy28.htm#28.

77. Shmuel A 16:14, *Jewish Publication Society Bible*, http://www.hareidi.org/bible/1_Samuel16.htm#14.

78. Shmuel A 18:10, *Jewish Publication Society Bible*, http://www.breslov.com/ bible/1_Samuel18.htm#10.

79. Shmuel B 1:6, *Jewish Publication Society Bible*, http://www.hareidi.org/bible/2_Samuel1.htm#6 .

80. Daniyel 4:30, *Jewish Publication Society Bible*, http://www.hareidi.org/bible/Daniel4.htm#30.

81. Daniyel 4:31, *Jewish Publication Society Bible*, http://www.hareidi.org/bible/Daniel4.htm#31.

82. Miller, L. 1975. Israel and the Jews. In *World History of Religion*, ed. J. G. Howells. New York: Brunner/Mazel; and Armstrong, K. 1993. *A History of God: The 4000-Year Quest of Judaism, Christianity, and Islam*. New York: Alfred A. Knopf.

83. Berger, N., ed. 1995. *Jews and Medicine: Religion, Culture*. Philadelphia: Jewish Publication Society.

84. Dorff, E. N. 1998. The Jewish tradition. In *Caring and Curing: Health and Medicine in the Western Religious Traditions*, ed. R. L. Numbers and D. W. Amundsen. Baltimore: John Hopkins University Press, 14.

85. Numbers and Amundsen, *Caring and Curing*, 25.

86. Jewish Values and Mental Health. See Web site http://www.rac.org/issues/issuemh.html.

87. Feldman, D. M. 1986. *Health and Medicine in the Jewish Tradition*. New York: Crossroad.

88. Rosner, F. 1996. Moses, Maimonides and prophetic medicine. *Journal of the History of Medicine and Allied Sciences* 51:313–24.

89. Marx, J. H., and S. L. Spray. 1969. Religious biographies and professional characteristics of psychotherapists. *Journal of Health and Social Behavior* 10:275–88.

90. Bergin, A. E., and J. P. Jensen. 1990. Religiosity and psychotherapists: A national survey. *Psychotherapy and Psychosomatics* 27:3–7.

91. Larson, D. B., M. J. Donahue, et al. 1989. Religious affiliations in mental health research samples as compared with national samples. *Journal of Nervous and Mental Disease* 177 (2): 109–11.

92. Armstrong, *A History of God*.

93. Easwaran, E. 1987. *The Upanishads*. Tomales, CA: Nilgiri Press.

94. Juthani, N. V. 1998. Understanding and treating Hindu patients. In *Handbook of Religion and Mental Health*, ed. H. G. Koenig. San Diego: Academic Press, 272.

95. Ibid., 273.

96. Rao, A. V. 1975. India. In *World History of Religion*, ed. J. G. Howells. New York: Brunner/Mazel.

97. Parkar, S. R., V. S. Dawani, and J. S. Apte. 2001. History of psychiatry in India. *J Postgrad Med* 47:73–76.

98. Parkar et al., ibid., 74.

99. Rao, A. V. 1975. India. In *World History of Religion*, ed. J. G. Howells. New York: Brunner/Mazel.

100. Parkar et al., History of psychiatry in India, 76.

101. See Web site http://buddhism.about.com/cs/theeightfoldpath/index.htm.

102. See Web site http://english.huayenworld.org/HYB_FAQ_021_Mahayana.htm.

103. What Mahayana Buddhists Believe. See Web site http://www.beliefnet.com/story/80/story_8045_1.html.

104. Unshuld, P. U. 1979. *Medical Ethics and Imperial China—a Study in Historical Anthropology*. Berkeley, CA: University of California Press.

105. Veith, I. 1975. The Far East: reflections on the psychological foundations. In *World History of Religion*, ed. J. G. Howells. New York: Brunner/Mazel.

106. Ibid.

107. Scotton, B. W. 1998. Treating Buddhist patients. In *Handbook of Religion and Mental Health*, ed. H. G. Koenig. San Diego: Academic Press.

CHAPTER 3: RELIGION, COPING, AND POSITIVE EMOTIONS

1. Koenig, H, G., M. McCullough, and D. B. Larson. 2001. *Handbook of Religion and Health: A Century of Research Reviewed*. New York: Oxford University Press.

2. Ibid., 18.

3. Zinnbauer, B. J., K. I. Pargament, and B. Cowell. 1997. Religion and spirituality: Unfuzzying the fuzzy. *Journal for the Scientific Study of Religion* 36:549–64; Koenig, H. G., L. K. George, and P. Titus. 2004. Religion, spirituality and health in medically ill hospitalized older patients. *Journal of the American Geriatrics Society* (April).

4. The Gallup Organization: Poll Topics and Trends. See Web site http://www.gallup.com/poll/topics/religion.asp (last accessed 7/18/03).

5. Ibid.

6. Schuster, M. A., B. D. Stein, L. H. Jaycox, R. L. Collins, G. N. Marshall, M. N. Elliott, A. J. Zhou, D. E. Kanouse, J. L. Morrison, and S. H. Berry. 2001. A national survey of stress reactions after the September 11, 2001, terrorist attacks. *New England Journal of Medicine* 345:1507–12.

7. Biema, D. 2001. Faith after the fall. *Time Magazine* October 8, 2001. See Web site: http://www.time.com/time/archive/preview/0,10987,1000951,00.html.

8. Pargament, K. I., K. Ishler, E. Dubow, P. Stanik, R. Rouiller, P. Crowe, E. Cullman, M. Albert, and B. J. Royster. 1994. Methods of religious coping with the Gulf War: Cross-sectional and longitudinal analyses. *Journal for the Scientific Study of Religion* 33:347–61.

9. Pargament, K. I., B. W. Smith, H. G. Koenig, and L. Perez. 1998. Patterns of positive and negative religious coping with major life stressors. *Journal for the Scientific Study of Religion* 37:710–24.

10. Smith, B.W. 1996. Coping as a predictor of outcomes following the 1993 Midwest flood. *Journal of Social Behavior and Personality* 11:225–39.

11. Weinrich, S., S. B. Hardin, and M. Johnson. 1990. Nurses respond to hurricane Hugo victims' disaster stress. *Archives of Psychiatric Nursing* 4:195–205.

12. Maton, K. I. 1989. The stress-buffering role of spiritual support: cross-sectional and prospective investigations. *Journal for the Scientific Study of Religion* 28:310–23.

13. Cronan, T. A., R. M. Kaplan, L. Posner, E. Lumberg, and F. Kozin. 1989. Prevalence of the use of unconventional remedies for arthritis in a metropolitan community. *Arthritis and Rheumatism* 32:1604–7.

14. Samuel-Hodge, C. D., S. W. Headen, A. H. Skelly, A. F. Ingram, T. C. Keyserling, E. J. Jackson, A. S. Ammerman, and T. A. Elasy. 2000. Influences on day-to-day self-management of type 2 diabetes among African American women. *Diabetes Care* 23:928–33.

15. Tix, A. P., and P. A. Frazier. 1997. The use of religious coping during stressful life events. *Journal of Consulting and Clinical Psychology* 66:411–22.

16. O'Brien, M. E. 1982. Religious faith and adjustment to long-term hemodialysis. *Journal of Religion and Health* 21:68–80.

17. Schnoll, R. A., L. L. Harlow, and L. Brower. 2000. Spirituality, demographic and disease factors, and adjustment to cancer. *Cancer Practice* 8:298–304; Halstead, M.T., and J. I. Fernsler. 1994. Coping stratgies of long-term cancer survivors. *Cancer Nursing* 17 (2): 94–100.

18. Ai, A. L., R. E. Dunkle, C. Peterson, and S. F. Bolling. 1998. The role of private prayer in psychological recovery among midlife and aged patients following cardiac surgery (CABG). *Gerontologist* 38:591–601; Saudia, T. L., M. R. Kinney, K. C. Brown, and L. Young-Ward. 1991. Health locus of control and helpfulness of prayer. *Heart and Lung* 20:60–65.

19. Harris, R. C., M. A. Dew, A. Lee, M. Amaya, L. Buches, D. Reetz, and G. Coleman. 1995. The role of religion in heart transplant recipients' health and well-being. *Journal of Religion and Health* 34 (1): 17–32.

20. Matthees, B. J., Anantachoti Puree, M. J. Kreitzer, K. Savik, M. I. Hertz, and C. R. Gross. 2001. Use of complementary therapies, adherence, and quality of life in lung transplant recipients. *Heart and Lung* 30:258–68.

21. Avants, S. K., L. A. Warburton, and A. Margolin. 2001. Spiritual and religious support in recovery from addiction among HIV-positive injection drug users. *Journal of Psychoactive Drugs* 33:39–45; Ironson, G., G. F. Solomon, E. G. Balbin, C. O. Cleirigh, A. George, M. Kumar, D. Larson, and T. E. Woods. Spirituality and religiousness are associated with long survival, health behaviors, less distress, and lower cortisol in people living with HIV/AIDS: The IWORSHIP scale, its validity and reliability. *Annals of Behavioral Medicine* (forthcoming).

22. Stern, R. C., E. R. Canda, and C. F. Doershuk. 1992. Use of non-medical treatment by cystic fibrosis patients. *Journal of Adolescent Health* 13:612–15.

23. Cooper-Effa, M., W. Blount, N. Kaslow, R. Rothenberg, and J. Eckman 2001. Role of spirituality in patients with sickle cell disease. *Journal of the American Board of Family Practice* 14:116–22.

24. Murphy, P. L., S. M. Albert, C. M. Weber, M. L. Del Bene, and L. P. Rowland, 2000. Impact of spirituality and religiousness on outcomes in patients with ALS. *Neurology* 55:1581–84.

25. Keefe, F. J., G. Affleck, J. Lefebvre, L. Underwood, D. S. Caldwell, J. Drew, J. Egert, J. Gibson, and K. Pargament. 2001. Giving with rheumatoid arthritis: The role of daily spirituality and daily religious and spiritual coping. *Journal of Pain* 2 (2): 101–10.

26. Silber, T. J., and M. Reilly. 1985. Spiritual and religious concerns of the hospitalized adolescent. *Adolescence* 20 (77): 217–24.

27. Ramirez-Johnson, J., C. Fayard, C. Garberoglio, and C. M. Ramirez. 2002. Is faith an emotion? Faith as a meaning-making affective process: An example from breast cancer patients. *American Behavioral Scientist* 45 (12): 1839–53.

28. Koenig, H. G., K. I. Pargament, and J. Nielsen. 1998. Religious coping and health status in medically ill hospitalized older adults. *Journal of Nervous and Mental Disease* 186 (9): 513–21.

29. Idler, E. L., M. A. Musick, C. G. Ellison, L. K. George, N. Krause, M. G. Ory, K. I. Pargament, L. H. Powell, L. G. Underwood, and D. R. Williams. 2003. Measuring multiple dimensions of religion and spirituality for health research. *Research on Aging* 25:327–65 (note: original scores reported in paper were converted to scores on the same scale as the Koenig et al. 1998 study above, for comparison purposes).

30. Pargament, K. I., H. G. Koenig, N. Tarakeshwar, and J. Hahn. 2003. Religious coping methods as predictors of psychological, physical, and spiritual outcomes among medically ill elderly patients: A two-year longitudinal study. *Journal of Health Psychology* (in submission); Pargament, K. I., H. G. Koenig, N. Tarakeshwar, and J. Hahn. 2001. Religious struggle as a predictor of mortality among medically ill elderly patients: A two-year longitudinal study. *Archives of Internal Medicine* 161:1881–85; Fitchett, G., B. D. Rybarczyk, G. A.

DeMarco, and J. J. Nicholas. 1999. The role of religion in medical rehabilitation outcomes: A longitudinal study. *Rehabilitation Psychology* 44 (4): 333–53.

31. Rammohan, A., Kiran Rao, and D. K. Subbakrishna. 2002. Religious coping and psychological wellbeing in carers of relatives with schizophrenia. *Acta Psychiatrica Scandinavica* 105 (5): 356–62.

32. Shrimali, Swasti, and K. D. Broota. 1987. Effect of surgical stress on belief in God and superstition: An in situ investigation. *Journal of Personality and Clinical Studies* 3 (2): 135–38.

33. Pettersson, T. 1991. Religion and criminality: Structural relationships between church involvement and crime rates in contemporary Sweden. *Journal for the Scientific Study of Religion* 30:279–91; see World Values Survey: http://www.umich.edu/~newsinfo/Releases/1997/Dec97/r121097a.html.

34. Cederblad, M., L. Dahlin, and O. Hagnell. 1995. Coping with life span crises in a group at risk of mental and behavioral disorders: From the Lundby study. *Acta Psychiatrica Scandinavica* 91:322–30.

35. Dekker, P., and P. Ester. 1996. Depillarization, deconfessionalization, and de-ideologization: Empirical trends in Dutch society 1958–1992. *Review of Religious Research* 37:325–41.

36. Braam, A. W., A. T. F. Beekman, D. J. H. Deeg, J. H. Smith, and W. van Tilburg. 1997. Religiosity as a protective or prognostic factor of depression in later life; results from the community survey in the Netherlands. *Acta Psychiatrica Scandinavia* 96:199–205.

37. Princeton Religion Research Center. 1996. Religion in America: Will the vitality of the church be the surprise of the 21st century? Princeton, NJ: The Gallup Poll, 53.

38. Ringdal, G., K. Gotestam, S. Kaasa, S. Kvinnslaud, and K. Ringdal. 1995. Prognostic factors and survival in a heterogeneous sample of cancer patients. *British Journal of Cancer* 73:1594–99.

39. Kesselring, A., M. J. Dodd, A. M. Lindsey, and A. L. Strauss. 1986. Attitudes of patients living in Switzerland about cancer and its treatment. *Cancer Nursing* 9:77–85.

40. Loewenthal, K. M., M. Cinnirella, G. Evdoka, and P. Murphy. 2001. Faith conquers all?: Beliefs about the role of religious factors in coping with depression among different cultural-religious groups in the UK. *British Journal of Medical Psychology* 74 (3): 293–303.

41. Koenig, H. G., M. McCullough, and D. Larson. 2001. *Handbook of Religion and Health.* New York: Oxford University Press, 117, 519–22.

42. Rokeach, M. 1960. *The Open and Closed Mind.* New York: Basic Books; Dreger, R. M. 1952. Some personality correlates of religious attitudes as determined by projective techniques. *Psychological Monographs* 66:335; Hassan, M. K., and A. Khalique. 1981. Religiosity and its correlates in college students. *Journal of Psychological Researches* 25 (3): 129–36; Cowen, E. L. 1954. The negative concept as a personality measure. *Journal of Consulting Psychology* 18:138–42; and Wright, J. C. 1959. Personal adjustment and its relationship to religious attitude and certainty. *Religious Education* 54:521–23.

43. James, W. 1890. *The Principles of Psychology.* New York: Holt, 19.

44. Koenig, H. G. 1998. *Handbook of Religion and Mental Health.* San Diego: Academic Press, 97–117, 519–22.

45. Ellison, C. G., J. D. Boardman, D. R. Williams, and J. S. Jackson. 2001. Religious involvement, stress, and mental health: Findings from the 1995 Detroit Area Study. *Social Forces.* 80 (1): 215–49; Pargament, K. I., N. Tarakeshwar, C. G. Ellison, and K. M. Wulff. 2001. Religious coping among the religious: The relationships between religious coping and well-being in a national sample of Presbyterian clergy, elders, and members. *Journal for the Scientific Study of Religion* 40 (3): 497–513; Hammermeister, J., M. Flint, J. Havens, and M. Peterson. 2001. Psychosocial and health-related characteristics of religious well-being. *Psychological Reports* 89 (3): 589–94; Ferriss, A. L. 2002. Religion and the quality of life. *Journal of Happiness Studies* 3 (3): 199–215; Cohen, A. B. 2002. The importance of spirituality in well-being for Jews and Christians. *Journal of Happiness Studies* 3 (3): 287–310; Francis, L. J., M. Robbins, and A. White. 2003. Correlation between religion and happiness: A replication. *Psychological Reports* 92 (1): 51–52; Krause, N., and C. G. Ellison. 2003. Forgiveness by God, forgiveness of others, and psychological well-being in late life. *Journal*

for the Scientific Study of Religion 42 (1): 77–93; Francis, L. J., and P. Kaldor. 2002. The relationship between psychological well-being and Christian faith and practice in an Australian population sample. *Journal for the Scientific Study of Religion* 41 (1): 179–84; Wink, P., and M. Dillon. 2003. Religiousness, spirituality, and psychosocial functioning in late adulthood: Findings from a longitudinal study. *Psychology and Aging* 18 (4): 916–24; and Kim, Y., L. Seidlitz, Y. Ro, J. S. Evinger, and P. R. Duberstein. 2004. Spirituality and affect: A function of changes in religious affiliation. *Personality and Individual Differences* 37 (4): 861–70.

46. Tsuang, M. T., W. M. Williams, J. C. Simpson, and M. J. Lyons. 2002. Pilot study of spirituality and mental health in twins. *American Journal of Psychiatry* 159 (3): 486–88; and Diener, E., and D. Clifton. 2002. Life satisfaction and religiosity in broad probability samples. *Psychological Inquiry*, 13 (3): 206–09.

47. Hunsberger, B., M. Pratt, and S. Pancer. 2001. Religious versus nonreligious socialization: Does religious background have implications for adjustment? *International Journal for the Psychology of Religion* 11 (2): 105–28.

48. Fry, P. 2001. The unique contribution of key existential factors to the prediction of psychological well-being of older adults following spousal loss. *Gerontologist* 41 (1): 69–81.

49. Cook, J. M., B. S. Black, P. V. Rabins, and P. German. 2000. Life satisfaction and symptoms of mental disorder among older African American public housing residents. *Journal of Clinical Geropsychology* 6 (1): 1–14.

50. Ellison et al. 2001. Religious involvement, stress, and mental health.

51. Laurencelle, R. M., S. C. Abell, and D. J. Schwartz. 2002. The relation between intrinsic religious faith and psychological well-being. *International Journal for the Psychology of Religion* 12 (2): 109–23.

52. Francis and Kaldor, Relationship, 179–84

53. Hintikka, J., T. Koskela, O. Kontula, K. Koskela, H.-T. Koivumaa-Honkanen, and H. Viinamaeki. 2001. Religious attendance and life satisfaction in the Finnish general population. *Journal of Psychology and Theology* 29 (2): 158–64.

54. Chliaoutakis, J. E., I. Drakou, C. Gnardellis, S. Galariotou, H. Carra, and M. Chliaoutaki. 2002. Greek Christian Orthodox Ecclesiastical lifestyle: Could it become a pattern of health-related behavior? *Preventive Medicine* 34 (4): 428–35.

55. Iecovich, E. 2001. Religiousness and subjective well-being among Jewish female residents of old age homes in Israel. *Journal of Religious Gerontology* 13 (1): 31–46.

56. Shkolnik, T., C. Weiner, L. Malik, and Y. Festinger. 2001. The effect of Jewish religiosity of elderly Israelis on their life satisfaction, health, function and activity. *Journal of Cross-Cultural Gerontology* 16 (3): 201–19.

57. Thomas, L. 2001. The job hypothesis: Gerotranscendence and life satisfaction among elderly Turkish Muslims. In *Aging and the Meaning of Time: A Multidisciplinary Exploration*, ed. Susan H. McFadden and Robert C. Atchley. New York: Springer Publishing Co., 207–27.

58. Anjana, R., and S. Raju. 2003. Management of maladjustment: A study on reciters and non-reciters of the *Bhagavad Gita*. *Journal of Indian Psychology* 21 (1): 21–27.

59. Swinyard, W. R., A.-K. Kau, and H.-Y. Phua. 2001. Happiness, materialism, and religious experience in the US and Singapore. *Journal of Happiness Studies* 2 (1): 13–32.

60. Koenig, *Handbook of Religion and Health*, 215, 522–23.

61. Sethi, S., and M. E. P. Seligman. 1993. Optimism and fundamentalism. *Psychological Science* 4:256–59; and Sethi, S., and M. E. P. Seligman. 1994. The hope of fundamentalists. *Psychological Science* 5:58.

62. Sherman, A. C., S. Simonton, D. C. Adams, U. Latif, T. G. Plante, S. Burns, et al. 2001. Measuring religious faith in cancer patients: Reliability and construct validity of the Santa Clara Strength of Religious Faith Questionnaire. *Psycho-Oncology* 10 (5): 436–43.

63. Ai, A. L., C. Peterson, S. F. Bolling, and H. Koenig. 2002. Private prayer and optimism in middle-aged and older patients awaiting cardiac surgery. *Gerontologist* 42 (1): 70–81.

64. Murphy, P. E., J. W. Ciarrocchi, R. L. Piedmont, S. Cheston, M. Peyrot, and G. Fitchett. 2000. The relation of religious belief and practices, depression, and hopelessness in

persons with clinical depression. *Journal of Consulting and Clinical Psychology* 68 (6): 1102–6.

65. Markstrom, C. A. 1999. Religious involvement and adolescent psychosocial development. *Journal of Adolescence* 22 (2): 205–21.

66. Krause, N. 2002. Church-based social support and health in old age: Exploring variations by race. *Journal of Gerontology* 57B: S332–47.

67. Krause, N. 2004. Common facets of religion, unique facets of religion, and life satisfaction among older African Americans. *Journals of Gerontology* 59B: S109–17.

68. Mattis, J. S., D. L. Fontenot, and C. A. Hatcher-Kay. 2003. Religiosity, racism, and dispositional optimism among African Americans. *Personality and Individual Differences* 34 (6): 1025–38.

69. Freud, S. 1930. Civilization and its discontents. In *Standard Edition of the Complete Psychological Works of Sigmund Freud*, ed. and trans. J. Strachey. London: Hogarth Press (published in 1962), 25.

70. Koenig, *Handbook of Religion and Health*, 215, 523.

71. Steptoe, S. 2004. The man with the purpose. *Time Magazine* (March 29): 54–56.

72. Hughes, D. E., and T. H. Peake. 2002. Investigating the value of spiritual well-being and psychosocial development in mitigating senior adulthood depression. *Activities, Adaptation and Aging* 26 (3): 15–35.

73. Feher, S., and R. C. Maly. 1999. Coping with breast cancer in later life: The role of religious faith. *Psycho-Oncology* 8 (5): 408–16; and Westlake, C., and K. Dracup. 2001. Role of spirituality in adjustment of patients with advanced heart failure. *Progress in Cardiovascular Nursing* 16 (3): 119–25.

74. Krause, N. 2003. Religious meaning and subjective well-being in late life. *Journal of Gerontology* 58 (3): S160–70.

75. Moadel, A., C. Morgan, A. Fatone, J. Grennan, J. Carter, G. Laruffa, et al. 1999. Seeking meaning and hope: Self-reported spiritual and existential needs among an ethnically diverse cancer patient population. *Psycho-Oncology* 8 (5): 378–85.

76. Mattis, Jacqueline S. 2002. Religion and spirituality in the meaning-making and coping experiences of African American women: A qualitative analysis. *Psychology of Women Quarterly* 26 (4): 309–21.

77. Francis, L. J. 2000. The relationship between Bible reading and purpose in life among 13–15-year-olds. *Mental Health, Religion and Culture* 3 (1): 27–36.

78. MacDonald, D. A., and D. Holland. 2002. Spirituality and boredom proneness. *Personality and Individual Differences* 32 (6): 1113–19.

79. Sowell, R., L. Moneyham, M. Hennessy, J. Guillory, A. Demi, and B. Seals. 2000. Spiritual activities as a resistance resource for women with human immunodeficiency virus. *Nursing Research* 49 (2): 73–82.

80. Cotton, S. P., E. G. Levine, C. M. Fitzpatrick, K. H. Dold, and E. Targ. 1999. Exploring the relationships among spiritual well-being, quality of life, and psychological adjustment in women with breast cancer. *Psycho-Oncology* 8 (5): 429–38.

81. Fisch, M. J., M. L. Titzer, J. L. Kristeller, J. Shen, P. J. Loehrer, S. H. Jung, S. D. Passik, and L. H. Einhorn. 2003. Assessment of quality of life in outpatients with advanced cancer: The accuracy of clinician estimations and the relevance of spiritual well-being—A Hoosier Oncology Group study. *Journal of Clinical Oncology* 21:2754–59.

82. Idler, E. L. 1995. Religion, health, and nonphysical senses of self. *Social Forces* 74 (2): 683–704.

83. Ruo, B., J. S. Rumsfeld, M. A. Hlatky, H. Liu, W. S. Browner, and M. A. Whooley. 2003. Depressive symptoms and health-related quality of life: The heart and soul study. *JAMA* 290:215–21.

84. Bartlett, S. J., R. Piedmont, A. Bilderback, A. K. Matsumoto, and J. M. Bathon. 2003. Spirituality, well-being, and quality of life in people with rheumatoid arthritis. *Arthritis and Rheumatism* 49 (6): 778–83.

85. Lazarus, R. S., and B. N. Lazarus. 1994. *Passion and Reason: Making Sense of Our Emotions*. New York: Oxford University Press; M. E. McCullough, R. A. Emmons, and J.-A. Tsang. 2002. The grateful disposition: A conceptual and empirical topography. *Journal of*

Personality and Social Psychology 82 (1): 112–27; and Robert A. Emmons and Michael E. McCullough. 2003. Counting blessings versus burdens: An experimental investigation of gratitude and subjective well-being in daily life. *Journal of Personality and Social Psychology* 84 (2): 377–89.

86. McCullough, Grateful disposition, 112–27.

87. Kendler, K. S., X. Q. Liu, C. O. Gardner, M. E. McCullough, D. Larson, and C. A. Prescott. 2003. Dimensions of religiosity and their relationship to lifetime psychiatric and substance use disorders. *American Journal of Psychiatry* 160 (3): 496–503.

88. Krause, N., and C. G. Ellison. 2003. Forgiveness by God, forgiveness of others, and psychological well-being in late life. *Journal for the Scientific Study of Religion* 42:77–93; M. E. McCullough, C. G. Bellah, S. D. Kilpatrick, and J. L. Johnson. 2001. Vengefulness: Relationships with forgiveness, rumination, well-being, and the big five. *Personality and Social Psychology Bulletin* 27:601–10; and J. W. Berry, E. L. Worthington, Jr., L. Parrott, III, L. O'Connor, and N. G. Wade. 2001. Dispositional forgivingness: Development and construct validity of the Transgression Narrative Test of Forgivingness (TNTF). *Personality and Social Psychology Bulletin* 27:1277–90.

89. Witvliet, C. v. O., T. E. Ludwig, and K. L. Vander Laan. 2001. Granting forgiveness or harboring grudges: Implications for emotion, physiology, and health. *Psychological Science* 121:117–23; Shih-Tseng Tina Huang, and Robert D. Enright. 2000. Forgiveness and anger-related emotions in Taiwan: Implications for therapy. *Psychotherapy: Theory, Research, Practice, Training* 37 (1): 71–79; and K. A. Lawler, J. W. Younger, R. L. Piferi, E. Billington, R. Jobe, K. Edmondson, and W. H. Jones. 2003. A change of heart: Cardiovascular correlates of forgiveness in response to interpersonal conflict. *Journal of Behavioral Medicine* 26:373–93.

90. Witvliet, Granting forgiveness or harboring grudges.

91. Berry, J., and E. L. Worthington, Jr. 2001. Forgiveness, relationship quality, stress while imagining relationship events, and physical and mental health. *Journal of Counseling Psychology* 48:447–55.

92. Seybold, K.S., P. C. Hill, J. K. Neumann, and D. S. Chi. 2001. Physiological and psychological correlates of forgiveness. *Journal of Psychology and Christianity* 20:250–59.

93. Kendler, Dimensions of religiosity.

94. Gorsuch, R. L., and J. Y. Hao. 1993. Forgiveness: An exploratory factor analysis and its relationships to religious variables. *Review of Religious Research* 34:333–47; and N. Krause, and B. Ingersoll-Dayton. 2001. Religion and the process of forgiveness in late life. *Review of Religious Research* 42:252–76.

95. Gorsuch and Hao, Forgiveness.

96. Mullet, E., J. Barros, L. Frongia, V. Usai, F. Neto, and S. R. Shafighi. 2003. Religious involvement and the forgiving personality. *Journal of Personality* 71 (1): 1–19.

97. Rye, Mark S., and Kenneth I. Pargament. 2002. Forgiveness and romantic relationships in college: Can it heal the wounded heart? *Journal of Clinical Psychology* 58 (4): 419–41.

98. Maner, Jon K., Carol L. Luce, Steven L. Neuberg, Robert B. Cialdini, Stephanie Brown, and Bard J. Sagarin. 2002. The effects of perspective taking on motivations for helping: Still no evidence for altruism. *Personality and Social Psychology Bulletin* 28 (11): 1601–10.

99. O'Connor, Lynn E., Jack W. Berry, Joseph Weiss, and Paul Gilbert. 2002. Guilt, fear, submission, and empathy in depression. *Journal of Affective Disorders* 71 (1–3): 19–27.

100. Dulin, Patrick, Robert D. Hill, Jay Anderson, and Dwight Rasmussen. 2001. Altruism as a predictor of life satisfaction in a sample of low-income older adult service providers. *Journal of Mental Health and Aging* 7 (3): 349–60; Alice L. Williams, David Haber, Gayle D. Weaver, and Jean L. Freeman. 1998. Altruistic activity: Does it make a difference in the senior center? *Activities, Adaptation and Aging* 22 (4): 31–39; E. Midlarsky, and E. Kahana. 1994. *Altruism in Later Life*. Thousand Oaks, CA: Sage Publications; C. Schwartz, J. B. Beisenhelder, M. Yunsheng, and G. Reed. 2003. Altruistic social interest behaviors are associated with better mental health. *Psychosomatic Medicine* 65:778–85; K. I. Hunter and M.

W. Linn. 1980–1981. Psychosocial differences between elderly volunteers and non-volunteers. *International Journal of Aging in Human Development* 12:205–13; A. Omoto and M. Snyder. 1995. Sustained helping without obligation: Motivation, longevity of service, and perceived attitude change among AIDS volunteers. *Journal of Personality of Social Psychology* 16:152–66; and B. J. Seelig and W. H. Dobelle. 2001. Altruism and the volunteer: Psychological benefits from participating as a research subject. *Journal of the American Society of Artificial Internal Organs* 47:3–5.

101. Underwood, B. 1977. Attention, negative affect, and altruism: An ecological validation. *Personality and Social Psychology Bulletin* 3 (1): 54–58.

102. Brown, S. L., R. M. Nesse, A. D. Vinokur, and D. M. Smith. 2003. Providing social support may be more beneficial than receiving it: Results from a prospective study of mortality. *Psychological Science* 14 (4): 320–27; and D. Oman, C. E. Thoresen, and K. McMahon. 1999. Volunteerism and mortality among the community-dwelling elderly. *Journal of Health Psychology* 4:301–16.

103. Vaillant, G. E. 2002. *Aging Well*. Boston, MA: Little, Brown.

104. Luks, A. 1988. Helper's high: Volunteering makes people feel good, physically and emotionally. And like "runner's calm," it's probably good for your health. *Psychology Today* (October): 39, 42.

105. Batson, C., K. C. Oleson, J. L. Weeks, S. P. Healy, et al. 1989. Religious prosocial motivation: Is it altruistic or egoistic? *Journal of Personality and Social Psychology* 57 (5): 873–84; and C. Batson. 1990. Good samaritans—or priests and Levites? Using William James as a guide in the study of religious prosocial motivation. *Personality and Social Psychology Bulletin* 16 (4): 758–68.

106. Lai Ling Chau, Ronald C. Johnson, John K. Bowers, Thomas J. Darvill, et al. 1990. Intrinsic and extrinsic religiosity as related to conscience, adjustment, and altruism. *Personality and Individual Differences* 11 (4): 397–400; and A. Sappington and J. Baker. 1995. Refining religious belief behavior relations. *International Journal for the Psychology of Religion* 5 (1): 38–48.

107. Smith, H., A. Fabricatore, and M. Peyrot. 1999. Religiosity and altruism among African American males: The Catholic experience. *Journal of Black Studies* 29 (4): 579–97; and F. M. Bernt. 1999. Religious commitment, attributional style, and gender as predictors of undergraduate volunteer behavior and attitudes. *Journal of Psychology and Theology* 27 (3): 261–72.

108. Data from 2001 edition of *The New Non-Profit Almanac in Brief: Facts and Figures on the Independent Sector*. Washington, DC: The Independent Sector (http://www.independentsector.org/PDFs/inbrief.pdf).

109. Lawson, D. L. 1999. *More Give to Live: How Giving Can Change Your Life*. San Diego: ALTI Publishing, 17.

110. Oman, D., C. E. Thoresen, and K. McMahon. 1999. Volunteerism and mortality among the community-dwelling elderly. *Journal of Health Psychology* 4:301–16.

111. O'Laoire, S. 1997. An experimental study of the effects of distant, intercessory prayer on self-esteem, anxiety, and depression. *Alternative Therapies in Health and Medicine* 3 (6): 38–53; and Jennifer L. Jacobson. 2002. An exploratory study regarding the effects of praying for others on physical and mental health in older adults. *Dissertation Abstracts International: Section B: the Sciences and Engineering* 63 (5-B): 2587.

112. Coward, H. 1986. Intolerance in the world's religions. *Studies in Religion* 15:419–31.

113. Ellison, C. G., and L. K. George. 1994. Religious involvement, social ties, and social support in a southeastern community. *Journal for the Scientific Study of Religion* 33:46–61.

114. George, Linda K., Dan G. Blazer, Dana C. Hughes, and Nancy Fowler. 1989. Social support and the outcome of major depression. *British Journal of Psychiatry* 154:478–85; and L. K. George. 1992. Social factors and the onset and outcome of depression. In *Aging, Health Behaviors, and Health Outcomes*, ed. K. W. Schaie, J. S. House, and D. G. Blazer. Hillsdale, NJ: Lawrence Erlbaum, 137–59.

115. Cohen, S., B. H. Gottlieb, and L. G. Underwood. 2000. Social relationships and

health. In *Social Support Measurement and Intervention*, ed. S. Cohen, L. G. Underwood, and B. H. Gottlieb. New York: Oxford University Press, 3–28.

116. Koenig, *Handbook of Religion and Health*, 215–16, 525–26.

117. Ellison, C. G., and L. K. George. 1994. Religious involvement, social ties, and social support in a southeastern community. *Journal for the Scientific Study of Religion* 33:46–61; D. E. Bradley. 1995. Religious involvement and social resources: Evidence from the data set, "Americans' Changing Lives." *Journal for the Scientific Study of Religion* 34:259–67; H. G. Koenig, J. C. Hays, L. K. George, D. G. Blazer, D. B. Larson, and L. R. Landerman. 1997. Modeling the cross-sectional relationships between religion, physical health, social support, and depressive symptoms. *American Journal of Geriatric Psychiatry* 5:131–43; and S. T. Ortega, R. D. Crutchfield, and W. A. Rushing. 1983. Race differences in elderly personal well-being. *Research on Aging* 5:101–18.

118. Koenig, H. G., D. O. Moberg, and J. N. Kvale. 1988. Religious activities and attitudes of older adults in a geriatric assessment clinic. *Journal of the American Geriatrics Society* 36:362–74.

119. Ortega, S. T., R. D. Crutchfield, and W. A. Rushing. 1983. Race differences in elderly personal well-being. *Research on Aging* 5:101–18.

120. Fiala, W. E., J. P. Bjorck, and R. Gorsuch. 2002. The Religious support scale: Construction, validation and cross-validation. *American Journal of Community Psychology* 30 (6): 761–86.

121. Cloninger, C. R. 1987. A systematic method for clinical description and classification of personality. *Archives of General Psychiatry* 44:573–88.

122. Hamer, D. 2004. *The God Gene: How Faith Is Hardwired into Our Genes*. New York: Doubleday.

123. Kendler, Kenneth S., Charles O. Gardner, and Carol A. Prescott. 1997. Religion, psychopathology, and substance use and abuse: A multimeasure, genetic-epidemiologic study. *American Journal of Psychiatry* 154 (3): 322–29.

124. Comings, D. E., N. Gonzales, G. Saucier, J. P. Johnson, and J. P. MacMurray. 2000. The DRD4 gene and the spiritual transcendence scale of the character temperament index. *Psychiatric Genetics* 10 (4): 185–89.

125. Kurup, R. K., and P. A. Kurup. 2003. Hypothalamic digoxin, hemispheric chemical dominance, and spirituality. *International Journal of Neuroscience* 113 (3): 383–93.

126. Abrahamson, A. C., L. A. Baker, and A. Caspi. 2002. Rebellious teens? Genetic and environmental influences on the social attitudes of adolescents. *Journal of Personality and Social Psychology* 83 (6): 1392–1408.

127. Shuman, J., and K. G. Meador. 2003. *Heal Thyself: Spirituality, Medicine and the Distortion of Christianity*. New York: Oxford University Press.

128. Koenig, H. G., K. I. Pargament, and J. Nielsen. 1998. Religious coping and health outcomes in medically ill hospitalized older adults. *Journal of Nervous and Mental Disorders* 186:513–21.

129. Kark, J. D., S. Carmel, R. Sinnreich, N. Goldberger, and Y. Friedlander. 1996. Psychosocial factors among members of religious and secular kibbutzim. *Israel Journal of Medical Science* 32:185–94.

130. Fountain, D. E. 1986. How to assimilate the elderly into your parish: The effects of alienation on church attendance. *Journal of Religion and Aging* 2 (3): 45–55.

131. Okun, M. A. 1993. Predictors of volunteer status in a retirement community. *International Journal of Aging and Human Development* 36:57–74.

132. Gorsuch, R. L., and J. Y. Hao. 1993. Forgiveness: An exploratory factor analysis and its relationship to religious variables. *Review of Religious Research* 34:333–47.

133. Kivett, V. R. 1979. Religious motivation in middle age: Correlates and implications. *Journal of Gerontology* 34:106–15; and F. D. Wolinsky and T. E. Stump. 1996. Age and the sense of control among older adults. *Journal of Gerontology* 51B: S217–20.

134. Hassan, M. K., and A. Khalique. 1981. Religiosity and its correlates in college students. *Journal of Psychological Researches* 25 (3): 129–36.

135. Watson, P. J., R. J. Morris, and R. W. Hood. 1989. Sin and self-functioning, part 4: Depression, assertiveness, and religious commitments. *Journal of Psychology and Theology* 17:44–58.

136. Kahoe, R. D. 1974. Personality and achievement correlates of intrinsic and extrinsic religious orientations. *Journal of Personality and Social Psychology* 29:812–18.

137. Batson, C. D., S. J. Naifeh, and S. Pate. 1978. Social desirability, religious orientation, and racial prejudice. *Journal for the Scientific Study of Religion* 17:31–41.

138. Ramanaiah, N. V., J. K. Rielage, and J. Sharpe. 2001. Spiritual well-being and personality. *Psychological Reports* 89 (3): 662.

139. Koenig, H. G., I. C. Siegler, K. G. Meador, and L. K. George. 1990. Religious coping and personality in later life. *International Journal of Geriatric Psychiatry* 5:123–31.

140. Koenig, *Handbook of Religion and Health*, 514–54.

141. LaMothe, R. W. 1996. Hatred, hostility, and faith: A theological perspective. *Pastoral Psychology* 44 (3): 185–98; and J. A. Haught. 1994. *Holy Hatred: Religious Conflicts of the '90s*. Amherst, NY: Prometheus Books.

142. Weima, J. 1965. Authoritarianism, religious conservatism and socio-centric attitudes in Roman Catholic groups. *Human Relations* 18, 231–39; and G. W. Allport and J. M. Ross. 1967. Personal religious orientation and prejudice. *Journal of Personality and Social Psychology* 5:432–43.

143. Bottoms, B. L., P. R. Shaver, F. S. Goodman, and J. Qin. 1995. In the name of God: A profile of religion-related child abuse. *Journal of Social Issues* 51:85–112; and L. H. Bowker. 1988. Religious victims and their religious leaders: Services delivered to one thousand battered women by the clergy. In *Abuse and Religion: When Praying Isn't Enough*, ed. A. L. Horton and J. A. Williamson. Lexington, KY: Lexington Books, 229–34.

144. Hochman, J. 1990. Miracle, mystery, and authority: The triangle of cult indoctrination. *Psychiatric Annals* 20 (4): 179–84, 187.

145. Adorno, T. W., E. Frenkel-Brunswick, D. J. Levinseson, R. N. Sanford. 1950. *The Authoritarian Personality*. New York: Harper & Row; and B. R. Strickland and S. C. Weddell. 1971. Religious orientation, racial prejudice, and dogmatism: A study of Baptists and Unitarians. *Journal for the Scientific Study of Religion* 11:395–99.

146. Raphael, F. J., S. Rani, R. Bale, and L. M. Drummond. 1996. Religion, ethnicity and obsessive-compulsive disorder. *International Journal of Social Psychiatry* 42:38–44; and P. S. Gangdev. 1998. Faith-assisted cognitive therapy of obsessive-compulsive disorder. *Australian and New Zealand Journal of Psychiatry* 32:575–78.

147. Richards, P. S., L. Owen, and S. Stein. 1993. A religiously oriented group counseling intervention for self-defeating perfectionism: A pilot study. *Counseling and Values* 37:96–104.

148. Ellis, A. 1988. Is religiosity pathological? *Free Inquiry* 18:27–32.

149. Dreger, R. M. 1952. Some personality correlates of religious attitudes as determined by projective techniques. *Psychological Monographs* 66:335.

150. Bobgan, M. 1981. *The Psychological Way: The Spiritual Way*. Santa Barbara, CA: EastGate Publishers.

151. Bobgan, M., and D. Bobgan. 1989. *Prophets of Psychoheresy I*. Santa Barbara, CA: EastGate Publishers.

152. Domino, G. 1985. Clergy's attitudes toward suicide and recognition of suicide lethality. *Death Studies* 9 (3–4): 187–99.

153. Ruiz, P. 1998. The role of culture in psychiatric care. *American Journal of Psychiatry* 155:1763–65.

154. Ruiz, P. 1985. Cultural barriers to effective medical care among Hispanic-American patients. *Annual Review of Medicine* 36:63–71.

155. Haught, *Holy Hatred*.

156. Weima, Authoritarianism, religious conservatism and socio-centric attitudes in Roman Catholic groups.

157. Allport, G. W., and J. M. Ross. 1967. Personal religious orientation and prejudice. *Journal of Personality and Social Psychology* 5:432–43.

158. Bottoms et al., In the name of god.

159. Ellison, C. G., J. P. Bartkowski, and K. L. Anderson. 1999. Are there religious variations in domestic violence? *Journal of Family Issues* 20:87–113.

160. Bowker, Religious victims and their religious leaders.

161. Hochman, Miracle, mystery, and authority.
162. Strickland and Weddell, Religious orientation, racial prejudice, and dogmatism.
163. Raphael et al., Religion, ethnicity and obsessive-compulsive disorder.
164. Gangdev, Faith-assisted cognitive therapy.
165. Richards et al., A religiously oriented group counseling intervention.
166. Dreger, Some personality correlates of religious attitudes.
167. Koenig, *Handbook of Religion and Health*, 514–18.
168. Exline, J. J. 2002. Stumbling blocks on the religious road: Fractured relationships, nagging vices, and the inner struggle to believe. *Psychological Inquiry* 13:182–89.
169. Hood, R., B. Spilka, B. Hunsberger, and R. Gorsuch. 1996. *The Psychology of Religion*. 2nd ed. New York: Guilford.
170. Lehrer, E. L., and C. U. Chiswick. 1993. Religion as a determinant of marital stability. *Demography* 30:385–403.
171. Exline, Stumbling blocks.
172. Koenig, H. G., K. I. Pargament, and J. Nielsen. 1998. Religious coping and health status in medically ill hospitalized older adults. *Journal of Nervous and Mental Disease* 186 (9): 513–21; K. I. Pargament, H. G. Koenig, N. Tarakeshwar, and J. Hahn. 2001. Religious struggle as a predictor of mortality among medically ill elderly patients: A two-year longitudinal study. *Archives of Internal Medicine* 161:1881–85; and McClain, Effect of spiritual well-being on end-of-life despair.
173. Exline, J. J., A. M. Yali, and M. Lobel. 1999. When God disappoints: Difficulty forgiving God and its role in negative emotion. *Journal of Health and Psychology* 4:365–79.
174. Exline, Stumbling blocks.
175. Ibid.
176. Altemeyer, B., and B. Hunsberger. 1997. *Amazing Conversions: Why Some Turn to Faith and Others Abandoned Religion*. Amherst, NY: Prometheus.
177. Exline, Stumbling blocks.
178. Baumesiter, R. F. 1993. Lying to yourself: The paradox of self-deception. In *Lying and Deception in Everyday Life*, ed. M. Lewis and C. Saarni. New York: Guilford, 66–83.
179. Baumeister, R. F., E. Bratslavsky, M. Muraven, and D. M. Tice. 1998. Ego depletion: Is the active self a limited resource? *Journal of Personality and Social Psychology* 74:1252–65.
180. Exline, J. J., A. M. Yali, and W. C. Sanderson. 2000. Guilt, discord, and alienation: The role of religious strain in depression and suicidality. *Journal of Clinical Psychology* 56 (12): 1481–96.
181. Turner, J. A., and S. Clancy. 1986. Strategies for coping with chronic low back pain: Relationship to pain and disability. *Pain* 24:355–64; and F. J. Keefe, G. Affleck, J. Lefebvre, L. Underwood, D. S. Caldwell, J. Drew. J. Egert, J. Gibson, and K. Pargament. 2001. Giving with rheumatoid arthritis: The role of daily spirituality and daily religious and spiritual coping. *Journal of Pain* 2 (2): 101–10.

CHAPTER 4: RELIGION, PSYCHIATRIC
SYMPTOMS, AND DISORDERS

1. Koenig, H. G. 1998. *Handbook of Religion and Health*. San Diego: Academic Press, 144–55, 536–38.
2. Cooley, C. E., and J. B. Hutton. 1965. Adolescent response to religious appeal as related to IPAT anxiety. *Journal of Social Psychology* 56:325–27; P. A. Morris. 1982. The effect of pilgrimage on anxiety, depression and religious attitude. *Psychological Medicine* 12:291–94; R. F. Paloutzian. 1981. Purpose in life and value changes following conversion. *Journal of Personality and Social Psychology* 41:1153–60; and D. R. Williams, D. B. Larson, R. E. Buckler, R. C. Heckmann, and C. M. Pyle. 1991. Religion and psychological distress in a community sample. *Social Science and Medicine* 32:1257–62.
3. Azhar, M. Z., S. L. Varma, and A. S. Dharap. 1994. Religious psychotherapy in anxi-

ety disorder patients. *Acta Psychiatrica Scandinavica* 90:1–3; C. R. Carlson, P. E. Bacaseta, and D. A. Simanton. 1988. A controlled evaluation of devotional meditation and progressive relaxation. *Journal of Psychology and Theology* 16:362–68; J. Kabat-Zinn, A. O. Massion, J. Kristeller, L. G. Peterson, K. E. Fletcher, L. Pbert, W. R. Lenderking, and S. F. Santorelli. 1992. Effectiveness of a meditation-based stress reduction program in the treatment of anxiety disorders. *American Journal of Psychiatry* 149:936–43; J. J. Miller, K. Fletcher, and J. Kabat-Zinn. 1995. Three-year follow-up and clinical implications of mindfulness meditation-based stress reduction intervention in the treatment of anxiety disorders. *General Hospital Psychiatry* 17:192–200; S. M. Razali, C. I. Hasanah, K. Aminah, and M. Subramaniam. 1998. Religious-sociocultural psychotherapy in patients with anxiety and depression. *Australian and New Zealand Journal of Psychiatry* 32:867–72; and S. Xiao, D. Young, and H. Zhang. 1998. Taoistic cognitive psychotherapy for neurotic patients: A preliminary clinical trial. *Psychiatry and Clinical Neurosciences* 52: S238–41.

4. Baker, M., and R. Gorsuch. 1982. Trait anxiety and intrinsic-extrinsic religiousness. *Journal for the Scientific Study of Religion* 21:119–22.

5. Sturgeon, R. S., and R. W. Hamley. 1979. Religion and anxiety. *Journal of Social Psychology* 108:137–38; A. E. Bergin, K. S. Masters, and P. S. Richards. 1987. Religiousness and mental health: A study of an intrinsically religious sample. *Journal of Counsulting Psychology* 34 (2): 197–204; S. Tapanya, R. Nicki, and O. Jarusawad. 1997. Worry and intrinsic/extrinsic religious orientation among Buddhist (Thai) and Christian (Canadian) elderly persons. *International Journal of Aging and Human Development* 44:73–83; P. Watson, N. Ghorbani, H. Davison, M. N. Bing, R. W. Hood, and A. F. Ghramaleki. 2002. Negatively reinforcing personal extrinsic motivations: Religious orientation, inner awareness, and mental health in Iran and the United States. *International Journal for the Psychology of Religion* 12 (4): 255–76; and H.-S. Park, W. Murgatroyd, D. C. Raynock, and M. A. Spillett. 1998. Relationship between intrinsic-extrinsic religious orientation and depressive symptoms in Korean Americans. *Counseling Psychology Quarterly* 11 (3): 315–24.

6. Tapanya et al., Worry and intrinsic/extrinsic religious orientation.

7. Ibid., 80.

8. Roff, L. L., R. Butkeviciene, and D. L. Klemmack. 2002. Death anxiety and religiosity among Lithuanian health and social service professionals. *Death Studies* 26 (9): 731–42; J. Irene Harris, Sean W. Schoneman, and Stephanie R. Carrera. 2002. Approaches to religiosity related to anxiety among college students. *Mental Health, Religion and Culture* 5 (3): 253–65; A. M. Abdel-Khalek. 2002. Age and sex differences for anxiety in relation to family size, birth order and religiosity among Kuwaiti adolescents. *Psychological Reports* 90 (3, Pt 1): 1031–36; J. D. Hovey and C. G. Magana. 2002. Cognitive, affective, and physiological expressions of anxiety symptomatology among Mexican migrant farmworkers: Predictors and generational differences. *Community Mental Health Journal* 38 (3): 223–37; S. B. Goldstein, E. A. Dudley, C. M. Erickson, and N. L. Richer. 2002. Personality traits and computer anxiety as predictors of Y2K anxiety. *Computers in Human Behavior* 18 (3): 271–84; D. Edwards and E. Besseling. 2001. Relationship between depression, anxiety, sense of coherence, social support and religious involvement in a small rural community affected by industrial relations conflict. *South African Journal of Psychology* 31 (4): 62–71; and J. Scott Young, Craig S. Cashwell, and Julia Shcherbakova. 2000. The moderating relationship of spirituality on negative life events and psychological adjustment. *Counseling and Values* 45 (1): 49–57.

9. Abdel-Khalek, Age and sex differences.

10. Chang, B. H., K. M. Skinner, and U. Boehmer. 2001. Religion and mental health among women veterans with sexual assault experience. *International Journal of Psychiatry in Medicine* 31:77–96.

11. Chang, B. H., K. M. Skinner, C. Zhou, and L. E. Kazis. 2003. The relationship between sexual assault, religiosity and mental health among male veterans. *International Journal of Psychiatry in Medicine* 33 (3): 223–40.

12. Falsetti, S. A., P. A. Resick, and J. L. Davis. 2003. Changes in religious beliefs following trauma. *Journal of Traumatic Stress* 16 (4): 391–98.

13. Schuster, A national survey of stress reactions.

14. Fontana, A., and R. Rosenheck. 2004. Trauma, change in strength of religious faith, and mental health service use among veterans treated for PTSD. *Journal of Nervous and Mental Disease* 192:579–84.

15. Freud, S. 1907. *Obsessive Acts and Religious Practices*. In *Standard Edition of the Complete Psychological Works of Sigmund Freud*, trans. and ed. J. Strachey. London: Hogarth Press (published in 1962).

16. Abramowitz, J. S. 2001. Treatment of scrupulous obsessions and compulsions using exposure and response prevention: A case report. *Cognitive and Behavioral Practice* 8 (1): 79–85.

17. Steketee, G., S. Quay, and K. White. 1991. Religion and guilt in OCD patients. *Journal of Anxiety Disorders* 5:359–67.

18. Sica, C., C. Novara, and E. Sanavio. 2002. Religiousness and obsessive-compulsive cognitions and symptoms in an Italian population. *Behaviour Research and Therapy* 40 (7): 813–23.

19. Hermesh, Haggai, Ruth Masser-Kavitzky, and Ruth Gross-Isseroff. 2003. Obsessive-compulsive disorder and Jewish religiosity. *Journal of Nervous and Mental Disease* 191 (3): 201–03.

20. Greenberg, David, and Gaby Shefler. 2002. Obsessive compulsive disorder in ultra-orthodox Jewish patients: A comparison of religious and non-religious symptoms. *Psychology and Psychotherapy* 75 (2): 123–30; Cenk Tek and Berna Ulug. 2001. Religiosity and religious obsessions in obsessive-compulsive disorder. *Psychiatry Research* 104 (2): 99–108; and A. Okasha, F. Lotaief, A. M. Ashour, N. El Mahalawy, A. Seif El Dawla, and G. H. El-Kholy. 2000. The prevalence of obsessive compulsive symptoms in a sample of Egyptian psychiatric patients. *Encephale* 26 (4): 1–10.

21. Yossifova, M., and K. M. Loewenthal. 1999. Religion and the judgment of obsessionality. *Mental Health, Religion and Culture* 2 (2): 145–51.

22. Alonso, P., J. M. Menchon, J. Pifarre, D. Mataix-Cols, L. Torres, P. Salgado, et al. 2001. Long-term follow-up and predictors of clinical outcome in obsessive-compulsive patients treated with serotonin reuptake inhibitors and behavioral therapy. *Journal of Clinical Psychiatry* 62 (7): 535–40.

23. Mataix-Cols, D., I. M. Marks, J. H. Greist, K. A. Kobak, and L. Baer. 2002. Obsessive-compulsive symptom dimensions as predictors of compliance with and response to behaviour therapy: Results from a controlled trial. *Psychotherapy and Psychosomatics* 71 (5): 255–62.

24. Koenig, *Handbook of Religion and Health*, 118–43, 216–17, 527–35.

25. Braam, A. W., A. T. F. Beekman, D. J. H. Deeg, J. H. Smith, and W. van Tilburg. 1997. Religiosity as a protective or prognostic factor of depression in later life; results from the community survey in the Netherlands. *Acta Psychiatrica Scandinavia* 96:199–205.

26. Koenig, H. G., L. K. George, and B. L. Peterson. 1998. Religiosity and remission from depression in medically ill older patients. *American Journal of Psychiatry* 155:536–42.

27. Bosworth, H. B., K. W. Park, D. R. McQuoid, and D. C. Steffens. 2003. The impact of religious practice and coping on geriatric depression recovery. *International Journal of Geriatric Psychiatry* 18:905–14.

28. Koenig, *Handbook of Religion and Health*, 527–35.

29. Azhar, M. Z., and S. L. Varma. 1995. Religious psychotherapy in depressive patients. *Psychotherapy and Psychosomatics* 63:165–73; L. R. Propst. 1980. The comparative efficacy of religious and nonreligious imagery for the treatment of mild depression in religious individuals. *Cognitive Therapy and Research* 4:167–78; L. R. Propst, R. Ostrom, P. Watkins, T. Dean, and D. Mashburn. 1992. Comparative efficacy of religious and nonreligious cognitive-behavior therapy for the treatment of clinical depression in religious individuals. *Journal of Consulting and Clinical Psychology* 60:94–103; Y. M. Toh and S. Y. Tan. 1997. The effectiveness of church-based lay counselors: A controlled outcome study. *Journal of Psychology and Christianity* 16:260–67; and S. M. Razali, C. I. Hasanah, K. Aminah, and M. Subramaniam. 1998. Religious-sociocultural psychotherapy in patients with anxiety and depression. *Australian and New Zealand Journal of Psychiatry* 32:867–72.

30. Koenig, H. G., H. J. Cohen, D. G. Blazer, C. Pieper, K. G. Meador, F. Shelp, V. Goli,

and R. DiPasquale. 1992. Religious coping and depression in elderly hospitalized medically ill men. *American Journal of Psychiatry* 149:1693–1700; and H. G. Koenig, L. K. George, and B. L. Peterson. 1998. Religiosity and remission from depression in medically ill older patients. *American Journal of Psychiatry* 155:536–42.

31. Williams, D. R., D. B. Larson, R. E. Buckler, R. C. Heckmann, and C. M. Pyle. 1991. Religion and psychological distress in a community sample. *Social Science and Medicine* 32:1257–62; Kendler et al., Religion, psychopathology, and substance use and abuse; and C. Park, L. H. Cohen, and L. Herb. 1990. Intrinsic religiousness and religious coping as life stress moderators for Catholics versus Protestants. *Journal of Personality and Social Psychology* 59:562–74.

32. Chang, Skinner, and Boehmer, Religion and mental health among women veterans; Chang et al., The relationship between sexual assault, religiosity and mental health among male veterans.

33. Folkman, S. 1997. Positive psychological states and coping with severe stress. *Social Science and Medicine* 45:1207–21.

34. Rabins, P. V., M. D. Fitting, J. Eastham, and J. Fetting. 1990. The emotional impact of caring for the chronically ill. *Psychosomatics* 31:331–36; and P. V. Rabins, M. D. Fitting, J. Eastham, and J. Zabora. 1990. Emotional adaptation over time in care-givers for chronically ill elderly people. *Age and Aging* 19:185–90.

35. Maton, K. I. 1989. The stress-buffering role of spiritual support: Cross-sectional and prospective investigations. *Journal for the Scientific Study of Religion* 28:310–23.

36. Smith, B. W. 1996. Coping as a predictor of outcomes following the 1993 Midwest flood. *Journal of Social Behavior and Personality* 11:225–39.

37. Kalil, A., C. E. Born, J. Kunz, and P. J. Caudill. 2001. Life stressors, social support, and depressive symptoms among first-time welfare recipients. *American Journal of Community Psychology* 29 (2): 355–69.

38. Pearce, M. J., T. D. Little, and J. E. Perez. 2003. Religiousness and depressive symptoms among adolescents. *Journal of Clinical Child and Adolescent Psychology* 32 (2): 267–76.

39. Schapman, A. M., and H. M. Inderbitzen-Nolan. 2002. The role of religious behaviour in adolescent depressive and anxious symptomatology. *Journal of Adolescence* 25 (6): 631–43.

40. Miller, L., V. Warner, P. Wickramaratne, and M. Weissman. 1997. *Journal of the American Academy of Child and Adolescent Psychiatry* 36:1416–25.

41. Varon, S. R., and A. W. Riley. 1999. Relationship between maternal church attendance and adolescent mental health and social functioning. *Psychiatric Services* 50 (6): 799–805.

42. Horowitz, J. L., and J. Garber. 2003. Relation of intelligence and religiosity to depressive disorders in offspring of depressed and nondepressed mothers. *Journal of the American Academy of Child and Adolescent Psychiatry* 42 (5): 578–86.

43. Miller, L., and M. Gur. 2002. Religiosity, depression and physical maturation in adolescent girls. *Journal of the American Academy of Child and Adolescent Psychiatry* 41 (2): 206–14.

44. Miller, L., M. Weissman, M. Gur, and S. Greenwald. 2002. Adult religiousness and history of childhood depression: Eleven-year follow-up study. *Journal of Nervous and Mental Disease* 190 (2): 86–93.

45. Sorenson, A. M., C. F. Grindstaff, and R. J. Turner. 1995. Religious involvement among unmarried adolescent mothers: A source of emotional support? *Sociology of Religion* 56:71–81.

46. Nooney, J., and E. Woodrum. 2002. Religious coping and church-based social support as predictors of mental health outcomes: Testing a conceptual model. *Journal for the Scientific Study of Religion* 41 (2): 359–68.

47. Krause, N. 2002. Church-based social support and health in old age: Exploring variations by race. *Journal of Gerontology* 57B (6): S332–47.

48. Higgins, M. P. 2002. Parental bereavement and religious factors. *Omega—Journal of Death and Dying* 45 (2): 187–207.

49. Baetz, M., D. B. Larson, G. Marcoux, R. Bowen, and R. Griffin. 2002. Canadian psychiatric inpatient religious commitment: An association with mental health. *Canadian Journal of Psychiatry* 47 (2): 159–66.

50. Hintikka, J., H. Vinaemaki, H. Koivumaa-Honkanen, A. Tanskanen, and J. Lehtonen. 1998. Associations between religious attendance, social support, and depression in psychiatric patients. *Journal of Psychology and Theology* 26 (4): 351–57.

51. Strawbridge, W. J., S. J. Shema, R. D. Cohen, R. E. Roberts, and G. A. Kaplan. 1998. Religiosity buffers effects of some stressors on depression but exacerbates others. *Journal of Gerontology* 53: S118–26.

52. Branco, K. J. 2000. Religiosity and depression among nursing home residents: Results of a survey of ten states. *Journal of Religious Gerontology* 12 (1): 43–61.

53. Braam, A. W., A. T. F. Beekman, et al., Religious involvement and depression in older Dutch citizens. *Social Psychiatry and Psychiatric Epidemiology* 32:284–91; and A. W. Braam, A. T. F. Beekman, et al., Religiosity as a protective or prognostic factor of depression in later life.

54. Braam, A. W., P. Van Den Eeden, M. J. Prince, A. T. F. Beekman, et al. 2001. Religion as a cross-cultural determinant of depression in elderly Europeans: Results from the EURODEP collaboration. *Psychological Medicine* 31 (5): 803–14.

55. Nelson, C. J., B. Rosenfeld, W. Breitbart, and M. Galietta. 2002. Spirituality, religion, and depression in the terminally ill. *Psychosomatics* 43 (3): 213–20.

56. Pargament, K. I., H. G. Koenig, N. Tarakeshwar, and J. Hahn. 2001. Religious struggle as a predictor of mortality among medically ill elderly patients: A two-year longitudinal study. *Archives of Internal Medicine* 161:1881–85.

57. Simoni, J. M., M. G. Martone, and J. F. Kerwin. 2002. Spirituality and psychological adaptation among women with HIV/AIDS: Implications for counseling. *Journal of Counseling Psychology* 49 (2): 139–47; L. T. Flannelly and J. Inouye. 2001. Relationships of religion, health status and socioeconomic status to the quality of life of individuals who are HIV positive. *Issues in Mental Health Nursing* 22 (3): 253–72; G. Ironson, G. F. Solomon, E. G. Balbin, C. O'Cleirigh, A. George, and M. Kumar, et al. 2002. The Ironson-Woods Spirituality/Religiousness Index is associated with long survival, health behaviors, less distress, and low cortisol in people with HIV/AIDS. *Annals of Behavioral Medicine* 24 (1): 34–48; and K. Siegel and E. W. Schrimshaw. 2002. The perceived benefits of religious and spiritual coping among older adults living with HIV/AIDS. *Journal for the Scientific Study of Religion* 41 (1): 91–102.

58. Levin, J. 2002. Is depressed affect a function of one's relationship with God?: Findings from a study of primary care patients. *International Journal of Psychiatry in Medicine* 32 (4): 379–93.

59. Stack, S. 1992. Religiosity, depression, and suicide. In *Religion and Mental Health*, ed. J. F. Schumaker. New York: Oxford University Press, 87–97.

60. Simpson, M. E., and G. H. Conklin. 1989. Socioeconomic development, suicide, and religion: A test of Durkheim's theory of religion and suicide. *Social Forces* 67 (4): 945–64.

61. Kok, Lee-peng. 1988. Race, religion and female suicide attempters in Singapore. *Social Psychiatry and Psychiatric Epidemiology* 23 (4): 236–39; and Unni Wikan. 1988. Bereavement and loss in two Muslim communities: Egypt and Bali compared. *Social Science and Medicine* 27 (5): 451–60.

62. Greening, L., and L. Stoppelbein. 2002. Religiosity, attributional style, and social support as psychosocial buffers for African American and white adolescents' perceived risk for suicide. *Suicide and Life-Threatening Behavior* 32 (4): 404–17.

63. Cook, J. M., J. L. Pearson, R. Thompson, B. S. Black, and P. V. Rabins. 2002. Suicidality in older African Americans: Findings from the EPOCH study. *American Journal of Geriatric Psychiatry* 10 (4): 437–46.

64. McClain, C. S., B. Rosenfeld, and W. Breitbart. 2003. Effect of spiritual well-being on end-of-life despair in terminally ill cancer patients. *Lancet* 361 (9369): 1603–7.

65. Huline-Dickens, S. 2000. Anorexia nervosa: Some connections with the religious attitude. *British Journal of Medical Psychology* 73 (1): 67–76.

66. Griffin, J., and E. M. Berry. 2003. A modern day holy anorexia? Religious language in advertising and anorexia nervosa in the West. *European Journal of Clinical Nutrition* 57 (1): 43–51.

67. Forthun, L. F., B. W. Pidcock, and J. L. Fischer. 2003. Religiousness and disordered eating: Does religiousness modify family risk? *Eating Behaviors* 4 (1): 7–26.

68. Smith, F. T., R. K. Hardman, P. Richards, and L. Fischer. 2003. Intrinsic religiousness and spiritual well-being as predictors of treatment outcome among women with eating disorders. *Eating Disorders: the Journal of Treatment and Prevention* 11 (1): 15–26.

69. Vaillant, G. E. 1975. Sociopathy as a human process. *Archives of General Psychiatry* 32:173–83.

70. Koenig, *Handbook of Religion and Health*, 181–90, 218–19, 545–46.

71. Stark, R. 1996. Religion as context: Hellfire and delinquency one more time. *Sociology of Religion* 57:163–73.

72. Wallace, J. M., and T. A. Forman. 1998. Religion's role in promoting health and reducing the risk among American youth. *Health Education and Behavior* 25:721–41.

73. Johnson, B. R. 2003. *The Great Escape: How Religion Alters the Delinquent Behavior of High-Risk Adolescents*. Philadelphia: Center for Research on Religion and Urban Civil Society, University of Pennsylvania. Johnson now heads up the Center for Religious Inquiry across the Disciplines at Baylor University in Waco, Texas.

74. Johnson, B. R., S. J. Jang, D. B. Larson, and S. D. Li. 2001. Does adolescent religious commitment matter? A reexamination of the effects of religiosity on delinquency. *Journal of Research in Crime and Delinquency* 38 (1): 22–44.

75. Johnson, B. R. 2003. *The InnerChange Freedom Initiative: A Preliminary Evaluation of a Faith-Based Prison Program*. Philadelphia: Center for Research on Religion and Urban Civil Society, University of Pennsylvania.

76. Kleiman, M. 2003. Faith-based fudging. How a Bush-promoted Christian prison program fakes success by massaging data. Posted August 5. See MSN Web site: http://slate.msn.com/id/2086617.

77. Lamb, H. R., L. Weinberger, and B. Gross. 1999. Community treatment of severely mentally ill offenders under the jurisdiction of the criminal justice system: A review. *Psychiatric Services* 50:907–13.

78. Moody-Smithson, M. 2001. Religion's effects on health outcomes: A literature review. Presented at CSAT's Faith and Community Partners Initiative National Focus Group Meeting, July 26–27, 2001, Washington, D.C. Rockville, MD: Logicon/Row Sciences, Inc.

79. See Web site: http://www.casacolumbia.org/absolutenm/templates/PressReleases.asp?articleid=115andzoneid=48.

80. Koenig, *Handbook of Religion and Health*, 166–80, 218, 539–45.

81. Ibid.

82. Kendler, Kenneth S., Xiao-Qing Liu, Charles O. Gardner, Michael E. McCullough, David Larson, and Carol A. Prescott. 2003. Dimensions of religiosity and their relationship to lifetime psychiatric and substance use disorders. *American Journal of Psychiatry* 160 (3): 496–503; Thomas Ashby Wills, Alison M. Yaeger, and James M. Sandy. 2003. Buffering effect of religiosity for adolescent substance use. *Psychology of Addictive Behaviors* 17 (1): 24–31; and S. Kelly Avants, David Marcotte, Ruth Arnold, and Arthur Margolin. 2003. Spiritual beliefs, world assumptions, and HIV risk behavior among heroin and cocaine users. *Psychology of Addictive Behaviors* 17 (2): 159–62.

83. Szaflarski, M. 2001. Gender, self-reported health and health-related lifestyles in Poland. *Health Care for Women International* 22 (3): 207–27; T. Winter, S. Karvonen, and R. J. Rose. 2002. Does religiousness explain regional differences in alcohol use in Finland? *Alcohol and Alcoholism* 37 (4): 330–39; and L. C. Hope, and C. C. Cook. 2001. The role of Christian commitment in predicting drug use amongst church affiliated young people. *Mental Health, Religion and Culture* 4 (2): 109–17.

84. Szaflarski, Gender, self-reported health and health-related lifestyles.

85. Winter et al., Does religiousness explain regional differences in alcohol use in Finland?

86. Hope and Cook, The role of Christian commitment.

87. Kessler, R. C., R. M. Crum, L. A. Warner, C. B. Nelson, J. Schulenberg, and J. C. An-

thony. 1997. Lifetime co-occurrence of *DSM-III-R* alcohol abuse and dependence with other psychiatric disorders in the national comorbidity survey. *Archives of General Psychiatry* 54:313–21.

88. Musick, M. A., D. G. Blazer, and J. C. Hays. 2000. Religious activity, alcohol use, and depression in a sample of elderly Baptists. *Research on Aging* 22 (2): 91–116.

CHAPTER 5: RELIGION AND SEVERE,

PERSISTENT MENTAL ILLNESS

1. Numbers, R. L., and D. W. Amundsen. 1998. *Caring and Curing: Health and Medicine in the Western Religious Traditions*. Baltimore, MD: Johns Hopkins University Press; and L. E. Sullivan. 1989. *Healing and Restoring: Health and Medicine in the World's Religious Traditions*. New York: Macmillan Publishing Co.

2. Lindgren, K. N., and R. D. Coursey. 1995. Spirituality and serious mental illness: A two-part study. *Psychosocial Rehabilitation Journal* 18 (3): 93–111.

3. Tepper, L., S. A. Rogers, E. M. Coleman, and H. N. Malony. 2001. The prevalence of religious coping among persons with persistent mental illness. *Psychiatric Services* 52 (5): 660–65.

4. Sullivan, William P. 1993. "It helps me to be a whole person": The role of spirituality among the mentally challenged. *Psychosocial Rehabilitation Journal* 16 (3): 125–34.

5. Russinova, Z., N. J. Wewiorski, and D. Cash. 2002. Use of alternative health care practices by persons with serious mental illness: Perceived benefits. *American Journal of Public Health* 92 (10): 1600–1603.

6. Bussema, Kenneth E., and Evelyn F. Bussema. 2000. Is there a balm in Gilead? The implications of faith in coping with a psychiatric disability. *Psychiatric Rehabilitation Journal* 24 (2): 117–24.

7. Yangarber-Hicks, N. I. 2003. Religious coping styles and recovery from serious mental illness. *Dissertation Abstracts International*: Section B: The Sciences and Engineering 63 (7-B): 3487.

8. Wahass, S., and G. Kent. 1997. Coping with auditory hallucinations: A cross-cultural comparison between Western (British) and non-Western (Saudi Arabian) patients. *Journal of Nervous and Mental Disease* 185:664–68.

9. Ireland, R. 1988. *The Challenge of Secularization*. Melbourne, Australia: Collins Dove, 32–44.

10. D'Souza, R. 2002. Do patients expect psychiatrists to be interested in spiritual issues? *Australasian Psychiatry* 10 (1): 44–47.

11. Reger, G. M., and S. A. Rogers. 2002. Diagnostic differences in religious coping among individuals with persistent mental illness. *Journal of Psychology and Christianity* 21 (4): 341–48.

12. Watters, W. 1992. *Deadly Doctrine: Health, Illness, and Christian God-talk*. Buffalo, NY: Prometheus Books, 145–46.

13. Vlachos, I. O., S. Beratis, and P. Hartocollis. 1997. Magico-religious beliefs and psychosis. *Psychopathology* 30 (2): 93–99.

14. Kulhara, P., A. Avasthi, and A. Sharma. 2000. Magico-religious beliefs in schizophrenia: A study from North India. *Psychopathology* 33 (2): 62–68.

15. Srinivasan, T., and R. Thara. 2001. Beliefs about causation of schizophrenia: Do Indian families believe in supernatural causes? *Social Psychiatry and Psychiatric Epidemiology* 36 (3): 134–40.

16. Al-Faraj, A. M., and A. M. Al-Ansari. 2002. What family caregivers of schizophrenic and non-psychotic in-patients in Bahrain believe about mental illness. *Arab Journal of Psychiatry* 13 (1): 26–30.

17. Sheehan, W., and J. Kroll. 1990. Psychiatric patients' belief in general health factors and sin as causes of illness. *American Journal of Psychiatry* 147:112–13.

18. McAll, R. K. 1982. *Healing the Family Tree*. London: Sheldon Press.

19. Ibid.

20. Wilson, W. P. 1998. Religion and the psychoses. In *Handbook of Mental Health and Religion*, ed. H. G. Koenig. San Diego: Academic Press, 161–72.

21. Peck, M. S. 1983. *People of the Lie: The Hope for Healing Human Evil.* New York: Simon & Schuster.

22. Bull, D. L. 2001. A phenomenological model of therapeutic exorcism for dissociative identity disorder. *Journal of Psychology and Theology* 29 (2): 131–39.

23. Bowman, E. S. 2000. The assets and liabilities of conservative religious faith for persons with severe dissociative disorders. *Journal of Psychology and Christianity* 19 (2): 122–38.

24. Sedman, G., and G. Hopkinson. 1966. The psychopathology of mystical and religious conversion experiences in psychiatric patients. *Confinia Psychiatrica* 9 (1): 1–19.

25. Wootton, R. J., and D. F. Allen. 1983. Dramatic religious conversion and schizophrenic decompensation. *Journal of Religion and Health* 22:212–20.

26. Salzman, L. 1953. The psychology of religious and ideological conversion. *Psychiatry* 16:177–87.

27. James, W. 1902. *The Varieties of Religious Experience.* New York: New American Library.

28. Wilson, W. P., D. B. Larson, and P. D. Meier. 1983. Religious life of schizophrenics. *Southern Medical Journal* 76:1096–100.

29. Wilson, W. P. 1972. Mental health benefits of religious salvation. *Diseases of the Nervous System* 36:382–86.

30. Koenig, H. G. 1994. *Aging and God.* Binghamton, NY: Haworth Press, 424–33.

31. Heirich, M. 1977. Change of heart: A test of some widely held theories about religious conversion. *American Journal of Sociology* 83:653–80.

32. Indian Council of Medical Research. 1988. Multicentre collaborative study of factors associated with the course and outcome of schizophrenia. New Delhi: ICMR; and D. Bhugra, B. Corridan, S. Rudge, J. Leff, and R. Mallett. 1999. Early manifestations, personality traits and pathways into care for Asian and white first-onset cases of schizophrenia. *Social Psychiatry and Psychiatric Epidemiology* 34 (11): 595–99.

33. Bhugra et al., Early manifestations.

34. Gutierrez-Lobos, K., B. Schmid-Siegel, B. Bankier, and H. Walter. 2001. Delusions in first-admitted patients: Gender, themes and diagnoses. *Psychopathology* 34 (1): 1–7.

35. Smith, A. C. 1982. *Schizophrenia and Madness.* London: Allen & Unwin.

36. Matthew 5:29–30, New International Version of the Holy Bible.

37. Erol, S., and C. Kaptanoglu. 2000. Self-inflicted bilateral eye injury by a schizophrenic patient. *General Hospital Psychiatry* 22 (3): 215–16.

38. Kushner, A. W. 1967. Two cases of auto-castration due to religious delusions. *British Journal of Medical Psychology* 40 (3): 293–98.

39. Favazza, A. R. 1989. Why patients mutilate themselves. *Hospital and Community Psychiatry* 40 (2): 137–45.

40. Bible verse cited in baby's killing. *Durham Herald.* December 15, 2004.

41. Cothran, M. M., and P. D. Harvey. 1986. Delusional thinking in psychotics: Correlates of religious content. *Psychological Reports* 58:191–99.

42. Siddle, R., G. Haddock, N. Tarrier, and E. Faragher. 2002. Religious delusions in patients admitted to hospital with schizophrenia. *Social Psychiatry and Psychiatric Epidemiology* 37 (3): 130–38.

43. Siddle, R., G. Haddock, N. Tarrier, and E. Faragher. 2002. The validation of a religiosity measure for individuals with schizophrenia. *Mental Health, Religion and Culture* 5 (3): 267–84.

44. Getz, G. E., D. E. Fleck, and S. M. Strakowski. 2001. Frequency and severity of religious delusions in Christian patients with psychosis. *Psychiatry Research* 103 (1): 87–91.

45. Yip, K. 2003. Traditional Chinese religious beliefs and superstitions in delusions and hallucinations of Chinese schizophrenic patients. *International Journal of Social Psychiatry* 49 (2): 97–111.

46. Pierre, J. M. 2001. Faith or delusion: At the crossroads of religion and psychosis. *Journal of Psychiatric Practice* 7 (3): 163–72.

47. Clark, R. A. 1981. Self-mutilation accompanying religious delusions—A case report and review. *Journal of Clinical Psychiatry* 42:243–45; M. H. Spero. 1983. Religious patients in psychotherapy. *British Journal of Medical Psychology* 56:287–91; and R. D. Margolis and K. W. Elifson. 1983. Validation of a typology of religious experience and its relation to the psychotic experience. *Journal of Psychology and Theology* 11:135–41.

48. Yorston, G. A. 2001. Mania precipitated by meditation: A case report and literature review. *Mental Health, Religion and Culture* 4 (2): 209–13.

49. Neeleman, J., and G. Lewis. 1994. Religious identity and comfort beliefs in three groups of psychiatric patients and a group of medical controls. *International Journal of Social Psychiatry* 40:124–34.

50. Feldman, J., and J. Rust. 1989. Religiosity, schizotypal thinking, and schizophrenia. *Psychological Reports* 65:587–93.

51. Chu, C. C., and H. E. Klein. 1985. Psychosocial and environmental variables in outcome of black schizophrenics. *Journal of the National Medical Association* 77:793–96.

52. Verghese, A., J. K. John, S. Rajkumar, J. Richard, B. B. Sethi, and J. K. Trivedi. 1989. Factors associated with the course and outcome of schizophrenia in India: Results of a two-year multicentre follow-up study. *British Journal of Psychiatry* 154:499–503.

53. Brenda, B. B. 2002. Factors associated with rehospitalization among veterans in a substance abuse treatment program. *Psychiatric Services* 53:1176–78.

54. Chu and Klein, Psychosocial and environmental variables; Verghese et al., Factors associated with the course and outcome of schizophrenia.

55. Carson, V., and K. Huss. 1979. Prayer: An effective therapeutic and teaching tool. *Journal of Psychiatric Nursing and Mental Health Services* 17:34–37; K. N. Lindgren, and R. D. Coursey. 1995. Spirituality and serious mental illness: A two-part study. *Psychosocial Rehabilitation Journal* 18 (3): 93–111; and N. C. Kehoe. 1999. A therapy group on spiritual issues for patients with chronic mental illness. *Psychiatric Services* 50 (8): 1081–83.

56. Joseph, S., and D. Diduca. 2001. Schizotypy and religiosity in 13–18 year old school pupils. *Mental Health, Religion and Culture* 4 (1): 63–69.

57. Maltby, J., I. Garner, C. A. Lewis, and L. Day. 2000. Religious orientation and schizotypal traits. *Personality and Individual Differences* 28 (1): 143–51.

58. Maltby, J., and L. Day. 2002. Religious experience, religious orientation and schizotypy. *Mental Health, Religion and Culture* 5 (2): 163–74.

59. Joseph, S., D. Smith, and D. Diduca. 2002. Religious orientation and its association with personality, schizotypal traits and manic-depressive experiences. *Mental Health, Religion and Culture* 5 (1): 73–81.

60. Feldman and Rust, Religiosity, schizotypal thinking, and schizophrenia.

61. Armstrong, R. G., G. L. Larsen, S. A. Mourer. 1962. Religious attitudes and emotional adjustment. *Journal of Psychological Studies* 13:35–47.

62. Peters, E., S. Day, J. McKenna, and G. Orbach. 1999. Delusional ideation in religious and psychotic populations. *British Journal of Clinical Psychology* 38 (1): 83–96.

63. Bhugra, D. 2002. Self-concept: Psychosis and attraction of new religious movements. *Mental Health, Religion and Culture* 5 (3): 239–52.

64. Breier, A., and B. M. Astrachan. 1984. Characterization of schizophrenic patients who commit suicide. *American Journal of Psychiatry* 141:206–9.

65. Kirov, G., R. Kemp, K. Kirov, and A. S. David. 1998. Religious faith after psychotic illness. *Psychopathology* 31 (5): 234–45.

CHAPTER 6: INTEGRATING RELIGION INTO
MENTAL HEALTH TREATMENTS

1. Koenig, H. G., ed. 1998. *Handbook of Religion and Mental Health*. San Diego: Academic Press, 514–54.

2. Frankl, V. 1959. *Man's Search for Meaning*. New York: Simon & Schuster.

3. Romans 8:28, New International Version.

4. Koenig, *Handbook of Religion and Mental Health*, 219–20, 547–48.

5. Koenig, H. 2002. *Purpose and Power in Retirement*. Philadelphia: Templeton Foundation Press.

6. Schwartz, C. E., and M. Sendor. 1999. Helping others helps oneself: Response shift effects in peer support. *Social Science and Medicine* 48 (11): 1563–75.

7. Hainsworth, J., and J. Barlow. 2001. Volunteers' experiences of becoming arthritis self-management lay leaders: "It's almost as if I've stopped aging and started to get younger!" *Arthritis and Rheumatism* 45 (4): 378–83.

8. Emmons, R. A., and M. E. McCullough. 2003. Counting blessings versus burdens: An experimental investigation of gratitude and subjective well-being in daily life. *Journal of Personality and Social Psychology* 84 (2): 377–89.

9. Dickinson, Emily. 1924. *The Complete Poems of Emily Dickinson*. Boston: Little, Brown; Bartleby.com. 2000. www.bartleby.com/113/.

10. Matthew 19:26, New International Version.

11. Nouwen, H. 1979. *The Wounded Healer*. Garden City, NY: Image Books.

12. Lewis, C. S. 1962. *The Problem of Pain*. New York: Macmillan Publishing Co.

13. Koenig, *Handbook of Religion and Mental Health*, 514–54.

14. Azhar, M. Z., S. L. Varma, A. S. Dharap. 1994. Religious psychotherapy in anxiety disorder patients. *Acta Psychiatrica Scandinavica* 90:1–3; M. Z. Azhar and S. L. Varma. 1995. Religious psychotherapy in depressive patients. *Psychotherapy and Psychosomatics* 63:165–73; M. Z. Azhar and S. L. Varma. 1995. Religious psychotherapy as management of bereavement. *Acta Psychiatrica Scandinavica* 91:233–35; S. L. Varma, A. Zain, K. Kerian. 1997. Experiences in religious psychotherapy. *Australian and New Zealand Journal of Psychiatry* 31:147–49; M. Shams, P. R. Jackson. 1993. Religiosity as a predictor of well-being and moderator of the psychological impact of unemployment. *Journal of Medical Psychology* 66:341–52; S. M. Razali, C. I. Hasanah, K. Aminah, and M. Subramaniam. 1998. Religious-sociocultural psychotherapy in patients with anxiety and depression. *Australian and New Zealand Journal of Psychiatry* 32:867–72; M. L. Adelekan, O. A. Abiodun, A. O. Imouoklhome-Obayan, G. A. Oni, and O. O. Ogunremi. 1993. Psychosocial correlates of alcohol, tobacco and cannabis use: Findings from a Nigerian university. *Drug and Alcohol Dependence* 33:247–56; and R. J. E. Ndom and M. L. Adelekan. 1996. Psychosocial correlates of substance use among undergraduates in Ilorin University, Nigeria. *East African Medical Journal* 73:541–47.

15. Anson, O., S. Carmel, D. Y. Bonneh, A. Levenson, and B. Maoz. 1990. Recent life events, religiosity, and health: An individual or collective effect. *Human Relations* 43:1051–66; J. D. Kark, S. Carmel, R. Sinnreich, N. Goldberger, and Y. Friedlander. 1996. Psychosocial factors among members of religious and secular kibbutzim. *Israel Journal of Medical Science* 32:185–94; D. Stein, E. Witztum, and A. K. De-Nour. 1989. Adolescent attitudes toward suicide. *Israel Journal of Psychiatry and Related Sciences* 26 (1–2): 58–68; D. Stein, E. Witztum, and D. Brom. 1992. The association between adolescents' attitudes toward suicide and their psychosocial background and suicidal tendencies. *Adolescence* 27:949–59; M. Moore and S. Weiss. 1995. Reasons for non-drinking among Israeli adolescents of four religions. *Drug and Alcohol Dependence* 38:45–50; and L. Baider, S. M. Russak, S. Perry, K. M. Kash, M. K. Gronert, B. Fox, J. C. Holland, and A. Kaplan-Denour. 1999. The role of religious and spiritual beliefs in coping with malignant melanoma: An Israeli sample. *Psycho-oncology* 8:27–35.

16. Verghese, A., J. K. John, S. Rajkumar, J. Richard, B. B. Sethi, J. K. Trivedi. 1989. Factors associated with the course and outcome of schizophrenia in India: Results of a two-year multicentre follow-up study. *British Journal of Psychiatry* 154:499–503; E. Taub, S. S. Steiner, E. Weingarten, and K. G. Walton. 1994. Effectiveness of broad spectrum approaches to relapse prevention in severe alcoholism: A long-term randomized controlled-trial of transcendental meditation, EMG biofeedback, and electronic neurotherapy. *Alcoholism Treatment Quarterly* 11 (1/2): 187–220; and C. N. Alexander et al. 1994. Treating and preventing alcohol, nicotine, and drug abuse through transcendental meditation: A review and meta-analysis. *Alcoholism Treatment Quarterly* 11 (1/2): 13–87.

17. Tapanya et al., Worry and intrinsic/extrinsic religious orientation; T. Emavardhana and C. D. Tori. 1997. Changes in self-concept, ego defense mechanisms, and religiosity fol-

lowing seven-day Vipassana meditation retreats. *Journal for the Scientific Study of Religion* 36 (2): 194–206; M. Thananart, C. D. Tori, and T. Emavardhana. 2000. A longitudinal study of psychosocial changes among Thai adolescents participating in a Buddhist ordination program for novices. *Adolescence* 35 (138): 285–93; and J. Kabat-Zinn, A. O. Massion, J. Kristeller, L. G. Peterson, K. E. Fletcher, L. Pbert, W. R. Lenderking, and S. F. Santorelli. 1992. Effectiveness of a meditation-based stress reduction program in the treatment of anxiety disorders. *American Journal of Psychiatry* 149:936–43.

18. Xiao, S., D. Young, and H. Zhang. 1998. Taoistic cognitive psychotherapy for neurotic patients: A preliminary clinical trial. *Psychiatry and Clinical Neurosciences* 52: S238–41.

19. Altman, Dick, or Roberta Rothschild at Roper Starch Worldwide. Harrison, NY; see Web site: http://www.mcsweeneys.net/links/press99/happiness.html.

20. *The World Factbook*. 2000. Washington, D.C.: Government Printing Office. See Web site: http://www.odci.gov/cia/publications/factbook/.

21. Brown, W. 2002. Psychoneuroimmunology and Western religious traditions. In *The Link between Religion and Health*, ed. H. G. Koenig and H. J. Cohen. New York: Oxford University Press, 262–74.

22. Jha, P. K, K. P. Yadav, and U. Kumari. 1997. Gender-difference and religio-cultural variation in altruistic behaviour. *Indian Journal of Psychometry and Education* 28 (2): 105–8.

23. Fitchett, G., L. A. Burton, and A. B. Sivan. 1997. The religious needs and resources of psychiatric patients. *Journal of Nervous and Mental Disorder* 185:320–26.

24. Sheehan, W., and J. Kroll. 1990. Psychiatric patients' belief in general health factors and sin as causes of illness. *American Journal of Psychiatry* 147:112–13.

25. Propst, L. R., R. Ostrom, P. Watkins, T. Dean, and D. Mashburn. 1992. Comparative efficacy of religious and nonreligious cognitive-behavior therapy for the treatment of clinical depression in religious individuals. *Journal of Consulting and Clinical Psychology* 60:94–103; and L. R. Propst. 1980. The comparative efficacy of religious and nonreligious imagery for the treatment of mild depression in religious individuals. *Cognitive Therapy and Research* 4:167–78.

26. Nielsen, S. L., W. B. Johnson, and A. Ellis. 2001. *Counseling and Psychotherapy with Religious Persons: A Rational Emotive Behavior Therapy Approach.* Mahwah, NJ: Lawrence Erlbaum Associates.

27. Azhar, M. Z., S. L. Varma, and A. S. Dharap. 1994. Religious psychotherapy in anxiety disorder patients. *Acta Psychiatrica Scandinavica* 90:1–3; M. Z. Azhar and S. L. Varma. 1995. Religious psychotherapy in depressive patients. *Psychotherapy and Psychosomatics* 63:165–73; M. Z. Azhar and S. L. Varma. 1995. Religious psychotherapy as management of bereavement. *Acta Psychiatrica Scandinavica* 91:233–35; and S. M. Razali, C. I. Hasanah, K. Aminah, and M. Subramaniam. 1998. Religious-sociocultural psychotherapy in patients with anxiety and depression. *Australian and New Zealand Journal of Psychiatry* 32:867–72.

28. Xiao, S., D. Young, and H. Zhang. 1998. Taoistic cognitive psychotherapy for neurotic patients: A preliminary clinical trial. *Psychiatry and Clinical Neurosciences* 52: S238–41.

29. Propst et al., Comparative efficacy of religious and nonreligious cognitive-behavior therapy.

30. Azhar and Varma, Religious psychotherapy in depressive patients.

31. Azhar and Varma, Religious psychotherapy as management of bereavement.

32. Azhar et al., Religious psychotherapy in anxiety disorder patients.

33. Zhang, Y., D. Young, S. Lee, L. Li, H. Zhang, Z. Xiao, et al. 2002. Chinese Taoist cognitive psychotherapy in the treatment of generalized anxiety disorder in contemporary China. *Transcultural Psychiatry* 39 (1): 115–29.

34. Cooper, L. A., C. Brown, H. T. Vu, D. E. Ford, and N. R. Powe. 2001. How important is intrinsic spirituality in depression care? A comparison of white and African American primary care patients. *Journal of General Internal Medicine* 16 (9): 634–38.

35. Koenig, *Handbook of Religion and Mental Health*.

References

36. Fallot, R. D. 2001. Spirituality and religion in psychiatric rehabilitation and recovery from mental illness. *International Review of Psychiatry* 13 (2): 110–16.

37. Phillips, R. E., R. Lakin, and K. I. Pargament. 2002. Development and implementation of a spiritual issues psychoeducational group for those with serious mental illness. *Community Mental Health Journal* 38 (6): 487–95.

38. Kehoe, N. C. 1999. A therapy group on spiritual issues for patients with chronic mental illness. *Psychiatric Services* 50 (8): 1081–83. See also http://www.expandingconnections.com/contact.htm.

39. Lindgren, K. N., and R. D. Coursey. 1995. Spirituality in serious mental illness: A 2-part study. *Psychosocial Rehabilitation Journal* 18 (3): 93–111; and C. O'Rourke. 1997. Listening for the sacred: Addressing spiritual issues in the group treatment of adults with mental illness. *Smith College Studies in Social Work* 67 (2): 177–96.

40. Salib, E., and S. Youakim. 2001. Spiritual healing in elderly psychiatric patients: A case control study in an Egyptian psychiatric hospital. *Aging and Mental Health* 5 (4): 366–70.

41. Lindgren, K. N., and R. D. Coursey. 1995. Spirituality and serious mental illness: A two-part study. *Psychosocial Rehabilitation Journal* 18 (3): 93–111.

42. Carson, V., and K. Huss. 1979. Prayer: An effective therapeutic and teaching tool. *Journal of Psychiatric Nursing and Mental Health Services* 17:34–37.

43. Raguram, R., A. Venkateswaran, J. Ramakrishna, and M. G. Weiss. 2002. Traditional community resources for mental health: A report of temple healing from India. *British Medical Journal* 325 (7354): 38–40.

44. Jablensky. A. 2000. Epidemiology of schizophrenia: The global burden of disease and disability. *European Archives of Psychiatry and Clinical Neurosciences* 250:274–85.

45. Tsemberis, S., and A. Stefancic. 2000. The role of an espiritista in the treatment of a homeless, mentally ill Hispanic man. *Psychiatric Services* 51 (12): 1572–74.

46. Garrison, V. 1977. Doctor, espiritista, or psychiatrist? Help seeking behavior in a Puerto Rican neighborhood in New York City. *Medical Anthropology* 1:165–91.

47. Koenig, H. G. 2002. *Spirituality in Patient Care: Why, How, When, and What.* Philadelphia: Templeton Foundation Press.

48. Spero, M. H. 1981. Countertransference in religious therapists of religious patients. *American Journal of Psychotherapy* 35:565–75.

49. Katkin, S., V. Zimmerman, J. Rosenthal, and M. Ginsburg. 1975. Using volunteer therapists to reduce hospital readmissions. *Hospital and Community Psychiatry* 26:151–53.

50. Park, J. Z., and C. Smith. 2000. "To whom much has been given . . .": Religious capital and community voluntarism among churchgoing Protestants. *Journal for the Scientific Study of Religion* 39:272–86.

51. Hodgkinson, V. A. 1995. *Key factors influencing caring, involvement, and community.* In Schervish, Hodgkinson, Gates, and Associates, eds. San Francisco: Jossey-Bass, 21–50.

52. Midlarsky, E. 1991. Helping as coping: Prosocial behavior. *Review of Personality and Social Psychology* 12:238–64; and Vaillant, *Aging Well.*

53. Boyer, G., R. Hachey, R. and C. Mercier. 1998. Roles of persons with severe mental illness in the community: Past, present, and future. *International Journal of Mental Health* 27 (3): 46–64.

CHAPTER 7: CARING FOR THE EMOTIONALLY AND MENTALLY ILL

1. See Web site: http://bkaw.bravepages.com/socsci/0202/HistorySumm.doc.

2. See Web site: http://www.catholiccharitiesinfo.org/.

3. See Web site: http://www.ymca.net/index.jsp.

4. Mission statement: "[The Salvation Army is] an evangelical part of the universal Christian Church. Its message is based on the Bible. Its ministry is motivated by the love of

God. Its mission is to preach the gospel of Jesus Christ and to meet human needs in His name without discrimination." See Web site: http://www.salvationarmyusa.org/WWW_USN.nsf/vw_dynamic_arrays/DD0A2958A13379EE85256D2B006BC794?openDocument.

5. Mankiller, Wilma, ed. 1998. *Reader's Companion to U.S. Women's History*. Boston: Houghton Mifflin. See Web site: http://college.hmco.com/history/readerscomp/ women/html/wm_033300_settlementho.htm.

6. Ibid.

7. Rauenbusch, W. 1908. *Christianity and the Social Crisis*. New York: MacMillan.

8. See Web site: http://www.imb.org/core/default.asp. The mission statement is: "The International Mission Board (formerly Foreign Mission Board) is an entity of the Southern Baptist Convention, the nation's largest evangelical denomination, claiming more than 40,000 churches with nearly 16 million members. The board's main objective is presenting the gospel of Jesus Christ in order to lead individuals to saving faith in Him and result in church-planting movements among all the peoples of the world."

9. See Web site: http://www.sbc.net/bfm/bfm2000.asp#xv. No specific arm exists for providing social services.

10. See Web site: http://ag.org/top/about/about.cfm. The mission is: (1) To introduce the lost to Christ; (2) To provide an environment for worshiping God and fellowshipping with others who hold similar values and love for God; (3) To effectively train and nurture believers. No specific arm exists for providing social services.

11. Jewish groups in America, which usually do not actively proselytize but rather focus on the needs of the family and the community, formed several organizations including the Association of Jewish Family and Children's Agencies (1972), Association of Jewish Aging Services (1960), and United Jewish Communities to provide needed services to the poor and disadvantaged Jews in America.

12. See Web site: http://www.catholiccharitiesinfo.org/. Its mission is: "Catholic Charities USA is a national network of agencies, institutions and individuals who aim to reduce poverty, support families and empower communities."

13. See Web site: http://www.chausa.org/DEFAULT.ASP. Its mission is: "Catholic Health Association represents the combined strength of its members, more than 2,000 Catholic health care sponsors, systems, facilities, and related organizations. Founded in 1915, CHA unites members to advance selected strategic issues that are best addressed together rather than as individual organizations."

14. Wineburg, Bob. July 31, 2003. The underbelly of the faith-based initiative. *Sightings* See website: http://marty-center.uchicago.edu/sightings/archive_2003/0731.shtml.

15. Ibid.

16. Koenig, H. G., L. K. George, K. G. Meador, D. G. Blazer, and P. Dyke. 1994. Religious affiliation and psychiatric disorder in Protestant baby boomers. *Hospital and Community Psychiatry* 45:586–96.

17. Gray, A. J. 2001. Attitudes of the public to mental health: A church congregation. *Mental Health, Religion and Culture* 4 (1): 71–79.

CHAPTER 8: LOCAL RELIGIOUS CONGREGATIONS

1. U. S. Department of Labor. 1998 *Occupational Outlook Handbook: United States Department of Labor*. Washington, D.C.: Bureau of Labor Statistics.

2. Weaver, A. J. 1995. Has there been a failure to prepare and support parish-based clergy in their role as front-line community mental health workers? A review. *Journal of Pastoral Care* 49:129–49.

3. The idea for this comparison was developed by Andrew J. Weaver, Ph.D.

4. Figure includes students and continuing members. See Web site: http://www.apa.org/books/4030043.html.

5. Ebaugh, H. R. 1993. The growth and decline of Catholic religious orders of women worldwide. *Journal for the Scientific Study of Religion* 32:68–73.

6. Veroff, J., R. A. Kulka, and E. Douvan. 1981. *Mental Health in America: Patterns of Help Seeking from 1957 to 1976.* New York: Basic Books.

7. Larson, D. B., A. A. Hohmann, L. G. Kessler, K. G. Meador, J. H. Boyd, and E. McSherry. 1988. The couch and the cloth: The need for linkage. *Hospital and Community Psychiatry* 39:1064–69.

8. Lafuze, J. E., D. V. Perkins, and G. A. Avirappattu. 2002. Pastors' perceptions of mental disorders. *Psychiatric Services* 53 (7): 900–901.

9. Monahan, John. 2001. Major mental disorder and violence: Epidemiology and risk assessment. In *Clinical Assessment of Dangerousness: Empirical Contributions*, ed. Franck Georges and Linda Pagani. Cambridge: Cambridge University Press, 89–102.

10. Pilgrim, David. Mental disorder and violence: An empirical picture in context. *Journal of Mental Health* 12 (1): 7–18.

11. Binder, Renee L. 1999. Are the mentally ill dangerous? *Journal of the American Academy of Psychiatry and the Law* 27 (2): 189–201.

12. Bergman, Andrea J., Holly J. Zack, and Mark Serper. 2000. Violence and the severely mentally ill. *New York State Psychologist* 12 (1): 17–19.

13. Weisman, A. G. 2000. A mediator of Anglo-American and Mexican attributional differences toward symptoms of schizophrenia? *Journal of Nervous and Mental Disease* 188 (9): 616–21.

14. Lafuze et al., Pastors' perceptions of mental disorders.

15. Neighbors, H. W. 1985. Seeking professional help for personal problems: Black Americans' use of health and mental health services. *Community Mental Health Journal* 21:156–66.

16. Thomas, S. B., S. C. Quinn, A. Billingsley, and C. H. Caldwell. 1994. The characteristics of northern black churches with community health outreach programs. *American Journal of Public Health* 84:575–79.

17. Taylor, R. J., C. G. Ellison, L. M. Chatters, J. S. Levin, and K. D. Lincoln. 2000. Mental health services in faith communities: The role of clergy in black churches. *Social Work* 45 (1): 73–87.

18. Veroff, Kulka, and Douvan, *Mental Health in America.*

19. Neighbors, H. W., J. S. Jackson, P. J. Bowman, and G. Gurin. 1983. Stress, coping, and black mental health: Preliminary findings from a national study. *Prevention in Human Services* 2 (3): 5–29.

20. Neighbors, H. W., M. A. Musick, and D. R. Williams. 1998. The African American minister as a source of help for serious personal crises: Bridge or barrier to mental health care? *Health, Education and Behavior* 25:759–77.

21. Mollica, R. R., F. J. Streets, J. Boscarino, and F. C. Redlich. 1986. A community study of formal pastoral counseling activities of the clergy. *American Journal of Psychiatry* 143:323–28.

22. Weaver, Has there been a failure to prepare and support parish-based clergy in the role as front-line community mental health workers?

23. Gottlieb, J. F., and M. Olfson. 1987. Current referral practices of mental health providers. *Hospital and Community Psychiatry* 38:1171–81.

24. Mollica et al., A community study of formal pastoral counseling activities of the clergy.

25. Taylor et al., Mental health services in faith communities.

26. Mays, B. E., and J. W. Nicholson. 1933. *The Negroe's Church.* New York: Russell & Russell.

27. Caldwell, C. H., L. M. Catters, A. Billingsley, and R. J. Taylor. 1995. Church-based support programs for elderly black adults: Congregational and clergy characteristics. In *Handbook on Religion, Spirituality and Aging*, ed. M. A. Kimble, S. H. McFadden, J. W. Ellor, and J. Seeber. Minneapolis: Augsburg Press; and C. E. Lincoln and L. H. Mmamiya. 1990. *The Black Church in the African American Experience.* Durham, NC: Duke University Press.

28. Taylor et al., Mental health services in faith communities.

29. Billingsley, A., and C. H. Caldwell. 1991. The church, the family, and the school in the African American community. *Journal of Negro Education* 60:427–40; and C. H. Cald-

well, A. D. Green, and A. Billingsely. 1994. Family support programs in black churches: A new look at old functions. In *Putting Families First*, ed. L. S. J. Kagan and B. Weissbourd. New York: Jossey-Bass.

30. See Web site: http://www.surgeongeneral.gov/library/mentalhealth/chapter2/sec8.html.

31. Hispanics are persons who report they are Mexican, Puerto Ricans, Cuban, Central or South American, or some other Latino origin; according to the March 2000 Census of U.S. Population, Hispanics number 32.8 million compared to blacks who number 35.5 million.

32. Abraido-Lanza, A. F., C. Guier, and T. A. Revenson. 1996. Coping and social support resources among Latinas with arthritis. *Arthritis Care and Research* 9 (6): 501–8; M. D. Mailick, G. Holden, and V. N. Walther. 1994. Coping with childhood asthma: Caretakers' views. *Health and Social Work* 19 (2): 103–11; and J. R. Mickley and K. Soeken. 1993. Religiousness and hope in Hispanic- and Anglo-American women with breast cancer. *Oncology Nursing Forum* 20:1171–77.

33. de Leon Siantz, M. L. 1994. The Mexican-American migrant farmworker family: Mental health issues. *Nursing Clinics of North America* 29 (1): 65–72; and M. Delgado. 1982. Ethnic and cultural variations in the care of the aged Hispanic elderly and natural support systems: A special focus on Puerto Ricans. *Journal of Geriatric Psychiatry*, 239–55.

34. Zaldivar, A., and J. Smolowitz. 1994. Perceptions of the importance placed on religion and folk medicine by non-Mexican-American Hispanic adults with diabetes. *The Diabetes Educator* 20:303–6; P. Ruiz and J. Langrod. 1976. The role of folk healers in community mental health services. *Community Mental Health Journal* 12 (4): 392–98; and P. Ruiz. 1998. The role of culture in psychiatric care. *American Journal of Psychiatry* 155:1763–65.

35. For more information, e-mail: SuFamilia@hispanichealth.org or call 1-866-SU-FAMILIA (783-2645).

36. See Web site: http://www.baylor.edu/~Charles_Kemp/hispanic_health.htm.

37. Data from the Catholic Diocese of Dallas. Personal communication, Maria del Carmen Uceda-Gras.

38. See Web site: http://www.lasobras.org/.

39. Mark DeHaven can be reached by e-mail at Mark.DeHaven@UTSouthwestern.edu; Maria del Carmen Uceda-Gras can be contacted at maria.uceda@lasobras.org.

40. Contact Diane Engster for a copy. Telephone: 703-360-1992. E-mail: dengster@aol.com.

41. Personal communication. Interview conducted by telephone, 2003.

42. Contact Jeri Fields at Mount Vernon Presbyterian Church to get a copy of the program description entitled "Agape Reservoir: A Ministry of Wholeness for Individuals Affected by Emotional or Mental Disorders" (JERIF@aol.com).

43. Duane Glasscock's e-mail is kkayduane@aol.com.

CHAPTER 9: NETWORKING AND ADVOCACY ORGANIZATIONS

1. Carole Wills, NAMI-Indianapolis, Faith Communities Education Committee. Telephone: 317-299-4570. E-mail: CaroleJWills@aol.com.

2. Gunnar Christiansen can be reached at gunnar@cox.net.

3. See Web site: http://www.faithnetnami.org/.

4. See Web site: http://www.interfaithcompeer.org/.

5. See Web site: http://www.compeer.org/.

6. Katkin, S., V. Zimmerman, J. Rosenthal, and M. Ginsburg. 1975. Using volunteer therapists to reduce hospital readmissions. *Hospital and Community Psychiatry* 26:151–53.

7. To learn more about this local program, contact Executive Director Nancy Karges at nancy@interfaithcompeer.org. See Web site: http://www.compeer.org/1/a1.asp.

8. See Faith in Action Web site at www.fiavolunteers.org to learn more about how to apply.

9. Faith groups that are linked with Pathways to Promise on their Web site include: American Baptist Churches in the USA, Disciples of Christ, Christian Reformed Church in America, Church of God (Anderson, IL), Episcopal Church, Evangelical Lutheran Church in-America, Lutheran Church-Missouri Synod, Mennonite Church, National Catholic Office for Persons with Disabilities, Presbyterian Church USA, Union of American Hebrew Congregations, United Church of Christ, United Methodist Church, and United Synagogue of America. See Web site: www.pathways2promise.org.

10. Harris, M. L., D. Engster, and P. B. Dornan. 1989. *New Models for Ministry: Serious Mental Illness and the Faith Community.* Washington, D.C.: New York Avenue Presbyterian Church. Contact Diane Engster to find out how a copy can be obtained (telephone: 703-360-1992; e-mail: dengster@aol.com).

11. Sareyan, A. 1993. *The Turning Point: How Persons of Conscience Brought about Major Change in the Care of America's Mentally Ill.* Washington, D.C.: American Psychiatric Press.

12. Margaret Ann Holt's e-mail is vicomim@excite.com, and the Web site is http://www.vaumc.org/gm/micom.htm.

13. See Web site: http://www.vaumc.org/gm/micom.htm.

14. Contact Gunnar Christianen at Gunnarc@deltanet.com on how to locate Ms. Gales.

CHAPTER 10: MISSION-DRIVEN FAITH-BASED SERVICES

1. See Web site: http://www.catholiccharitiesusa.org/who/stats.htm.

2. Information obtained from Jane Stenson, director of community services, Catholic Charities U.S.A., Alexandria, VA. Web site: http://www.catholiccharitiesusa.org/states/index.htm.

4. Information obtained from Bob Mills at Cssrmills@aol.com.

5. See November 2001 issue of *The NonProfit Times.* Top 100 revenues zoom to $49 million (by M. Sinclair); See Web site: http://www.nptimes.com/Nov01/sr1.html.

6. Web site for Lutheran Services in America: http://www.lutheranservices.org/whoweare.htm.

7. Contact Jill Schumann by telephone at 800-664-3848 or by e-mail at jschumann@lutheranservices.org.

8. Lutheran Services in America, 1999 Annual Survey Results. Based on feedback from 80% of member organizations.

9. Contact Brent Diers at 708-771-7180 (ext. 283) or by e-mail: BDiersLCFS@aol.com.

10. Contact Bruce Strade by e-mail at bstrade@lfsnorthwest.org.

11. Contact Charles Lockwood at 724-452-4453 (ext. 100); e-mail: ctlglade@sgi.net.

12. Harris, M. L., D. Engster, and P. B. Dornan. 1989. *New Models for Ministry: Serious Mental Illness and the Faith Community.* Washington, D.C.: New York Avenue Presbyterian Church. Contact Diane Engster to find out how a copy can be obtained (telephone: 703-360-1992; e-mail: dengster@aol.com).

13. See Web site: www.mma-online.org.

14. Contact Robert Blake, director, 1451 Dundee Avenue, Elgin, IL 60120.

15. See Web site: www.king-view.org.

16. See Web site: info@oaklawn.org.

17. See Web site: www.meadowlarkinc.org.

18. Call 316-284-6400.

19. See Web site: www.brooklane.org.

20. See Web site: www.adriel.com.

21. See Web site: www.pennfoundation.org.

22. See Web site: www.philhaven.com.

23. See Web site: www.flrc.org.

24. Call 717-656-7358.

25. *The Columbia Encyclopedia.* 6th ed.. 2001.

26. Winston, D. 1999. *Red-Hot and Righteous: The Urban Religion of the Salvation Army.* Cambridge: Harvard University Press.

27. See Web site: http://www1.salvationarmy.org/ihq/www_sa.nsf/vw-dynamic-index/5F180AE9ED2270FE80256D4B0044DBA2?openDocument.
28. See Web site: http://www1.salvationarmy.org/ihq/www_sa.nsf/vw-sublinks/E5C6EB09E25BC2A080256D4B004CEF40?openDocument.
29. See Web site: http://www1.salvationarmy.org/ihq/www_sa.nsf/vw-sublinks/D46980EA862CD1FD80256D4F00411840?openDocument.
30. Roger Fallot, Ph.D., is co-director of Community Connections in Washington, D.C., a private, not-for-profit mental health agency, which since 1984 has worked with persons with severe mental illness to assist them toward stable, integrated community living. He is the editor of *New Directions for Mental Health Services, Spirituality and Religion in Recovery from Mental Illness* (Jossey-Bass, 1998).
31. The president and CEO of AFCA is Bert Goldberg, and he can be reached at 1-800-634-7346 or by e-mail at skupfer@ajfca.org.
32. See Web site: http://www.ajfca.org/facts.html.

CHAPTER 11: FAITH-INTEGRATED COUNSELING

1. Gibbons, J. L., J. Thomas, L. VandeCreek, and A. K. Jessen. 1991. The value of hospital chaplains: Patient perspectives. *Journal of Pastoral Care* 45 (2): 117–25.
2. Koenig, H. G., L. K. George, B. L. Peterson, and C. F. Pieper. 1997. Depression in medically ill hospitalized older adults: Prevalence, correlates, and course of symptoms based on six diagnostic schemes. *American Journal of Psychiatry* 154:1376–83.
3. Koenig, H. G., L. K. George, and K. G. Meador. 1997. Use of antidepressants by non-psychiatrists in the treatment of hospitalized medically ill depressed elderly patients. *American Journal of Psychiatry* 154:1369–75.
4. Kanapaux, W. 2004. Many needs but few psychiatric services for seniors in long-term care. *Psychiatric Times* 23 (November 13): 1.
5. Parkum, K. H. 1985. The impact of chaplaincy services in selected hospitals in the eastern United States. *Journal of Pastoral Care* 39:262–69.
6. Florell, J. L. 1973. Crisis-intervention in orthopedic surgery: Empirical evidence of the effectiveness of a chaplain working with surgery patients. *Bulletin of the American Protestant Hospital Association* 37 (2): 29–36.
7. Florell, Crisis-intervention in orthopedic surgery; and J. R. Bliss, E. McSherry, and J. Fassett. 1995. Chaplain intervention reduces costs in major DRGs: An experimental study. In *Proceedings NIH Clinical Center Conference on Spirituality and Health Care Outcomes*, ed. H. Heffernan, E. McSherry, and R. Fitzgerald.
8. Sharp, C. G. 1991. The use of chaplaincy in the neonatal intensive care unit. *Southern Medical Journal* 84 (12): 1482–86.
9. VandeCreek, L., and M. Lyon. 1994/1995. The general hospital chaplain's ministry: Analysis of productivity, quality and cost. *The Caregiver Journal* 11 (2): 3–13.
10. Personal communication with Dr. James Harper, director of pastoral care, Health Midwest, Kansas City, MO; e-mail: James.Harper3@hcamidwest.com.
11. VandeCreek, L. 2000. How has health care reform affected professional chaplaincy programs and how are department directors responding? *Journal of Health Care Chaplaincy* 10 (1): 7–17.
12. Carter, H. G. Save prison, mental hospital chaplains. *The Atlanta Constitution*, September 12, 1991.
13. See Web site: http://www.acpe.edu/.
14. See Web site: http://www.acpe.edu/brochure.htm.
15. Special issue: Contract pastoral care and education: The trend of the future? *Journal of Health Care Chaplaincy* 9 (1/2).
16. HealthCare Chaplaincy Web site: www.healthcarechaplaincy.org.
17. For more information about HVCP, contact Anne Marie Lardeau at amlardeau@earthlink.net or go to their Web site at: http://www.la4seniors.com/hvcp.htm.
18. See Web site: http://www.aapc.org/.

19. See Web site: http://www.aapc.org/history.htm.

20. Contact Roy Woodruff, executive director of AAPC, for more information: 703-385-6967; e-mail: roy@aapc.org.

21. Doug Ronsheim, director of PPI and recent president of AAPC. E-mail: PPI6324DR@aol.com.

22. See Samaritan Web site: http://www.samaritan-institute.org/information/default.asp?NavPageID=12028.

23. For more information contact NICSHC at 417-885-2735.

24. See Web site: http://www.he.net/~joes/home/Christ_Community/.

25. See Web site: http://www.pinerest.org/.

26. The Teen Challenge International, U.S.A. Accreditation Revision Committee, Springfield, MS, June 5, 1992; revision by Dave Scotch, accreditation manager, January 2002.

27. More information about location can be obtained from their Web site at www.teenchallenge.com.

28. An evaluation of the Teen Challenge treatment program. *National Institute on Drug Abuse, Services Research Reports.* No. 78-440, 1977, 14, US: DHEW.

29. See Web site: http://www.raphacare.com/.

30. Minirth, F. B., P. Meier, and P. D. Tournier. 1994. *Happiness Is a Choice: The Symptoms, Causes, and Cures of Depression.* New York: Baker.

31. See Web site: http://webserver.fni.com/heritage/may96/MinMeier.html.

32. See Web site: http://www.rapidnet.com/~jbeard/bdm/Psychology/self-est/rapha.htm.

33. See Web site: http://www.raphacare.com/.

34. Brian Nystrom's e-mail address is Nystroms@uswest.net.

35. See Web site: http://www.nystromcounseling.com.

36. See Web site: http://www.aacc.net/aboutaacc.html.

37. See Web site: http://www.caps.net/about.htm.

38. See Web site: http://www.actheals.org/.

39. See Web site: http://www.cmdahome.org/.

40. Jerry Stromberg's e-mail address is cchf@cchf.org.

41. Canning, S. S., M. K. Neal, R. Fine, and K. J. Meese. 2002. Mental health resources: The "hole" in holistic, Christian, community-based health care? *Health and Development,* a journal published by the Christian Community Health Fellowship CCHF, cchf@cchf.org.

42. Contact Sally Schwer Canning at Wheaton College (Sally.S.Canning@wheaton. edu).

CHAPTER 12: NON-CHRISTIAN
FAITH-BASED SERVICES

1. *Yearbook of American and Canadian Churches.* 1997. New York: National Council of Churches, 1, 252–58. This number may or may not include children.

2. Earle, K. A. 1996. Effects of cultural factors on mental health care for American Indians living in New York state. *Dissertation Abstracts International, A (Humanities and Social Sciences)* 57 (4-A): 1844.

3. Garrett, J. T., and M. W. Garrett. 1998. The path of good medicine: Understanding and counseling Native American Indians. In *Counseling American Minorities,* ed. Donald R. Atkinson, George Morten, et al. 5th ed. New York: McGraw-Hill, 183–92.

4. Contact the editor by e-mail: wellnations@dtgnet.com.

5. See Web site: http://wings.buffalo.edu/publications/mcjrnl/v6n1/native.html.

6. American Indian Counseling Center, Rio Hondo Mental Health Building, 17707 Studebaker Rd., Cerritos, CA 90703; telephone 562-402-0677.

7. See Web site: http://www.frc.merced.k12.ca.us/frcweb/crd2001web/CRDWeb_1Page7.html. Telephone: 209-742-6642.

8. Kurian, G. T., T. M. Johnson, and D. B. Barrett, eds. 2001. *World Christian Encyclopedia: A Comparative Survey of Churches and Religions AD 30–AD 2200.* New York: Oxford University Press.

9. Much of the following section is based on a conversation that I had with Dr. Basit early in 2002. Abdul Basit's e-mail is ABasit97@aol.com.

10. Basit, A. 1997. *The Essence of the Quran: Commentary and Interpretation of Surah Al-Fatihah*. Lahore, Pakistan: Kazi Publishers.

11. The contact person for the four mosques participating in this project is Sharifa Alkhateeb (telephone: 703-759-7698) in Great Falls, VA.

12. Contact Salma Abugideiri by home phone: 703-430-6175; by work phone: 571-203-8900; or by e-mail: Selkadi@aol.com.

13. See Web site: http://www.communityhealingcenters.org ; the contact person there is Jamal Granick (phone: 415-499-1115; e-mail: jlgranick@mindspring.com).

14. See Web site: http://www.hammoude.com/Ihhs.html. The contact person there is Judith Muhammad, who is the staff psychologist and clinical director. Her cell phone number is 248-789-0214 and e-mail address is Smuslim@aol.com.

15. *Yearbook of American and Canadian Churches*, 1, 252–58

16. See Web site: http://www.jewishfellowshipcenter.org/.

17. See Web site: http://jewishcounselingservice.com/.

18. A private online chat costs $45 for 30 minutes and $90 for 60 minutes; e-mail therapy is offered for $35 per e-mail or $125 for four e-mails; and telephone consultations are offered at $60 per 30-minute session and $90 per 60-minute session.

19. Fabrega, H., Jr. 2001. Mental health and illness in traditional India and China. *Psychiatric Clinics of North America* 24 (3): 555–67.

20. *Yearbook of American and Canadian Churches*, 1, 252–58

21. Reverend Chhean's e-mail address is KChhean@dmh.co.la.ca.us.

22. Shapiro, S. C. 2001. People who are making a difference. *Long Beach Press-Telegram*, December 9, 2001, A13; T. Manzer. Seeking heaven: The passageway consists of strict moral and religious guidelines to fulfill an enlightened state of being. *Long Beach Press-Telegram*, December 8, 2001, A21.

23. Manzer, Seeking heaven, A22.

24. See Web site: http://www.apctc.org/about_us.htm.

25. See Web site: http://members.aol.com/uparatana/index.html.

CHAPTER 13: BARRIERS TO RESEARCH AND IMPLEMENTATION

1. More information on workshops can be obtained from Harold G. Koenig (koenig@geri.duke.edu); dates are posted on www.dukespiritualityandhealth.org in the Presentations section of the Web site.

2. Hill, P. C., and R. Hood. 1999. *Measures of Religiosity*. Chattanooga, TN: Religious Education Press.

3. Koenig, H. G., K. G. Meador, and G. Parkerson. 1997. Religion index for psychiatric research. *American Journal of Psychiatry* 154 (6): 885–86.

4. Multidimensional measurement of religiousness/spirituality for use in health research: A report of the Fetzer Institute/National Institute on Aging Working Group. 1999. Kalamazoo, MI: Fetzer Institute.

5. Hall, D. E., H. G. Koenig, and K. G. Meador. 2004. Conceptualizing "Religion": How language shapes and constrains knowledge in the study of religion and health. *Perspectives in Biology and Medicine* 47 (3): 386–401.

6. Propst, L. R. 1987. *Psychotherapy in a Religious Framework: Spirituality in the Emotional Healing Process*. New York: Human Sciences Press.

7. Larson, E. J., and L. Witham. 1997. Scientists are still keeping the faith. *Nature* 386 (6624): 435–36.

8. Larson, E. J., and L. Witham. 1998. Leading scientists still reject God. *Nature* 394 (6691): 313.

9. Princeton Religion Research Center. 1996. *Religion in America: Will the Vitality of the Church Be the Surprise of the 21st Century?* Princeton, NJ: The Gallup Poll, 22.

10. Bergin, A. E., and J. P. Jensen. 1990. Religiosity and psychotherapists: A national survey. *Psychotherapy* 27:3–7; and H. G. Koenig, M. Hover, L. B. Bearon, and J. L. Travis. 1991. Religious perspectives of doctors, nurses, patients and families: Some interesting differences. *Journal of Pastoral Care* 45:254–67.

11. Comment made at the Spirituality at End-of-Life Conference sponsored by the NIA, NINR, Fetzer Institute, and other NIH departments on October 22, 2001, at the NIH campus, Bethesda, MD.

12. Koenig, H. G., ed. 1998. *Handbook of Religion and Mental Health*. San Diego: Academic Press, 74.

13. Larson, D. B., E. M. Pattison, D. G. Blazer, A. R. Omran, and B. H. Kaplan. 1986. Systematic analysis of research on religious variables in four major psychiatric journals, 1978–1982. *American Journal of Psychiatry* 143:329–34.

14. Weaver, A. J., J. A. Samford, D. B. Larson, L. A. Lucas, H. G. Koenig, and V. Patrick. 1998. A systematic review of research on religion in four major psychiatric journals: 1991–1995. *Journal of Nervous and Mental Disease* 186:187–90.

15. Greg Fricchione's e-mail address is gfricch@emory.edu.

16. Carson, V. B., and H. G. Koenig. 2002. *Parish Nursing: Stories of Service and Care*. Philadelphia, PA: Templeton Foundation Press.

17. Contact Jill Schumann at 800-664-3848 or by e-mail at jschumann@lutheranservices.org.

18. Contact Brent Diers by phone at 708-771-7180 (ext. 283) or by e-mail at BDiersLCFS@aol.com.

CHAPTER 14: IDENTIFYING POSSIBLE SOLUTIONS

1. More information on workshops can be obtained from Harold G. Koenig (koenig@geri.duke.edu); dates are posted on www.dukespiritualityandhealth.org. See the Presentations section of the Web site.

2. DeHaven, M. J., I. B. Hunter, L. Wilder, J. W. Walton, and J. Berry. 2004. Health programs in faith-based organizations: Are they effective? Could they provide predictable care for those in need? *American Journal of Public Health* 94 (6): 1030–1036.

3. Toh, Y. M., S. Y. Tan, C. D. Osburn, and D. E. Faber. 1994. The evaluation of a church-based lay counseling program: Some preliminary data. *Journal of Psychology and Christianity* 13 (3): 270–75; and Y. M. Toh and S. Y. Tan. 1997. The effectiveness of church-based lay counselors: A controlled outcome study. *Journal of Psychology and Christianity* 16 (3): 260–67.

4. A copy of this report can be obtained from Byron Johnson. His e-mail address is byronj@sas.upenn.edu.

5. Taylor, R. J., C. G. Ellison, L. M. Chatters, J. S. Levin, and K. D. Lincoln. 2000. Mental health services in faith communities: The role of clergy in black churches. *Social Work* 45 (1): 73–87.

6. Ibid.

7. Contact Roy Woodruff, executive director of AAPC, for more information: call 703-385-6967, or e-mail: roy@aapc.org.

GLOSSARY

1. Koenig, H. G., ed. 1998. *Handbook of Religion and Mental Health*. San Diego: Academic Press, 18.

2. Ibid.

ADDITIONAL RESOURCES

1. Additional contact information: 806-359-6362, e-mail: westcliff@amaonline.com.

INDEX